Annual Update in Intensive Care and Emergency Medicine

The series *Annual Update in Intensive Care and Emergency Medicine* is the continuation of the series entitled *Yearbook of Intensive Care and Emergency Medicine* in Europe and *Intensive Care Medicine: Annual Update* in the United States.

More information about this series at http://link.springer.com/bookseries/8901

Jean-Louis Vincent
Editor

Annual Update in Intensive Care and Emergency Medicine 2022

Springer

Editor
Jean-Louis Vincent
Department of Intensive Care
Erasme University Hospital
Université libre de Bruxelles
Brussels, Belgium
jlvincent@intensive.org

ISSN 2191-5709 ISSN 2191-5717 (electronic)
Annual Update in Intensive Care and Emergency Medicine
ISBN 978-3-030-93432-3 ISBN 978-3-030-93433-0 (eBook)
https://doi.org/10.1007/978-3-030-93433-0

This Springer imprint is published by the registered company Springer Nature Switzerland AG
The registered company address is: Gewerbestrasse 11, 6330 Cham, Switzerland

Contents

Part I Sepsis and the Immune Response

1 **The Role of Mitochondria in the Immune Response in Critical Illness** 3
Y. Wang and A. S. McLean

2 **Immunomodulation by Tetracyclines in the Critically Ill: An Emerging Treatment Option?** 13
A. Sauer, C. Putensen, and C. Bode

3 **Hit Early: Blocking Interleukin-1 in the Treatment of COVID-19 Pneumonia** 29
E. J. Giamarellos-Bourboulis, M. Mouktaroudi, and M. G. Netea

4 **Hemoadsorption Therapy During ECMO: Emerging Evidence** 39
A. Supady, T. Wengenmayer, and D. Brodie

Part II Respiratory Issues

5 **The Forgotten Circulation and Transpulmonary Pressure Gradients** 51
E. Bowcock, S. R. Orde, and A. S. McLean

6 **Oxygen: Origin, Physiology, Pathophysiology, and Use in the Critically Ill** 67
H. P. M. M. Gelissen, H. J. de Grooth, and A. M. E. de Man

7 **Nebulized Therapeutics for COVID-19 Pneumonia in Critical Care** 81
J. Dhanani and M. C. Reade

Part III Mechanical Ventilation

8 **Positive End-Expiratory Pressure in Invasive and Non-invasive Ventilation of COVID-19 Acute Respiratory Distress Syndrome** 101
L. Weaver, D. G. Bates, and L. Camporota

9 **Personalized Mechanical Ventilation Settings: Slower Is Better!** 113
P. L. Silva, P. R. M. Rocco, and P. Pelosi

10 **Spontaneous Breathing in Acute Respiratory Failure** 129
E. Chiodaroli and D. Chiumello

11 **Laryngeal Injury: Impact on Patients in the Acute and Chronic Phases** 137
E. Kelly, S. Wallace, and Z. Puthucheary

Part IV Fluids and Electrolytes

12 **Fluid Responsiveness as a Physiologic Endpoint to Improve Successful Weaning** 151
R. Castro, P. Born, and J. Bakker

13 **Tidal Volume Challenge Test: Expanding Possibilities** 161
S. N. Myatra, N. Prabu, and J.-L. Teboul

14 **Fluid Management in COVID-19 ICU Patients** 173
R. Shi, X. Monnet, and J.-L. Teboul

15 **Electrolytes in the ICU** 183
A. Reintam Blaser, A. R. H. van Zanten, and A. M. E. de Man

Part V Renal Failure

16 **Hemodynamic Instability During Continuous Renal Replacement Therapy: Is It All About Fluid?** 203
S. M. T. Nasser, N. Boyer, and L. G. Forni

17 **How to Prolong Filter Life During Continuous Renal Replacement Therapy?** 213
Y. Tsujimoto and T. Fujii

18 **Prevention of Acute Kidney Injury After Cardiac Surgery** 223
M. Ostermann, K. Weerapolchai, and N. Lumlertgul

Part VI Circulatory Shock

19 **Contrast-Enhanced Renal Ultrasound for Assessment of Renal Perfusion in Critically Ill Patients** 237
J. Watchorn, K. Bramham, and S. Hutchings

20 **Focused Clinical Hemodynamic Assessment in Septic Shock** 249
E. Kattan, G. Hernández, and J. Bakker

21 **Vasopressor Choice and Timing in Vasodilatory Shock** 259
P. M. Wieruszewski and A. K. Khanna

Part VII Cardiac Arrest

22 Advanced Life Support Update 273
G. D. Perkins and J. P. Nolan

23 Brain Injury Biomarkers for Predicting Outcome After Cardiac Arrest 285
J. Humaloja, N. J. Ashton, and M. B. Skrifvars

Part VIII Neurocritical Care and Neuromonitoring

24 The Emerging Role of the Microbiota in Neurocritical Care 301
D. Battaglini, P. Pelosi, and C. Robba

25 Brain–Multiorgan Cross-Talk in Critically Ill Patients with Acute Brain Injury 317
K. Kotfis, D. Siwicka-Gieroba, and W. Dąbrowski

26 The Importance of Neuromonitoring in Non Brain Injured Patients 333
D. Battaglini, P. Pelosi, and C. Robba

Part IX Artificial Intelligence

27 Artificial Intelligence in Critical Care Medicine 353
J. H. Yoon, M. R. Pinsky, and G. Clermont

28 Artificial Intelligence in Infection Management in the ICU 369
T. De Corte, S. Van Hoecke, and J. De Waele

Part X Quality of Care

29 Acute Medical Rehabilitation in Intensive Care 385
H. M. Buyruk, Y. Buyruk, and C. Ince

30 Sepsis Performance Improvement Programs: From Evidence Toward Clinical Implementation 397
M. Schinkel, P. W. B. Nanayakkara, and W. J. Wiersinga

Index 409

Abbreviations

AKI	Acute kidney injury
APACHE	Acute physiology and chronic health evaluation
ARDS	Acute respiratory distress syndrome
COVID	Coronavirus disease
CRP	C-reactive protein
CRRT	Continuous renal replacement therapy
CT	Computed tomography
DAMP	Damage-associated molecular pattern
DO_2	Oxygen delivery
ECMO	Extracorporeal membrane oxygenation
EHR	Electronic health record
GCS	Glasgow Coma Scale
ICU	Intensive care unit
IFN	Interferon
IL	Interleukin
LV	Left ventricular
MAP	Mean arterial pressure
NO	Nitric oxide
NOS	Nitric oxide synthase
PAMP	Pathogen-associated molecular pattern
PEEP	Positive end-expiratory pressure
RBC	Red blood cell
RCT	Randomized controlled trial
RRT	Renal replacement therapy
RV	Right ventricular
SARS-CoV-2	Severe acute respiratory syndrome coronavirus-2
SOFA	Sequential organ failure assessment
TBI	Traumatic brain injury
TNF	Tumor necrosis factor
VILI	Ventilator-induced lung injury
V_T	Tidal volume

Part I

Sepsis and the Immune Response

The Role of Mitochondria in the Immune Response in Critical Illness

1

Y. Wang and A. S. McLean

1.1 Introduction

Immune dysregulation, characterized by an imbalance between a systemic inflammatory response syndrome and a compensatory anti-inflammatory response syndrome, is often observed in critically ill patients [1, 2]. This imbalance between the pro- and anti-inflammatory responses frequently leads to immunoparalysis in critically ill patients, rendering them more susceptible to further infections, and is associated with increased mortality [3]. Currently, no effective treatments are available to restore immune homeostasis and reduce mortality in these patients, largely due to the heterogeneity in patients' immune status and more importantly the lack of understanding of the underlying cause of such immune dysfunction [2, 4]. Immune response is not a standalone process but is interconnected with other cellular activities, a very important one of which is cellular metabolism. Metabolic pathways and immune response are tightly intertwined both in health and in disease [5]. The link between immune cell function and mitochondrial function is now well recognized and a field known as "immunometabolism" is dedicated to understanding the relationship between immune and metabolic pathways [6–8]. Mitochondria play a crucial role in regulating not only the growth, but also the function, of immune cells. In addition to providing energy to support the synthesis of the macromolecules essential for immune cell proliferation, mitochondria also act as signaling organelles, driving

Y. Wang (✉)
Department of Intensive Care Medicine, Nepean Hospital, Kingswood, NSW, Australia

Centre for Immunology and Allergy Research, Westmead Institute for Medical Research, Westmead, NSW, Australia
e-mail: ya.wang@sydney.edu.au

A. S. McLean
Department of Intensive Care Medicine, Nepean Hospital, Kingswood, NSW, Australia

J.-L. Vincent (ed.), *Annual Update in Intensive Care and Emergency Medicine 2022*, Annual Update in Intensive Care and Emergency Medicine,
https://doi.org/10.1007/978-3-030-93433-0_1

activation of immune cells via metabolic intermediates, mitochondrial DNA (mtDNA), and reactive oxygen species (ROS). In addition, mitochondrial dynamics (fusion and fission), biogenesis (synthesis of new mitochondria), and mitophagy (degradation of damaged mitochondria) also play important roles in regulating immune cell functions. Knowledge in immunometabolism in critical illness, in particularly sepsis, opens up a new paradigm in patient care. Potential therapies targeting metabolic pathways, instead of solely immune-related pathways, might be the way to repair cellular function and restore immune homeostasis [4]. The other aspect of immunometabolism—looking at how immune responses influence metabolic pathways—is equally important, but beyond the scope of this review. Interaction between metabolism and immune response at the organ level has been reviewed elsewhere [6].

1.2 Mitochondrial Machinery That Mediates and Regulates Immune Responses in Critical Illness

Apart from being the powerhouse of the cell, the mitochondrion has emerged as a signaling hub that shapes and modulates how the immune system responds to infection or trauma. Mitochondrial dysfunction is evident in leukocytes from critically ill patients, and is believed to be the underlying cause of immunoparalysis and may account for the development of organ dysfunction [7–9]. Early recovery of mitochondrial function correlates with improved recovery in critically ill patients [10].

1.2.1 Metabolic Reprogramming

The immune-regulating mitochondrial machinery is a complex network involving many pathways and mechanisms that diverge and converge at various levels. Metabolic reprogramming is one mechanism that has been well studied in both innate and adaptive immune cells. Immune cells at different activation states (quiescent vs. activated), or with different functions (pro-inflammatory vs. anti-inflammatory), and different cell types (granulocytes, macrophages, dendritic cells, T- and B-lymphocytes), make use of different metabolic pathways (e.g., glycolysis, oxidative phosphorylation, fatty acid metabolism) to produce ATP [11]. The choice of different metabolic pathways, supports the energy demand of cells at different activation state. For example, upon infection or stimulation, immune cells become activated and produce cytokines and hence tend to favor glycolysis over oxidative phosphorylation for fast turnaround of ATP. Although the same amount of starting material, such as glucose, is used, oxidative phosphorylation generates 18 times more ATP than glycolysis, although is a lot slower. On the other hand, the choice of metabolic pathway determines the fate of the immune cells, i.e., naïve or memory, effector or regulatory, etc. However, the environment that the cells are in in the first place, triggers the changes in the metabolic pathways. The overall trend is that neutrophils, inflammatory macrophages (M1 macrophages), activated effector T cells, and dendritic cells rely more on aerobic glycolysis, whereas alternatively polarized macrophages (M2 macrophages), regulatory T cells (Tregs), and memory T cells prefer oxidative phosphorylation and fatty acid oxidation for energy production [8, 11, 12]. Metabolic reprogramming serves an important role in catering for the immune cells' energy demand at different phases of their activation and proliferation. However, imbalance across the metabolic pathways could have serious pathological impact. One example may be the hyperlactatemia often seen in critically ill patients. Increased aerobic glycolysis in the activated immune cells during the initial hyper-inflammatory response is believed to contribute to the increase in blood lactate levels in sepsis [13, 14].

1.2.2 Mitochondrial ROS and mtDNA

Metabolic reprogramming sets the scene for the immune response, which is then subjected to many more modifications and regulations by factors that are directly or indirectly related to mitochondrial metabolism. Two important mitochondria-related immune regulators that have been well studied are mitochondrial ROS and mtDNA. Mitochondrial ROS are produced in healthy mitochondria, as a by-product of oxidative phosphorylation. At low dose, mitochondrial ROS serve important signaling functions, especially in the innate immune response. They are known to mediate NLRP3 inflammasome activation, leading to production of the pro-inflammatory cytokines, interleukin (IL)-1β and IL-18 [8, 15]. Mitochondrial ROS also induce a type-I interferon (IFN) response via mitochondrial antiviral-signaling (MAVS) and the IFN regulatory factor 3 (IRF3) pathway [16]. However, the level of mitochondrial ROS needs to be tightly regulated by the antioxidant system. Excessive mitochondrial ROS can cause oxidative damage to proteins/enzymes involved in oxidative phosphorylation and create mutations in mtDNA, contributing to the immune dysregulations as seen in critical illness [17]. Like mitochondrial ROS, mtDNA also plays an important role in innate immunity [12]. In healthy cells, mtDNA is located in the matrix of mitochondria, encoding 13 proteins, all of which are components of oxidative phosphorylation. mtDNA is released to the cytosol upon mitochondrial dysfunction which involves changes to the integrity or permeability of the mitochondrial membrane. mtDNA, released into the cytosol, can activate the NLRP3 inflammasome with release of IL-1β and IL-18. Due to its bacterial origin, cytosolic mtDNA also serves as a damage-associated molecular pattern (DAMP), which can be recognized by intracellular pattern recognition receptors (PRRs), such as Toll-like receptor 9 (TLR9), and initiate the nuclear factor-kappa B (NF-κB)-dependent pro-inflammatory signaling pathway. In addition, cytosolic mtDNA can also be sensed by cyclic GMP-AMP synthase (cGAS) and activate the cGAS/stimulator of IFN genes (cGAS/STING) pathway and its downstream IFN response [18]. mtDNA can also be released into the circulation and cause systemic inflammation. Circulating mtDNA has been associated with mortality in critically ill patients [19].

1.2.3 Succinate and Itaconate

In addition to mitochondrial ROS and mtDNA, metabolites such as succinate and itaconate have also emerged as part of immune-regulating mitochondrial machinery [4, 20]. Both succinate and itaconate are intermediates from the tricarboxylic acid (TCA) cycle with opposite effects on the immune response. The TCA cycle generates nicotinamide adenine dinucleotide (NADH) and flavin adenine dinucleotide ($FADH_2$), providing electrons to fuel oxidative phosphorylation. Succinate accumulation occurs under conditions such as hypoxia or inflammation. It can be released from mitochondria into the cytosol and functions as a signal transducer promoting pro-inflammatory gene expression via hypoxia-inducible factor 1α (HIF-1α) activation. Accumulation and oxidation of succinate by succinate dehydrogenase (SDH) in the mitochondria also leads to increased production of mitochondrial ROS via a process called reverse electron transport. This further enhances the pro-inflammatory effect of succinate. Like ROS, the level of succinate needs to be carefully regulated due to its inflammation aggravating effect. Plasma succinate has been proposed as a predictor of mortality for critically ill patients who are severely injured [21]. Itaconate, which is derived from cis-aconitate of the TCA cycle, is a succinate-regulating factor. It is shown to counteract the pro-inflammatory effect of succinate by inhibiting SDH. Itaconate can also be released into the cytosol and activate transcription factor NF-E2 p45-related factor 2 (Nrf2), a master regulator of antioxidant and anti-inflammatory responses [22]. Recently, itaconate has also been shown to inhibit the inflammatory response in macrophages through activating transcription factor 3 (ATF3).

1.2.4 Mitochondrial Dynamics

The above mentioned immune-regulating mitochondrial factors are centered around the biochemical aspect of mitochondrial biology. Another important aspect of immune-regulating mitochondrial machinery is mitochondrial dynamics, which is to maintain and provide infrastructural support for the immune response. The size and shape of mitochondria undergo constant change through fusion and fission, which is important for maintaining the health and function of mitochondria. First, fusion incorporates newly synthesized mitochondria (from mitochondrial biogenesis) into the current mitochondrial network. Second, fusion also allows for mixing of proteins and/or mtDNA between the existing mitochondria, which on one hand enhances the metabolic capacity of the mitochondria, and on the other enables the damaged proteins and/or mutated mtDNA to be segregated from the healthy ones. Finally, segregation is achieved via fission and the damaged mitochondria can be destroyed through a process known as mitophagy. The proportion of mitochondria with damaged proteins or mutated mtDNA is kept below a critical threshold level through this process to maintain mitochondrial function [23, 24]. In addition to quality control, mitochondrial fusion and fission also participate in immune regulation. In activated T cells, there is an increase in fission, which creates round and fragmented mitochondria with loose cristae, favoring aerobic glycolysis. And in memory T cells, increased fusion generates elongated mitochondria which favors oxidative phosphorylation and fatty acid oxidation [8, 25].

1.3 Immunometabolism: The Perfect World Scenario vs. the Critical Illness Scenario

So far, we have presented a list of mitochondrial components that are thought to play important roles in regulating the immune response. Our list is far from complete, but does highlight a few mechanisms that could relate to the development of immune dysregulation in critical illness. Figure 1.1 illustrates what we think would

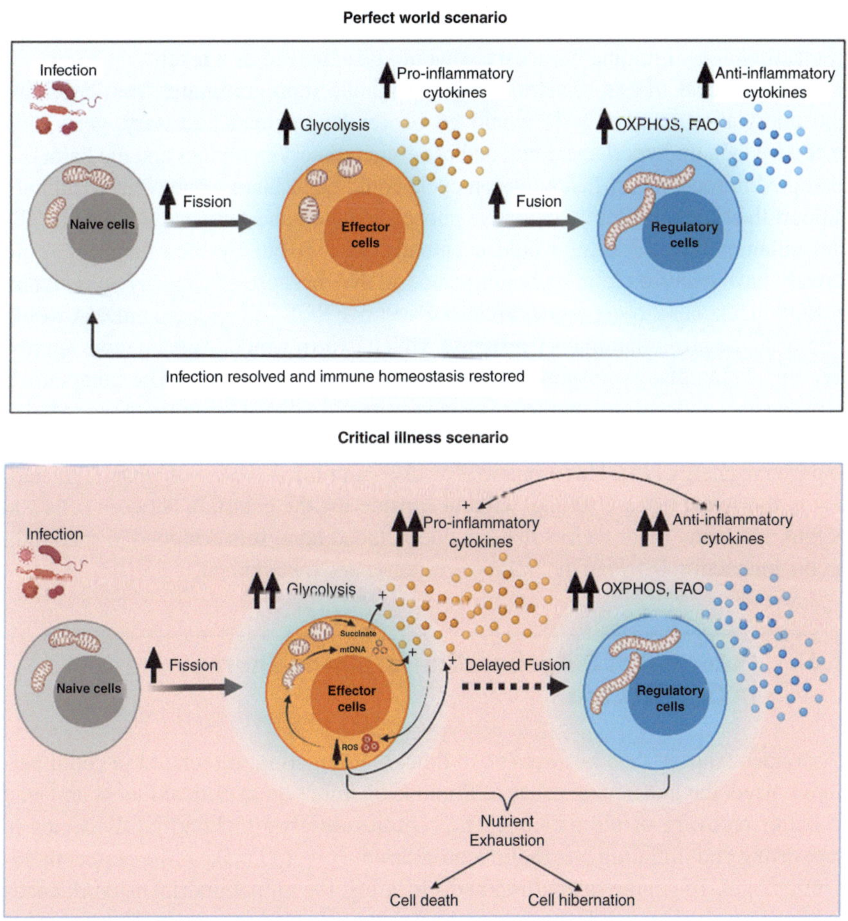

Fig. 1.1 Immunometabolism in the 'perfect world scenario' vs. the 'critical illness scenario'. *OXPHOS* oxidative phosphorylation, *FAO* fatty acid oxidation

happen to the immune response when metabolism was in perfect control (the perfect world scenario) and when it became inconsistent and changeable (the critical illness scenario). In the perfect world scenario, the presence of an insult (e.g., infection or a trauma-related stress signal), would trigger metabolic reprogramming, switching from oxidative phosphorylation to glycolysis. This would enable activation of immune cells and production of pro-inflammatory cytokines and other mediators. At the same time, mitochondrial fission would increase to keep up with the metabolic reprogramming. The slightly elevated mitochondrial ROS and succinate in response to initial insult or cytokines would promote the pro-inflammatory response. Once the insult was eliminated, mitochondrial fusion would increase to create fused elongated mitochondria that favor oxidative phosphorylation and fatty acid oxidation. This would allow activation of regulatory immune cells and production of anti-inflammatory cytokines and other mediators. And itaconate would counteract the effect of succinate, activate the Nrf2-mediated antioxidant pathway to dampen down mitochondrial ROS, and activate ATF3 to inhibit the inflammatory response in macrophages. Immune homeostasis would be achieved as a result.

In the critical illness scenario, initial metabolic reprogramming from oxidative phosphorylation to glycolysis would go on for longer than necessary, generating excessive lactate (hyperlactatemia) and pro-inflammatory cytokines and mediators. A disrupted mitochondrial fusion/fission cycle could be to blame, one which could not support the timely switch to oxidative phosphorylation and fatty acid oxidation. The anti-inflammatory response would eventually kick in but by then damage would already have occurred to mitochondria and mtDNA because of excessive production of ROS in response to stress or cytokines. Excessive ROS and released mtDNA would aggravate the pro-inflammatory response, which in turn would trigger a more aggressive anti-inflammatory response to try and salvage the situation. The competition between pro- and anti-inflammatory responses would exhaust the nutrients and lead to shutdown of the whole metabolic system. Cells would either die or go into hibernation to preserve energy [26]. This scenario is an over-simplified version of what might happen in the actual disease setting, without considering the crosstalk between cells and organs and many other factors that are not included here. It is designed to shed light on the interaction between the immune response and metabolism.

1.4 Potential of Mitochondria-Targeting Therapy in Critical Care

Our understanding thus far leads us to think that targeting mitochondria could perhaps correct the underlying cause of immune dysfunction in critical illness and lead to better recovery of the patients. The central role of mitochondrial dynamics in supporting and initiating metabolic reprogramming would make it the perfect therapeutic target. To get the fusion/fission cycle going, the mitochondrial network needs to be replenished by newly synthesized mitochondria via biogenesis. Therapies that could potentially boost mitochondrial biogenesis are mitochondrial transplantation, metformin, nitric oxide (NO), and carbon monoxide. Mitochondrial transplantation has been used successfully in pediatric patients with myocardial ischemia-reperfusion injury [27]. Metformin can activate peroxisome proliferator-activated receptor (PPAR)-gamma coactivator-1α (PGC-1α), and Nrf2, the master regulator of mitochondrial biogenesis and antioxidant systems [28]. Premorbid use of metformin is associated with lower mortality in sepsis [29]. NO and carbon monoxide can also enhance mitochondrial biogenesis [30–32]. Dietary nitrite has been trialed in patients with coronary artery disease (ClinicalTrials.gov Identifier: NCT00069654). Other therapies, such as mitochondria-targeted antioxidant (MitoQ) [33], could also be beneficial in protecting mtDNA and oxidative phosphorylation from oxidative damage. MitoQ has been trialed in people with Parkinson's disease (ClinicalTrials.gov Identifier: NCT00329056).

1.5 Challenges of Applying Mitochondria-Targeting Therapy in Critical Care

There are challenges to overcome before mitochondria-targeting therapy would be possible. First, how do we assess mitochondrial dysfunction in the clinic and identify patients who would benefit from such therapy? A few possible ways could be considered. Non-invasive assessment of mitochondrial oxygen metabolism using a novel device called the COMET monitor was tested on 40 patients during the acute phase of sepsis. This device is based on the protoporphyrin IX-triplet state lifetime technique (PpIX-TSLT) and has been shown to be feasible [33]. This technology is still in its early phase of clinical application but does offer some hope. Another possible biomarker that could potentially be used for assessing mitochondrial dysfunction is plasma mtDNA, but its sensitivity and specificity need further investigation [19, 34, 35]. Furthermore, we could consider using immune response markers as a surrogate markers, one such example could be IFNα inducible protein 27 (IFI27) [36]. If we could overcome the first challenge, the second would be how to deliver mitochondria-targeting therapies to the right organ at the right time.

1.6 Conclusion

In this chapter, we have demonstrated the important role of mitochondria in regulating the immune response and proposed a scenario that explains immune–metabolism crosstalk in the context of critical illness. We have highlighted the role of mitochondrial dynamics in overseeing and supporting metabolic reprogramming during immune cell activation. Mitochondrial ROS can be friend or foe when it comes to immune regulation. Two TCA intermediates—succinate and itaconate—with opposite effects have emerged as important players of the immune-regulating mitochondrial machinery. Our understanding in immunometabolism could take us to the next era of critical care: mitochondria-targeting therapy.

References

1. Duggal NA, Snelson C, Shaheen U, Pearce V, Lord JM. Innate and adaptive immune dysregulation in critically ill ICU patients. Sci Rep. 2018;8:10186.
2. Surbatovic M, Vojvodic D, Khan W. Immune response in critically ill patients. Mediat Inflamm. 2018;2018:9524315.
3. Frazier WJ, Hall MW. Immunoparalysis and adverse outcomes from critical illness. Pediatr Clin N Am. 2008;55:647–68.
4. Koutroulis I, Batabyal R, McNamara B, Ledda M, Hoptay C, Freishtat RJ. Sepsis immunometabolism: from defining sepsis to understanding how energy production affects immune response. Crit Care Explor. 2019;1:e0061.
5. Faas MM, de Vos P. Mitochondrial function in immune cells in health and disease. Biochim Biophys Acta Mol basis Dis. 2020;1866:165845.
6. Lercher A, Baazim H, Bergthaler A. Systemic immunometabolism: challenges and opportunities. Immunity. 2020;53:496–509.
7. McBride MA, Owen AM, Stothers CL, et al. The metabolic basis of immune dysfunction following sepsis and trauma. Front Immunol. 2020;11:1043.
8. Angajala A, Lim S, Phillips JB, et al. Diverse roles of mitochondria in immune responses: novel insights into immuno-metabolism. Front Immunol. 2018;9:1605.
9. Cheng SC, Scicluna BP, Arts RJ, et al. Broad defects in the energy metabolism of leukocytes underlie immunoparalysis in sepsis. Nat Immunol. 2016;17:406–13.
10. Carré JE, Orban JC, Re L, et al. Survival in critical illness is associated with early activation of mitochondrial biogenesis. Am J Respir Crit Care Med. 2010;182:745–51.
11. Pearce EL, Pearce EJ. Metabolic pathways in immune cell activation and quiescence. Immunity. 2013;38:633–43.
12. Sack MN. Mitochondrial fidelity and metabolic agility control immune cell fate and function. J Clin Invest. 2018;128:3651–61.
13. Haji-Michael PG, Ladrière L, Sener A, Vincent JL, Malaisse WJ. Leukocyte glycolysis and lactate output in animal sepsis and ex vivo human blood. Metabolism. 1999;48:779–85.
14. Gibot S. On the origins of lactate during sepsis. Crit Care. 2012;16:151.
15. Zhou R, Yazdi AS, Menu P, Tschopp J. A role for mitochondria in NLRP3 inflammasome activation. Nature. 2011;469:221–5.
16. Agod Z, Fekete T, Budai MM, et al. Regulation of type I interferon responses by mitochondria-derived reactive oxygen species in plasmacytoid dendritic cells. Redox Biol. 2017;13:633–45.
17. Abilés J, de la Cruz AP, Castaño J, et al. Oxidative stress is increased in critically ill patients according to antioxidant vitamins intake, independent of severity: a cohort study. Crit Care. 2006;10:R146.
18. Riley JS, Tait SW. Mitochondrial DNA in inflammation and immunity. EMBO Rep. 2020;21:e49799.
19. Harrington JS, Huh JW, Schenck EJ, Nakahira K, Siempos II, Choi AMK. Circulating mitochondrial DNA as predictor of mortality in critically ill patients: a systematic review of clinical studies. Chest. 2019;156:1120–36.
20. Murphy MP, O'Neill LAJ. Krebs cycle reimagined: the emerging roles of succinate and itaconate as signal transducers. Cell. 2018;174:780–4.
21. D'Alessandro A, Moore HB, Moore EE, Reisz JA, Wither MJ, Ghasasbyan A, et al. Plasma succinate is a predictor of mortality in critically injured patients. J Trauma Acute Care Surg. 2017;83:491–5.
22. Mills EL, Ryan DG, Prag HA, et al. Itaconate is an anti-inflammatory metabolite that activates Nrf2 via alkylation of KEAP1. Nature. 2018;556:113–7.
23. Garbern JC, Lee RT. Mitochondria and metabolic transitions in cardiomyocytes: lessons from development for stem cell-derived cardiomyocytes. Stem Cell Res Ther. 2021;12:177.

24. Carelli V, Maresca A, Caporali L, Trifunov S, Zanna C, Rugolo M. Mitochondria: biogenesis and mitophagy balance in segregation and clonal expansion of mitochondrial DNA mutations. Int J Biochem Cell Biol. 2015;63:21–4.
25. Mills EL, Kelly B, O'Neill LAJ. Mitochondria are the powerhouses of immunity. Nat Immunol. 2017;18:488–98.
26. Singer M. The role of mitochondrial dysfunction in sepsis-induced multi-organ failure. Virulence. 2014;5:66–72.
27. McCully JD, Cowan DB, Emani SM, Del Nido PJ. Mitochondrial transplantation: from animal models to clinical use in humans. Mitochondrion. 2017;34:127–34.
28. Katila N, Bhurtel S, Park PH, Choi DY. Metformin attenuates rotenone-induced oxidative stress and mitochondrial damage via the AKT/Nrf2 pathway. Neurochem Int. 2021;148:105120.
29. Tan K, Simpson A, Huang S, Tang B, McLean A, Nalos M. The association of premorbid metformin exposure with mortality and organ dysfunction in sepsis: a systematic review and meta-analysis. Crit Care Explor. 2019;1:e0009.
30. Nisoli E, Clementi E, Paolucci C, et al. Mitochondrial biogenesis in mammals: the role of endogenous nitric oxide. Science. 2003;299:896–9.
31. Shiva S, Sack MN, Greer JJ, et al. Nitrite augments tolerance to ischemia/reperfusion injury via the modulation of mitochondrial electron transfer. J Exp Med. 2007;204:2089–102.
32. Lancel S, Hassoun SM, Favory R, Decoster B, Motterlini R, Neviere R. Carbon monoxide rescues mice from lethal sepsis by supporting mitochondrial energetic metabolism and activating mitochondrial biogenesis. J Pharmacol Exp Ther. 2009;329:641–8.
33. Lowes DA, Thottakam BM, Webster NR, Murphy MP, Galley HF. The mitochondria-targeted antioxidant MitoQ protects against organ damage in a lipopolysaccharide-peptidoglycan model of sepsis. Free Radic Biol Med. 2008;45:1559–65.
34. Faust HE, Reilly JP, Anderson BJ, et al. Plasma mitochondrial DNA levels are associated with ARDS in trauma and sepsis patients. Chest. 2020;157:67–76.
35. Mao JY, Li DK, Zhang HM, Wang XT, Liu DW. Plasma mitochondrial DNA levels are associated with acute lung injury and mortality in septic patients. BMC Pulm Med. 2021;21:66.
36. Tang BM, Shojaei M, Parnell GP, et al. A novel immune biomarker IFI27 discriminates between influenza and bacteria in patients with suspected respiratory infection. Eur Respir J. 2017;49:1602098.

Immunomodulation by Tetracyclines in the Critically Ill: An Emerging Treatment Option?

2

A. Sauer, C. Putensen, and C. Bode

2.1 Introduction

Sepsis and acute respiratory distress syndrome (ARDS) are still the most common causes of death in critically ill patients. Although our knowledge of the underlying immunopathogenesis has grown tremendously and we have made substantial advances in supportive care, the overall mortality for sepsis and ARDS remains high [1, 2]. In 2016, sepsis was redefined as life-threatening organ dysfunction caused by a dysregulated host response to infection. Hyperinflammation occurring concurrently with immunosuppression puts patients at risk for developing fatal secondary infections and chronic critical illness syndrome [1]. An extension of sepsis in terms of pathogenesis has made ARDS similarly resistant to therapy and the prognosis for patients with this syndrome remains equally dismal [2]. Despite over 30 years of preclinical and clinical trials, no effective pharmacotherapies exist to improve outcomes in patents with sepsis or ARDS [1, 2]. New therapeutic agents are desperately needed, even more so in the light of the ongoing coronavirus disease 2019 (COVID-19) pandemic.

Tetracyclines are a family of bacteriostatic antibiotics that inhibit protein synthesis by reversibly binding to the bacterial ribosome. Upon binding they allosterically prevent the binding of the amino acyl-tRNA to the mRNA ribosome complex. They exhibit broad-spectrum antibacterial activity against a wide-range of Gram-positive and Gram-negative bacteria as well as atypical pathogens, such as chlamydiae, spirochaetes, and rickettsiae [3]. Additionally, tetracyclines exert pleiotropic immunomodulatory effects that may be able to rebalance immune homeostasis in critically ill patients. Their beneficial anti-inflammatory effects have been reported for chronic

A. Sauer · C. Putensen · C. Bode (✉)
Department of Anesthesiology and Intensive Care Medicine, University Hospital Bonn, Bonn, Germany
e-mail: christian.bode@ukbonn.de

J.-L. Vincent (ed.), *Annual Update in Intensive Care and Emergency Medicine 2022*, Annual Update in Intensive Care and Emergency Medicine,
https://doi.org/10.1007/978-3-030-93433-0_2

pulmonary diseases, chronic inflammatory skin diseases, autoimmune disorders, as well as neurodegenerative diseases, and they have become a standard of care in the treatment of periodontitis, acne, and rosacea [3, 4]. Recently, evidence has emerged that tetracyclines could potentially be beneficial in ARDS and sepsis [5–7].

In this chapter, we provide an overview of the current preclinical and clinical studies on the immunomodulatory effects of tetracyclines in the critical care setting (Tables 2.1 and 2.2). We elucidate the underlying mechanisms of the immunomodulatory properties of tetracyclines that may have therapeutic effects in sepsis and ARDS. Finally, we discuss future research perspectives including the role of non-antibiotic tetracyclines.

2.2 Immunopathogenesis of Sepsis

Sepsis is a heterogenous syndrome characterized by an unbalanced hyperinflammatory state and profound immunosuppression. Pathogen-associated molecular patterns (PAMPs) released by sepsis-inducing microorganisms activate pattern recognition receptors (PRRs) expressed by various immune cells and trigger a strong innate immune response. The best known PAMPs include lipopolysaccharide (LPS), lipoteichoic acid (LPA), and microbial DNA. PRRs can also sense cell injury-associated endogenous molecules referred to as damage-associated molecular patterns (DAMPs), such as ATP, mitochondrial DNA, hyaluronan, heat shock proteins, and fibrinogen [1, 8]. Upon ligand binding, activation of downstream signalling pathways (e.g., nuclear factor kappa-B [NF-κB] and mitogen-activated protein kinase [MAPK]) leads to the transcription of genes encoding pro-inflammatory cytokines and chemokines such as tumor necrosis factor (TNF)-α, interleukin (IL)-1ß, IL-8, IL-18 and interferons (IFN). The expression of IL-1ß and IL-18 is tightly regulated by inflammasomes, which execute a unique form of programmed cell-death called pyroptosis. In most cases, these processes aid in neutralizing invading pathogens and apoptotic cells. However, in sepsis they can lead to an unbalanced host response that can potentially trigger a life-threatening "cytokine storm" [1, 9]. Another hallmark of the innate immune response in sepsis is the activation of the complement system, which results in the recruitment of leukocytes, endothelial cells, and platelets and ultimately in sepsis-induced endothelial barrier dysfunction. Loss of vascular integrity leads to tissue edema and reduced microvascular perfusion. Coagulation activation is tightly interconnected with complement activation and predisposes patients to disseminated intravascular coagulation (DIC), microvascular immunothrombosis, and hemorrhage.

The initial hyperinflammatory state is counterbalanced by immunosuppression which involves both innate and adaptive immunity. One key phenomenon is the apoptosis of B and CD4+ and CD8+ T cells and dendritic cells causing an acquired immune deficiency syndrome linked to an unfavorable prognosis. Depletion of T cells is further augmented by increased expression of programmed cell death 1 (PD1) and upregulation of its ligand (PDL1) on various immune and epithelial cells. The reprogramming of antigen-presenting cells results in reduced human leukocyte

Table 2.1 Immunomodulatory effects of tetracyclines in preclinical and clinical models of acute respiratory distress syndrome (ARDS)

Author	Year	Tetracycline	Model	Stimulants or pathogens	Immune response
Peukert et al. [5]	2021	Tetracycline	Mouse, human (*ex vivo*)	LPS, H1N1 influenza virus (mouse); viral, bacterial, and non-pulmonary ARDS (human)	IL-1ß, IL-18, caspase-1 activation, neutrophil influx ↓, survival ↑
Zhang et al. [20]	2019	Doxycycline	Mouse	Paraquat	MMP-9, MPO, neutrophil influx ↓
Wang et al. [24]	2014	Doxycycline	Rat	Cardiopulmonary bypass	TNF-α, IL-1ß, MMP-9 ↓
Zhang et al. [17]	2014	Doxycycline	Dog	Cardiopulmonary bypass	MMP-9, MPO, neutrophil influx ↓
Roy et al. [16]	2012	CMT-3	Pig	Ischemia by clamping of SMA, placement of fecal clot in peritoneum	TNF-α, IL-1ß, Il-6, IL-8, IL-10 ↓, MMP-2, -9, NE, survival ⇔
Ng et al. [27]	2012	Doxycycline	Mouse	H3N2 influenza virus	MMP-2, MMP-9, T1-α, thrombomodulin, neutrophil influx ↓
Moon et al. [22]	2012	Doxycycline	Mouse	LPS	Syndecan-1 (MMP-7 substrate), neutrophil influx ↓
Zhou et al. [25]	2010	CMT-3	Sheep	3rd degree burn, smoke inhalation, barotrauma	MMP-2 ↓, MMP-9 ⇔, survival ↑
Sochor et al. [21]	2009	Doxycycline	Rat	Acute pancreatitis (intraductal glycodeoxycholic acid, cerulein)	MMP-9, neutrophil influx ↓
Fujita et al. [26]	2007	Doxycycline	Mouse	LPS or *Streptococcus pneumoniae*	MMP-2, -9, neutrophil influx ↓, survival ↑
Kim et al. [14]	2006	CMT-3	Rat	Ventilation	MMP-9, MPO, neutrophil influx ↓
Fujita et al. [28]	2006	Doxycycline	Mouse	Bleomycin	MMP-2, -9, neutrophil influx ↓
Steinberg et al. [19]	2005	CMT-3	Pig	Ischemia by clamping of SMA, placement of fecal clot in peritoneum	IL-6, IL-8, IL-10, NE ↓, IL-1, MMP-2, -9, neutrophil influx ⇔, survival ↑
Steinberg et al. [15]	2003	CMT-3	Rat	Cecal ligation and puncture	MMP-2, MMP-9 ↓, survival ↑
Carney et al. [23]	2001	CMT-3	Pig	LPS	MMP-2, MMP-9, neutrophil influx ↓
McCann et al. [29]	1999	CMT-3	Pig	Cardiopulmonary bypass, LPS	Neutrophil influx ↓
Carney et al. [13]	1999	CMT-3	Pig	Cardiopulmonary bypass, LPS	MMP-2, MMP-9, NE, neutrophil influx ↓, survival ↑

↑ significant increase, ↓ significant decrease, ⇔ no significant difference, *CMT-3* chemically modified tetracycline 3, *IL* interleukin, *LPS* lipopolysaccharide, *MMP* metalloproteinase, *MPO* myeloperoxidase, *NE* neutrophil elastase, *SMA* superior mesenteric artery, *TNF-α* tumor necrosis factor alpha, *T1-α* membrane protein of alveolar type I epithelium

Table 2.2 Immunomodulatory effects of tetracyclines in preclinical and clinical models of sepsis

Author	Year	Tetracycline	Model	Stimulants or pathogens	Immune response
Colaço et al. [6]	2021	Doxycyline	Mouse	*E. coli*, H1N1 influenza virus, *C. albicans*, *Plasmodium berghei*	Liver, lung, kidney injury ↓, mitochondrial protein synthesis ↓; FAO, steroid sensitivity, survival ↑
Patel et al. [7]	2020	Doxycycline	Mouse	Cecal ligation and puncture	TNF-α, IL-1ß, IL-6, MPO ↓, survival ↑
Sun et al. [35]	2020	Minocycline	Human THP-1 monocytes	LPS	TNF-α, IL-8, MIP-1α, MIP-1ß ↓, modulated NF-κB-, p38-, ERK1/2-pathways
Sun et al. [34]	2015	Minocycline, tigecycline, doxycycline	Human THP-1 monocytes	LPS	Autophagy ↑ by inhibiting mTOR; TNF-α, IL-8 ↓
Nukarinen et al. [48]	2015	Doxycycline	RCT	Severe sepsis or septic shock	MMP-8, -9, TIMP-1 ⇔
Fredeking et al. [47]	2015	Doxycycline	RCT	Dengue virus	IL-6, TNF-α, mortality ↓
Bode et al. [45]	2014	Doxycycline	Human THP-1 monocytes, PBMCs (*ex vivo*)	LPS, E. coli	Phagocytosis, IL-1ß, IL-6 ↓, TLR-1, TLR-4, TLR-6 ↓
Tai et al. [41]	2013	Minocycline	Human THP-1 monocytes	LPS	TNF-α, IL-6, IFN-γ, IL-8, IP-10, MCP-1, MIP-1α, MIP-1ß, RANTES, eotaxin ↓, IKKα/β phosphorylation inhibited
Pang et al. [33]	2012	Minocycline	Human monocytes (*ex vivo*)	LPS	TNF-α, IL-1ß, IL-6, COX-2, PGE_2 ↓, LOX-1, NF-κB, LITAF, Nur77, PI3K/Akt-, p38-MAPK pathway ↓
Castro et al. [46]	2011	Tetracycline, doxycycline	RCT	Dengue virus	IL-6, Il-1ß, TNF-α ↓, IL-1ra ↑, TNF-R1 ⇔
Maitra et al. [40]	2005	CMT-3	Rat	Cecal ligation and puncture	Liver injury, MMP-9, MMP-2, TGF-ß1, caspase-3 ↓, survival ↑
Maitra et al. [38]	2004	CMT-3	Rat	Cecal ligation and puncture	TNF-α ↓, p38-, p42/44–MAPK activation inhibited, survival ↑
Maitra et al. [39]	2003	CMT-3	Rat	Cecal ligation and puncture	Liver injury, NO, MMP-9 ↓, survival ↑

Table 2.2 (continued)

Author	Year	Tetracycline	Model	Stimulants or pathogens	Immune response
D'Agostino et al. [44]	2001	CMTs,	Murine J774 macrophages	LPS	TNF-α, IL-10 ⇔, iNOS, nitrite, NO, Il-12 ↓, cytotoxity ↑
Patel et al. [42]	1999	CMTs, minocycline	Murine RAW 264.7 cells, human A 549 cells	LPS	PGE_2, nitrite ↓ (CMT-3)
D'Agostino et al. [36]	1998	Doxycycline	Mouse, murine macrophages	LPS	NO ↓, survival ↑
Amin et al. [43]	1997	CMTs, doxycycline	Murine macrophages	LPS	iNOS mRNA accumulation and protein expression ↓
Milano et al. [37]	1997	Tetracycline	Mouse, murine macrophages	LPS	TNF-α, IL-1α, nitrate, iNOS activity ↓, macrophages: NO ↓, TNF-α, IL-1α ⇔, survival ↑

↑ significant increase, ↓ significant decrease, ⇔ no significant difference, *C. albicans Candida albicans*, *CMT-3* chemically modified tetracycline 3, *COX-2* cyclooxygenase 2, *E. coli Escherichia coli, ERK* extracellular-signal regulated kinases, *FAO* fatty acid oxidation, *IFN* interferon, *IKK* inhibitor of nuclear factor kappa B kinase, *IL* interleukin, *IL-1ra* interleukin-1 receptor antagonist, *iNOS* inducible nitric oxide synthase, *IP-10* interferon gamma induced protein 10, *LITAF* lipopolysaccharide induced TNF factor, *LPS* lipopolysaccharide, *LOX-1* lectin-like oxidized low density lipoprotein receptor-1, *MMP* metalloproteinase, *MAPK* mitogen-activated protein kinase, *MCP* monocyte chemoattractant protein, *MIP* macrophage inflammatory protein, *MPO* myeloperoxidase, *mTOR* mammalian target of rapamycin, *NF-κB* nuclear factor kappa-light-chain-enhancer of activated B-cells, *NO* nitric oxide, *PBMCs* peripheral blood mononuclear cells, *PGE_2* prostaglandin E_2, *PI3k* phosphatidylinositol-3-kinase, *RANTES* regulated upon activation, normal T cell expressed and presumably secreted, *RCT* randomized controlled trial, *TGF-β1* transforming growth factor beta 1, *TIMP-1* tissue inhibitor of metalloproteinase-1, *TLR* toll-like receptor, *TNF-α* tumor necrosis factor alpha, *TNF R1* tumor necrosis factor receptor 1

antigen-antigen D related (HLA-DR) expression on monocytes and impaired production of pro-inflammatory mediators, including TNF-α, IL-6, Il-1ß, and IFN-γ referred to as "immunoparalysis". Although these compensatory mechanisms attempt to restore immune homeostasis, a subtype of patients develops persistent inflammation, immunosuppression, and catabolism syndrome (PICS), which is predictive of a poor outcome. It is most likely caused by persistent inflammation through a constant release of DAMPs driving organ injury [1].

2.3 Immunopathogenesis of ARDS

Sepsis and ARDS have similar underlying mechanisms: ARDS, defined as a life-threatening form of respiratory failure, is driven by an uncontrolled inflammatory host response induced by direct (pulmonary) or indirect (extrapulmonary) insults.

The most common causes include sepsis, viral and bacterial pneumonia, aspiration of gastric contents, and major trauma [2].

Inflammasome activation plays a central role in the development of ARDS [5]. In general, inflammasomes are multiprotein complexes that consist of a sensor NOD-, LRR- and pyrin domain-containing protein 3 (NLRP3), an adaptor apoptosis-associated speck-like protein containing a CARD (ASC), and an effector (caspase-1) [10]. Inflammasome activation generates IL-1ß and IL-18 which both drive the inflammatory cascade forward and are linked to an unfavorable prognosis [5]. This process involves two signals. Inflammasomes assemble downstream of PRRs in response to PAMPs and DAMPs. For example, LPS binding to Toll-like receptor 4 (TLR4) leads to the translocation of NF-κB into the nucleus and the transcription of pro-inflammatory mediators and inflammasome components including pro-caspase-1, pro–IL-1β, and pro-IL-18 (signal 1). Various stimuli such as ATP, viral RNA, and pore-forming toxins activate the sensor NLRP3, resulting in inflammasome assembly via ASC oligomerization (signal 2). Active capase-1 converts pro-IL-1β and pro-IL-18 into their mature forms causing pyroptotic cell death [5, 10, 11]. Inflammation and pyroptosis mediate substantial epithelial and endothelial injury with a subsequent loss of the alveolar-capillary barrier integrity, leading to influx of protein-rich edema fluid and immune cells into the alveoli [2]. This exudative edema causes dysfunctional surfactant and atelectasis, which in turn can predispose patients to biophysical injury of the lungs [2].

The influx of immune cells (especially neutrophils) triggered by the activation of TLRs on alveolar type II cells and resident macrophages is a salient feature of ARDS [12]. As neutrophils begin their transepithelial migration into the lungs, they become primed to phagocytose invading microbes and release toxic mediators including reactive oxygen species (ROS), neutrophil elastase, proteases, and nitric oxide (NO). Proteases such as metalloproteinases (MMPs) contribute to the disruption of the barrier integrity and lung parenchyma by degrading collagen [12–15]. Both neutrophil elastase and MMPs are known to promote lung injury in patients with ARDS [15]. Lastly, persistent inflammation and unbalanced immune homeostasis can further intensify existing lung damage and cause lasting injury and fibrosis [2].

2.4 Mechanisms of Action of Tetracyclines in ARDS

In vitro and *in vivo* studies have highlighted the wide-range of immunomodulatory effects of tetracyclines in models of ARDS, pneumonia, and sepsis [7, 16, 17]. They improve survival and organ injury by modulating a plethora of inflammatory pathways that become dysregulated in critically ill patients [1, 5, 6, 18]. In ARDS, tetracyclines decrease a variety of inflammatory mediators, including inflammasome-dependent IL-1ß and IL-18 secretion, which drives ARDS development [5, 16, 19]. Furthermore, they impair the breakdown of extracellular matrix components and inhibit neutrophil infiltration [14, 17, 20–23] (Fig. 2.1).

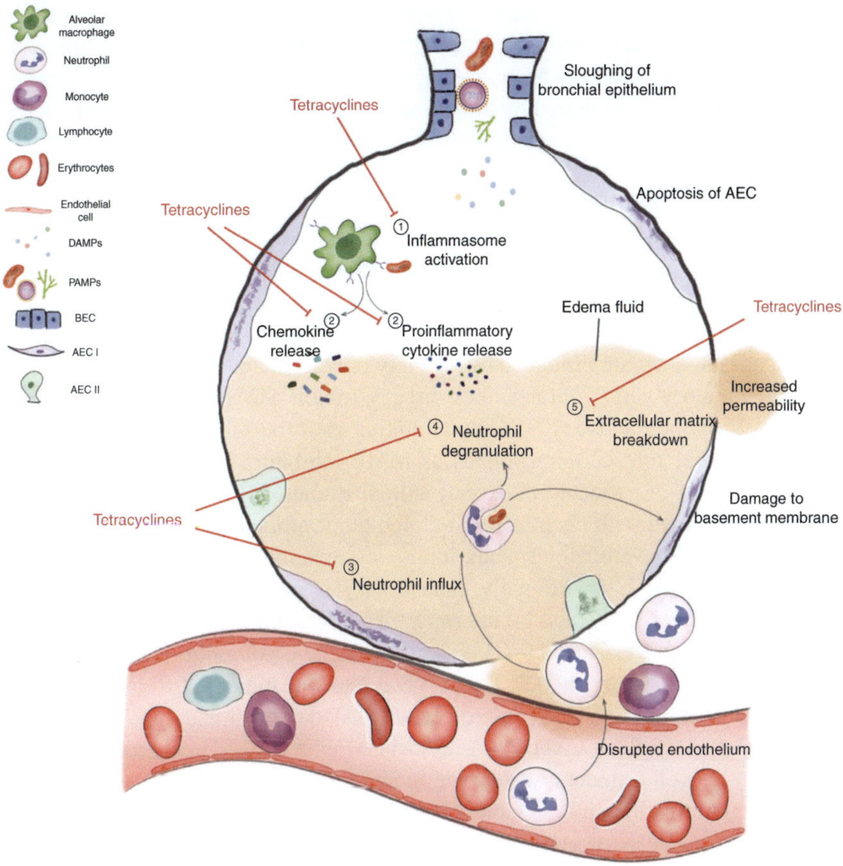

Fig. 2.1 The immunomodulatory effects of tetracyclines in ARDS. ① By sensing pathogen-associated molecular patterns (PAMPs) and damage-associated molecular patterns (DAMPs), Toll-like receptors (TLRs) become activated, thereby triggering the activation of the NLRP3 inflammasome. Tetracyclines inhibit the activation of nuclear factor-kappa B (NF-κB) and the NLRP3 inflammasome and subsequent ② release of proinflammatory cytokines and chemokines causes impaired ③ chemotaxis of immune cells including neutrophils. Tetracyclines further block ④ neutrophil degranulation and ⑤ extracellular matrix breakdown. ⊥ inhibition, *AEC I* type I alveolar epithelial cell, *AEC II* type II alveolar epithelial cell, *BEC* bronchial epithelial cell

2.4.1 *In Vivo* Models

2.4.1.1 Effects on Inflammatory Cytokines and NLRP3 Inflammasome Caspase-1 Signaling

Tetracyclines significantly reduce the secretion of pro-inflammatory cytokines, including TNF-α, IL-1ß, IL-6, and IL-8, thereby improving survival and lung injury in indirect models of ARDS [16, 19, 24].

Current research suggests that a key mechanism underlying the immunomodulatory effects of tetracyclines is the inhibition of the secretion of the pro-inflammatory cytokines IL-1ß and Il-18 via the NLRP3 inflammasome pathway. In a recent study, tetracycline significantly reduced both LPS- and influenza-induced lung injury in mice by inhibiting inflammasome-caspase-1 dependent IL-1ß and IL-18 production. This effect was mediated by direct inhibition of caspase-1 activation by tetracycline [5].

2.4.1.2 Effects on MMPs

The best described property of tetracyclines is the inhibition of MMPs in ARDS. MMPs are a family of zinc-dependent endopeptidases that degrade the basement membrane as well as extracellular matrix components and are involved in numerous pathological conditions including inflammation, tissue remodeling, and tumorigenesis. They are produced by a variety of cells including stromal, epithelial, and inflammatory cells. Tetracyclines directly inhibit MMP activity by chelating Zn^{2+} ions from their active site and by inhibiting their transcription [3].

The potential role of tetracyclines as MMP inhibitors in the pathogenesis of ARDS has been investigated in several animal studies. Carney et al. [23] showed that pigs pretreated with chemically modified tetracycline 3 (CMT-3) 12 h prior to intravenous LPS developed less lung injury, less edema and hypoxia by inhibiting MMP-9 and MMP-2. Additionally, plateau airway pressure was decreased [23]. Similar results were achieved by the same group through the inhibition of gelatinases and neutrophil elastase by CMT-3 in a porcine cardiopulmonary bypass and LPS-induced lung injury model. The survival rate was increased from 60 to 100% by CMT-3 treatment [13]. Steinberg et al. [15] demonstrated that blockage of MMP-2 and MMP-9 by CMT-3 was associated with less edema and histological lung injury as well as increased survival in an indirect model of ARDS in rats subjected to cecal ligation and puncture. Of note, CMT-3 prevented all the histopathological changes seen in ARDS [15]. Although not statistically significant, the authors observed a 64% reduction in MMP-2 activity and a 34% reduction in MMP-9 activity in bronchoalveolar lavage (BAL) fluid in a porcine model of ARDS [19]. Furthermore, administration of CMT-3 improved hemodynamics, gas exchange, lung histology, and survival through the inhibition of MMP-2 in an ovine ARDS model induced by third-degree burns, smoke inhalation and barotrauma injuries [25]. MMP-9 levels were not affected by CMT-3 but levels were only measured in plasma and not in BAL fluid as opposed to in the studies described earlier [25]. Levels of MMP-2, MMP-9, and neutrophil elastase measured in plasma were also not affected by CMT-3 in a cecal ligation and puncture-induced ARDS model [16]. The authors concluded that this might be due to the use of ketamine, which has been shown to weaken the effects of cecal ligation and puncture in rats via the inhibition of NF-κB.

Doxycycline has also been described as another potent MMP inhibitor in various animal models of primary and secondary ARDS [17, 20, 21, 24, 26, 27]. In a pancreatitis-induced ARDS model, doxycycline reduced MMP-9 levels which correlated with decreased pulmonary edema and hemorrhage [21]. Similar results were reproduced in cardiopulmonary bypass-induced ARDS models [20, 24]. The positive influence of doxycycline on endothelial barrier integrity was also demonstrated by decreased levels of endothelial protein. Not only were MMP-2 and MMP-9 levels in BAL fluid reduced in a H3N2 influenza-induced ARDS model, so were concentrations of endothelial protein thrombomodulin and T1-α, a membrane protein of alveolar type I epithelium, indicating less alveolar capillary membrane damage [27]. Furthermore, doxycycline might attenuate the development of pulmonary fibrosis in ARDS through the inhibition of gelatinases [28].

2.4.1.3 Effects on Neutrophil Transmigration

One of the hallmarks of ARDS is the influx of neutrophils into the lungs. Tetracyclines attenuate neutrophil infiltration and thereby prevent ARDS, an effect possibly linked to the concomitant decrease of MMP levels [13, 14, 23, 26]. In a ventilation-induced lung injury (VILI) model, pretreatment with CMT-3 decreased neutrophil infiltration and myeloperoxidase levels, which correlated significantly with MMP-9 activity. The role of MMP-9 during neutrophil migration is, however, not well defined. As a proteinase, MMP-9 could potentially degrade the basement membrane and thereby facilitate migration [14]. In an *in vitro* experiment, neutrophil transmigration across Matrigel and MMP-9 levels in the Matrigel invasion chamber were reduced by doxycycline [21].

Pretreatment with CMT-3 inhibited neutrophil influx in models of bacterial- and cardiopulmonary bypass-induced ARDS [13, 23, 29]. Additionally, doxycycline prevented neutrophil infiltration in models of viral-, bacterial-, cardiopulmonary bypass- and pancreatitis-induced ARDS [17, 21, 22, 27, 30].

2.4.2 Human Data

Recently, Peukert et al. described the effect of tetracycline on the NLRP3 inflammasome pathway in patients with direct ARDS (Fig. 2.1). Human alveolar leukocytes were isolated within 24 h of onset of direct ARDS. Cultured leukocytes continued to produce IL-1ß and IL-18 suggesting that the NLRP3 inflammasome pathway remained intact. Tetracycline inhibited the production of IL-1ß and IL-18 by alveolar leukocytes in a dose-dependent manner. This study indicates that the inhibition of caspase-1-dependent IL-1ß and IL-18 by tetracyclines might be a new therapeutic approach in patients with direct ARDS [5].

A randomized clinical trial is currently investigating whether doxycycline can limit the NF-κB dependent release of pro-inflammatory cytokines and thereby prevent evolution towards ARDS in patients with COVID-19 (ClinicalTrials.gov Identifier: NCT04371952). In 89 high-risk COVID-19 patients living in long-term care facilities, it was recently shown that the administration of doxycycline within 12 h after symptom onset was associated with early clinical recovery, decreased hospitalization and reduced mortality [31]. These findings contradict the results of a randomized controlled trial which suggested doxycycline was not effective for suspected COVID-19 [32]. In this study, 798 participants received doxycycline compared to 994 participants randomized to standard care. However, the trial had several limitations: first, the trial included participants recruited within 14 days after symptom onset. Second, almost half of the participants were accrued without PCR-confirmed severe acute respiratory syndrome coronavirus 2 (SARS-CoV-2) infection [32]. Because the inflammasome-caspase-1 pathway is activated early in ARDS [5, 8], this might explain why doxycycline was not beneficial.

2.5 Mechanisms of Action of Tetracyclines in Sepsis

Tetracyclines exert their pleiotropic immunomodulatory effects via several inflammatory pathways such as NF-κB and MAPKs downstream of PRRs whereby they inhibit the secretion of inflammatory mediators including cytokines, chemokines, MMPs, prostaglandin E_2 (PGE_2), and NO [7, 33–38]. They also ameliorate sepsis-induced liver injury by inhibiting apoptotic pathways [39, 40]. Mild perturbation of mitochondrial function by tetracyclines can install disease tolerance mechanisms like tissue repair and metabolic reprogramming [6].

2.5.1 *In Vitro* Models

2.5.1.1 Effects on Cytokine and Chemokine Production

An uncontrolled host response to infection can trigger a so-called cytokine storm which is one of the main characteristics of sepsis [1]. Mounting evidence has identified autophagy as an important regulator of excessive inflammation. Sun et al. [35] have shown that minocycline, which induces autophagy by inhibiting the mammalian target of rapamycin (mTOR) signaling pathway, suppresses cytokine production and cell proliferation, and protects human THP-1 cells from LPS-toxicity. Additionally, the study suggests that the IKK/NF-κB signal pathway was linked to minocycline-induced autophagy [35]. A previous study also demonstrated that minocycline decreased cytokine and chemokine production by inhibiting IKKα/β phosphorylation in LPS-stimulated THP-1 cells [41]. The influence of tetracyclines on certain signaling pathways was further characterized by Sun et al. [34]. The modulated phosphorylation of the NF-κB-, p38- and ERK1/2-pathways by doxycycline, minocycline, and tigecycline significantly inhibited the expression of TNF-α, IL-8, macrophage inflammatory protein 1α (MIP-1α) and MIP-1ß by LPS-stimulated THP-1 cells [34].

2.5.1.2 Effects on Arachidonic Acid Metabolites and NO Production

Metabolites of arachidonic acid, such as PGE_2 and NO, are inhibited by tetracyclines and play a role in inflammatory processes [42]. CMT-3 inhibited both nitrite and the cyclooxygenase 2 (COX-2) mediated PGE_2 accumulation in murine macrophages stimulated with LPS [42]. Moreover, tetracyclines regulate inducible NO synthase (iNOS) at the post-transcriptional level, thereby decreasing NO levels in LPS-stimulated murine macrophages [36, 37, 43, 44].

2.5.2 *In Vivo* Models

2.5.2.1 Effects on MAPK Signaling Pathways and Inflammatory Mediators

Doxycycline ameliorated systemic and pulmonary inflammation in a murine sepsis model induced by cecal ligation and puncture [7]. By decreasing levels of IL-1ß, IL-6, TNF-α, myeloperoxidase (MPO), and the antioxidant glutathione in plasma and lung homogenates, doxycycline improved survival. The anti-inflammatory effect of CMT-3 is possibly mediated through the inhibition of MAPKs. In rats subjected to cecal ligation and puncture, pretreatment with CMT-3 inhibited TNF-α secretion and activation of p38 and p42/44–MAPK pathways, thereby preventing the progression to septic shock [38].

Tetracyclines also act as inhibitors of NO synthesis. In mice injected intraperitoneally with LPS, doxycycline prevented septic shock by inhibiting nitrate production by an IL-10 independent mechanism [36]. Furthermore, tetracyclines caused a decrease in iNOS activity in a similar sepsis model [37].

2.5.2.2 Effects on Organ Dysfunction

Maitra et al. [39] showed that CMT-3 improved survival and was hepatoprotective in rats subjected to sepsis by cecal ligation and puncture. They demonstrated that the underlying mechanisms by which CMT-3 improved survival and hepatic injury were the CMT-3 induced reduction of MMP-9 and NO. The hepatoprotective effect of CMT-3 was further characterized by the same group. Administration of CMT-3 in septic rats caused decreased levels of MMP-9 and increased the expression of tissue inhibitor of metalloproteinase-1 (TIMP-1), which is an *in vivo* inhibitor of MMP-9. Furthermore, transforming growth factor beta-1 (TGF-ß1) and caspase-3 were reduced, thereby preventing liver injury and increasing survival in septic rats [40]. Recently, Colaço et al. [6] demonstrated how doxycycline can protect against sepsis by inducing disease tolerance without diminishing bacterial load in a mouse model of bacterial sepsis. In this study, tissue damage of the liver, lungs, and kidneys on a molecular and histopathological level was reduced by treatment with doxycycline. Furthermore, the authors demonstrated similar protective effects in influenza-induced sepsis in contrast to fungal- or cerebral malaria-induced infection models. Bulk RNA sequencing showed that doxycycline altered the expression of genes involved in epithelial cell differentiation suggesting more effective lung repair without the development of lung fibrosis. Functional analysis found a cluster of down-regulated genes related to decreased liver collagen production indicating that doxycycline potentially plays a role in limiting liver fibrosis. During infection, livers of septic mice accumulated acylcarnitines and steroids. Administration of doxycycline partially decreased this accumulation suggesting that it might reverse the block in mitochondrial import of fatty acids during sepsis. It also increased the activation of glucocorticoid receptors through serine phosphorylation. Furthermore, it was shown that mild perturbation of mitochondrial function, like the electron transport chain, by doxycycline can activate disease tolerance mechanisms, such as tissue repair and metabolic reprogramming in sepsis. One of the underlying mechanisms could be the doxycycline-induced sensitization to adrenergic agonists that reduces lipid accumulation in the liver. This elegant study demonstrates how doxycycline may rebalance immune homeostasis in sepsis [6].

2.5.3 Human Data

Minocycline significantly ameliorated the LPS-induced inflammatory response in human monocytes obtained from healthy volunteers by decreasing the production of TNF-α, IL-1ß, IL-6, COX-2, and PGE_2, as well as reducing activation of lectin-like oxidized low density lipoprotein receptor-1 (LOX-1), TNF-α factor (LITAF), and Nur77 nuclear receptor. The immunomodulatory effects of minocycline were mediated through the blocked activation of NF-κB, p38 MAPK, and phosphoinositide 3-kinase (PI3K)/Akt pathways [33]. Consistent with this, another study demonstrated that doxycycline reduced the LPS-induced gene expression of IL-1ß and IL-6 as well as phagocytosis of heat-inactivated *Escherichia coli* by monocytes [45].

The Fredeking group investigated the impact of tetracyclines on the inflammatory response in patients with dengue hemorrhagic fever in two randomized controlled trials [46, 47]. In the first trial, hospitalized patients received usual care or usual care combined with doxycycline or tetracycline. Serum cytokine and cytokine receptor levels were determined on days 1, 3, and 7 of treatment. Doxycycline was significantly more effective in modulating levels of IL-6, IL-1ß, TNF-α, IL-1 receptor antagonist (IL-1ra) and TNF-R1 than tetracycline. In the second trial with 231 participants, doxycycline treatment was associated with lower mortality, which positively correlated with reduced levels of pro-inflammatory cytokines. Patients in the doxycycline arm had a 46% lower mortality than those in the usual care arm [47].

In a prospective randomized placebo-controlled pilot trial, intravenous doxycycline did not have an impact on MMP-8, MMP-9, or TIMP-1 in patients with severe sepsis or septic shock [48]. This finding might be explained by the small sample size and large variance of disease severity that made it nearly impossible to detect a statistical significance. Only 23 patients were included in the analysis of this pilot trial. The studied population was also very heterogenous in terms of disease severity and disease onset, which was reflected in the detected variation in baseline concentrations and activities of MMP-8, MMP-9, and TIMP-1 [48].

2.6 Future Research Perspectives

ARDS and sepsis are both heterogenous syndromes characterized by significant variability in the degree of immune dysregulation, disease severity, and prognosis. As described in this chapter, tetracyclines modulate immunity at multiple levels involving the inhibition of concurrent pro- and anti-inflammatory pathways. Although our knowledge of the underlying mechanisms has increased, we need more clinical trials before we can adopt tetracyclines as routine treatment in sepsis and ARDS.

To prevent the development of antibiotic resistance, we need to further investigate the use of non-antibacterial tetracycline derivatives such as CMT-3; their effectiveness has already been observed in preclinical trials [5, 16, 25]. Furthermore, research should focus on developing tetracyclines with minimal adverse effects and on augmenting certain immunomodulatory effects.

Most clinical trials of novel sepsis and ARDS therapies have focused on large patient cohorts without considering the heterogenous nature of both syndromes and the varying immune responses of each patient. This has likely contributed to the fact that immunomodulatory drugs have not been demonstrated to have a clinical benefit in the past. Each patient needs to be longitudinally evaluated by using biomarkers and establishing baseline immune cell responsiveness [1]. In other words, immune profiling is necessary to stratify critical care patients in future trials and to identify biological subphenotypes in ARDS and sepsis. Calfee et al. [49] have described differential responses to treatment according to phenotype in ARDS. Predictive enrichment strategies are recommended to promote the efficiency of clinical trials and to enable precision medicine.

2.7 Conclusion

In summary, tetracyclines have been shown to be potent drugs with pleiotropic immunomodulatory effects inhibiting multiple inflammatory pathways that trigger an uncontrolled immune response in ARDS and sepsis. In preclinical studies, tetracyclines have been described as promising immunomodulatory agents that seem to have the potential to correct the unbalanced immune homeostasis present in critically ill individuals. Future trials need to further investigate tetracyclines in terms of dosing and side effects as well as focus on preventing antibiotic resistance. Finally, the extent of inflammation and immunosuppression varies between each patient explaining why so many trials have failed to show a survival benefit for immunomodulatory drugs in the past. We need to identify subphenotypes of ARDS and sepsis that will respond to adjunctive tetracycline treatment.

References

1. Steinhagen F, Schmidt SV, Schewe JC, Peukert K, Klinman DM, Bode C. Immunotherapy in sepsis—brake or accelerate? Pharmacol Ther. 2020;208:107476.
2. Matthay MA, Zemans RL, Zimmerman GA, et al. Acute respiratory distress syndrome. Nat Rev Dis Prim. 2019;5:18.
3. Griffin MO, Fricovsky E, Ceballos G, Villarreal F. Tetracyclines: a pleitropic family of compounds with promising therapeutic properties. Review of the literature. Am J Physiol Cell Physiol. 2010;299:C539–48.
4. Smith-Norowitz TA, Weaver D, Norowitz YM, et al. Doxycycline suppresses Chlamydia pneumoniae induced interferon-gamma responses in peripheral blood mononuclear cells in children with allergic asthma. J Infect Chemother. 2018;24:470–5.

5. Peukert K, Fox M, Schulz S, et al. Inhibition of caspase-1 with tetracycline ameliorates acute lung injury. Am J Respir Crit Care Med. 2021;204:53–63.
6. Colaço HG, Barros A, Neves-Costa A, et al. Tetracycline antibiotics induce host-dependent disease tolerance to infection. Immunity. 2021;54:53–67.e7.
7. Patel A, Khande H, Periasamy H, Mokale S. Immunomodulatory effect of doxycycline ameliorates systemic and pulmonary inflammation in a murine polymicrobial sepsis model. Inflammation. 2020;43:1035–43.
8. Opitz B, van Laak V, Eitel J, Suttorp N. Innate immune recognition in infectious and noninfectious diseases of the lung. Am J Respir Crit Care Med. 2010;181:1294–309.
9. Zarrin AA, Bao K, Lupardus P, Vucic D. Kinase inhibition in autoimmunity and inflammation. Nat Rev Drug Discov. 2021;20:39–63.
10. Guo H, Callaway JB, Ting JPY. Inflammasomes: mechanism of action, role in disease, and therapeutics. Nat Med. 2015;21:677–87.
11. Hornung V, Latz E. Critical functions of priming and lysosomal damage for NLRP3 activation. Eur J Immunol. 2010;40:620–3.
12. Zemans RL, Matthay MA. What drives neutrophils to the alveoli in ARDS? Thorax. 2017;72:1–3.
13. Carney DE, Lutz CJ, Picone AL, et al. Matrix metalloproteinase inhibitor prevents acute lung injury after cardiopulmonary bypass. Circulation. 1999;100:400–6.
14. Kim JH, Suk MH, Yoon DW, et al. Inhibition of matrix metalloproteinase-9 prevents neutrophilic inflammation in ventilator-induced lung injury. Am J Physiol Lung Cell Mol Physiol. 2006;291:L580–7.
15. Steinberg J, Halter J, Schiller HJ, et al. Metalloproteinase inhibition reduces lung injury and improves survival after cecal ligation and puncture in rats. J Surg Res. 2003;111:185–95.
16. Roy SK, Kubiak BD, Albert SP, et al. Chemically modified tetracycline 3 prevents acute respiratory distress syndrome in a porcine model of sepsis + ischemia/reperfusion-induced lung injury. Shock. 2012;37:424–32.
17. Zhang C, Gong W, Liu H, Guo Z, Ge S. Inhibition of matrix metalloproteinase-9 with low-dose doxycycline reduces acute lung injury induced by cardiopulmonary bypass. Int J Clin Exp Med. 2014;7:4975–82.
18. Halter JM, Pavone LA, Steinberg JM, et al. Chemically modified tetracycline (COL-3) improves survival if given 12 but not 24 hours after cecal ligation and puncture. Shock. 2006;26:587–91.
19. Steinberg J, Halter J, Schiller H, et al. Chemically modified tetracycline prevents the development of septic shock and acute respiratory distress syndrome in a clinically applicable porcine model. Shock. 2005;24:348–56.
20. Zhang F, Hu L, Wu YX, et al. Doxycycline alleviates paraquat-induced acute lung injury by inhibiting neutrophil-derived matrix metalloproteinase 9. Int Immunopharmacol. 2019;72:243–51.
21. Sochor M, Richter S, Schmidt A, Hempel S, Hopt UT, Keck T. Inhibition of matrix metalloproteinase-9 with doxycycline reduces pancreatitis-associated lung injury. Digestion. 2009;80:65–73.
22. Moon A, Gil S, Gill SE, Chen P, Matute-Bello G. Doxycycline impairs neutrophil migration to the airspaces of the lung in mice exposed to intratracheal lipopolysaccharide. J Inflamm (Lond). 2012;9:31.
23. Carney DE, McCann UG, Schiller HJ, et al. Metalloproteinase inhibition prevents acute respiratory distress syndrome. J Surg Res. 2001;99:245–52.
24. Wang CT, Zhang L, Wu HW, Wei L, Xu B, Li DM. Doxycycline attenuates acute lung injury following cardiopulmonary bypass: involvement of matrix metalloproteinases. Int J Clin Exp Pathol. 2014;7:7460–8.
25. Zhou X, Wang D, Ballard-Croft CK, Simon SR, Lee HM, Zwischenberger JB. A tetracycline analog improves acute respiratory distress syndrome survival in an ovine model. Ann Thorac Surg. 2010;90:419–26.

26. Fujita M, Harada E, Ikegame S, et al. Doxycycline attenuated lung injury by its biological effect apart from its antimicrobial function. Pulm Pharmacol Ther. 2007;20:669–75.
27. Ng HH, Narasaraju T, Phoon MC, Sim MK, Seet JE, Chow VT. Doxycycline treatment attenuates acute lung injury in mice infected with virulent influenza H3N2 virus: involvement of matrix metalloproteinases. Exp Mol Pathol. 2012;92:287–95.
28. Fujita M, Ye Q, Ouchi H, et al. Doxycycline attenuated pulmonary fibrosis induced by bleomycin in mice. Antimicrob Agents Chemother. 2006;50:739–43.
29. McCann UG, Gatto LA, Searles B, et al. Matrix metalloproteinase inhibitor: differential effects on pulmonary neutrophil and monocyte sequestration following cardiopulmonary bypass. J Extra Corpor Technol. 1999;31:67–75.
30. Liu J, Zhong X, He Z, et al. Effect of low-dose, long-term roxithromycin on airway inflammation and remodeling of stable noncystic fibrosis bronchiectasis. Mediat Inflamm. 2014;2014:708608.
31. Alam MM, Mahmud S, Rahman MM, Simpson J, Aggarwal S, Ahmed Z. Clinical outcomes of early treatment with doxycycline for 89 high-risk COVID-19 patients in long-term care facilities in New York. Cureus. 2020;12:e9658.
32. Butler CC, Yu LM, Dorward J, et al. Doxycycline for community treatment of suspected COVID-19 in people at high risk of adverse outcomes in the UK (PRINCIPLE): a randomised, controlled, open-label, adaptive platform trial. Lancet Respir Med. 2021;9:1010–20.
33. Pang T, Wang J, Benicky J, Saavedra JM. Minocycline ameliorates LPS-induced inflammation in human monocytes by novel mechanisms including LOX-1, Nur77 and LITAF inhibition. Biochim Biophys Acta. 2012;1820:503–10.
34. Sun J, Shigemi H, Tanaka Y, Yamauchi T, Ueda T, Iwasaki H. Tetracyclines downregulate the production of LPS-induced cytokines and chemokines in THP-1 cells via ERK, p38, and nuclear factor-κB signaling pathways. Biochem Biophys Rep. 2015;4:397–404.
35. Sun J, Shigemi H, Cao M, et al. Minocycline induces autophagy and inhibits cell proliferation in LPS-stimulated THP-1 cells. Biomed Res Int. 2020;2020:5459209.
36. D'Agostino P, La Rosa M, Barbera C, et al. Doxycycline reduces mortality to lethal endotoxemia by reducing nitric oxide synthesis via an interleukin-10-independent mechanism. J Infect Dis. 1998;177:489–92.
37. Milano S, Arcoleo F, D'Agostino P, Cillari E. Intraperitoneal injection of tetracyclines protects mice from lethal endotoxemia downregulating inducible nitric oxide synthase in various organs and cytokine and nitrate secretion in blood. Antimicrob Agents Chemother. 1997;41:117–21.
38. Maitra SR, Bhaduri S, Chen E, Shapiro MJ. Role of chemically modified tetracycline on TNF-α and mitogen-activated protein kinases in sepsis. Shock. 2004;22:478–81.
39. Maitra SR, Bhaduri S, Valane PD, Tervahartiala T, Sorsa T, Ramamurthy N. Inhibition of matrix metalloproteinases by chemically modified tetracyclines in sepsis. Shock. 2003;20:280–5.
40. Maitra SR, Shapiro MJ, Bhaduri S, El-Maghrabi MR. Effect of chemically modified tetracycline on transforming growth factor beta1 and caspase-3 activation in liver of septic rats. Crit Care Med. 2005;33:1577–81.
41. Tai K, Iwasaki H, Ikegaya S, Ueda T. Minocycline modulates cytokine and chemokine production in lipopolysaccharide-stimulated THP-1 monocytic cells by inhibiting IκB kinase α/β phosphorylation. Transl Res. 2013;161:99–109.
42. Patel R, Attur MG, Dave M, et al. A novel mechanism of action of chemically modified tetracyclines: inhibition of COX-2-mediated prostaglandin E2 production. J Immunol. 1999;163:3459–67.
43. Amin AR, Patel RN, Thakker GD, Lowenstein CJ, Attur MG, Abramson SB. Post-transcriptional regulation of inducible nitric oxide synthase mRNA in murine macrophages by doxycycline and chemically modified tetracyclines. FEBS Lett. 1997;410:259–64.
44. D'Agostino P, Ferlazzo V, Milano S, et al. Anti-inflammatory effects of chemically modified tetracyclines by the inhibition of nitric oxide and interleukin-12 synthesis in J774 cell line. Int Immunopharmacol. 2001;1:1765–76.

45. Bode C, Diedrich B, Muenster S, et al. Antibiotics regulate the immune response in both presence and absence of lipopolysaccharide through modulation of Toll-like receptors, cytokine production and phagocytosis in vitro. Int Immunopharmacol. 2014;18:27–34.
46. Castro JEZ, Vado-Solis I, Perez-Osorio C, Fredeking TM. Modulation of cytokine and cytokine receptor/antagonist by treatment with doxycycline and tetracycline in patients with dengue fever. Clin Dev Immunol. 2011;2011:370872.
47. Fredeking TM, Zavala-Castro JE, González-Martínez P, et al. Dengue patients treated with doxycycline showed lower mortality associated to a reduction in IL-6 and TNF levels. Recent Pat Antiinfect Drug Discov. 2015;10:51–8.
48. Nukarinen E, Tervahartiala T, Valkonen M, et al. Targeting matrix metalloproteinases with intravenous doxycycline in severe sepsis—a randomised placebo-controlled pilot trial. Pharmacol Res. 2015;99:44–51.
49. Wilson JG, Calfee CS. ARDS subphenotypes: understanding a heterogeneous syndrome. Crit Care. 2020;24:102.

Hit Early: Blocking Interleukin-1 in the Treatment of COVID-19 Pneumonia

3

E. J. Giamarellos-Bourboulis, M. Mouktaroudi, and M. G. Netea

3.1 Introduction

The rise of the pandemic by the novel severe acute respiratory syndrome coronavirus-2 (SARS-CoV-2) generated concern in the medical community for patients who are admitted to the intensive care unit (ICU) because of severe respiratory failure. The majority of these patients have unfavorable outcomes and this led to the consideration of how progression into severe respiratory failure and ICU admission may be prevented. The current approach for bacterial sepsis advocates that early initiation of treatment is a life-saving strategy [1]. This opinion was based on the observation that starting antimicrobials in the first hour from hypotension was associated with 79.1% survival and that every hour of delay impacted by 7.6% the relative increase in the odds for death [2]. What are the similarities between coronavirus disease 2019 (COVID-19) and sepsis that could indicate that the principles of early treatment may apply, and how feasible is this in COVID-19? One recent meta-analysis described that almost 80% of hospitalized patients with COVID-19 meet the Sepsis-3 definition using the Sequential Organ Failure Assessment (SOFA) score [3]. Despite the similarity in definition, the major obstacle for early treatment in COVID-19 would be the lack of extremely potent antiviral drugs, even though a recent retrospective analysis of 475 hospitalized patients showed that start of

E. J. Giamarellos-Bourboulis (✉) · M. Mouktaroudi
4th Department of Internal Medicine, National and Kapodistrian University of Athens Medical School, Athens, Greece
e-mail: egiamarel@med.uoa.gr

M. G. Netea
Department of Internal Medicine and Radboud Center for Infectious Diseases, Radboud University, Nijmegen, The Netherlands

Department of Immunology and Metabolism, Life and Medical Sciences Institute, University of Bonn, Bonn, Germany

J.-L. Vincent (ed.), *Annual Update in Intensive Care and Emergency Medicine 2022*, Annual Update in Intensive Care and Emergency Medicine,
https://doi.org/10.1007/978-3-030-93433-0_3

remdesivir in the first 3 days from positive testing for SARS-CoV-2 was associated with lower odds for death [4].

Early treatment of COVID-19 thus needs to rely on the early recognition of the activation of the pro-inflammatory cascade and of the immediate start of anti-inflammatory treatment aiming to prevent progression into severe respiratory failure and unfavorable outcome. The current chapter provides existing evidence about the kinetics of cytokines for disease progression, to suggest novel biomarkers for prognosis and to present clinical evidence on the strategy of early anti-inflammatory treatment for COVID-19, with a focus on interleukin (IL)-1-dependent pathways.

3.2 Cytokines and Disease Progression in COVID-19

Early since the beginning of the SARS-CoV-2 pandemic, it was realized that the more severe patients were suffering from hyperinflammation, which was associated with unfavorable outcome [5]. Since then, several prospective studies have been conducted to associate the concentrations of circulating cytokines with disease severity and disease prognosis. A PubMed search entering the keywords "plasma cytokines" and "COVID-19" on 22 October 2021 retrieved 697 results. Pre-prints, reviews, and case reports were excluded leaving 587 peer-reviewed articles. Following the reading of the abstracts, only studies associating plasma cytokines with disease severity and prognosis were retained. Some of these studies, summarized in Table 3.1, compare the circulating levels of cytokines with disease severity. It needs to be highlighted that not all existing cytokines were measured in all studies; however, one common denominator of the studies analyzed in Table 3.1 is that concentrations of IL-6 and IL-1 receptor antagonist (IL-1ra) increase with increasing disease severity [6–11].

Another set of studies tried to identify which of the circulating cytokines may be a biomarker of prognosis in COVID-19. All these studies used 30-day mortality as an endpoint and their results are summarized in Table 3.2. Most of the enrolled patients were severe on enrolment and analyses indicated that circulating concentrations of IL-6 and, to a lesser extent other cytokines, were increased from the day of

Table 3.1 Synopsis of studies measuring circulating cytokines in the plasma of patients with coronavirus disease 2019 (COVID-19) on the day of hospital admission

Ref.	Design	Study period	Country	Number of patients	Cytokines increased in severe/critical ICU patients
6	Single-center, biobank	NR	USA	36	M-CSF, IL-1ra, IP-10, MCP-1, IL-2, TNFα, IL-6,
7	Single-center, prospective	March–May 2020	Turkey	100	IL-1ra, IL-18
8	Prospective	NR	USA	15	IL-1ra, IL-6, IL-19
9	Prospective	NR	USA	40	IL-1β, IL-6, IL-10, sTNFR1
10	Prospective	February–March 2020	China	1472	IL-6
11	Prospective	February–May 2020	Italy	175	IL-2, IL-6, IL-8, IL-16, sTNFR1

IL interleukin, *TNF* tumor necrosis factor, *ICU* intensive care unit, *NR* not reported, *M-CSF* macrophage colony-stimulating factor, *IP* interferon-inducible protein, *MCP* monocyte chemoattractant protein, *IL-1ra* IL-1 receptor antagonist

Table 3.2 Synopsis of studies associating cytokine admission levels with unfavorable outcome in coronavirus disease 2019 (COVID-19)

Ref.	Design	Study period	Country	Number of patients	Disease severity	Cytokine greater in non-survivors	Suggested prognostic cut-off for unfavorable outcome
12	Single-center, prospective	April–May 2020	Italy	46	Stage I to III	IL-6	NR
13	Single-center, prospective	January–June 2020	China	31	Severe	IL-6, IL-8, IL-10	NR
14	Three centers, prospective	February 2020–July 2021	Japan	102	Moderate and severe	IL-6	49 pg/ml for IL-6
15	Three centers, prospective	March–April 2020	France	150	Severe	IL-6, CRP	212 pg/ml for IL-6
16	Single-center, prospective	March–April 2020	USA	1484	Mild to severe	IL-6, IL-8, TNF-α	70 pg/ml for IL-6, 50 pg/ml for IL-8; 35 pg/ml for TNF-α
17	Multicenter, prospective	March–May 2020	Greece	178	Severe	IL-6	30 pg/ml for IL-6

IL interleukin, *TNF* tumor necrosis factor, *CRP* C-reactive protein, *NR* not reported

admission among non-survivors [12–17]. However, the results of these studies need to be interpreted under the notion that the research question was "which measured cytokines predicted an unfavorable outcome among patients who were already either severe or critical?". None of these studies searched for a biomarker that could identify which patients with moderate illness will progress over time into severe or critical illness.

3.3 Contribution of Monocytes and Macrophages in Early Cytokine Response

The hyperinflammation of COVID-19 has features of cytokine storm syndrome or macrophage activation syndrome. Macrophage activation syndrome is often described as an auto-inflammatory entity due to sudden stimulation of tissue macrophages with over-production of IL-1β and the generation of a vicious cycle where IL-1β propagates further production of cytokines by macrophages through its receptor [18]. Inflammasomes play a central role in the production of IL-1β since they activate caspase-1, which cleaves inactive pro-IL-1β to active IL-1β.

There is scarce evidence regarding the participation of the NACHT, LRR, and PYD domains-containing protein (NLRP) inflammasome in the pathogenesis of COVID-19. In one post-mortem study of only four patients, lung sections were stained for components of the NLRP3 inflammasome mainly apoptosis-associated speck-like protein containing a caspase recruitment domain (ASC) and caspase-1; lung deposition was significantly higher than in control subjects [19]. It has been suggested that several particles of other coronaviruses may stimulate components of the NLRP3 inflammasome. More precisely, ORF3a binds to ASC and ORF8b binds to leucine-rich repeats and this stimulates the assembly of NLRP3 [20]. Although activation of NLRP3 leads to activation of the proteolytic activity of caspase-1, the excess production of IL-β is a dual process, because for caspase-1 to act, priming of the cell cytoplasm with pro-IL-1β is needed. It has been suggested that alarmins or damage-associated molecular patterns (DAMPs) that are released from the lung epithelial cells during rapid viral replication act on Toll-like receptor-4 (TLR4) and lead to intracellular accumulation of pro-IL-1β [21]. Indeed, increased levels of the DAMP S100A9 (also known as calprotectin) circulate in the plasma of patients with COVID-19 [11]. In parallel to the production of pro-IL-1β under the stimulation of DAMPs, one more cytokine of the IL-1 family is produced, namely IL-1α. This is already active and does not necessitate any further processing. Abundant release of IL-1α is described in lung infections, including COVID-19 [22].

Both IL-1α and IL-1β act on the IL-1 receptor in tissue macrophages and perpetuate the inflammatory process. In an attempt of the host to attenuate this phenomenon, IL-1ra is produced to limit the binding of IL-1α and IL-1β to their receptor and to minimize biological function [23]. There are three main observations that suggest that early production of IL-1α and IL-1β drives progression into severe respiratory failure:

- IL-1ra is increased in many severe cases of COVID-19 (Table 3.1).
- Treatment with anakinra, a recombinant human IL-1ra, has been associated with survival benefit in severe COVID-19 [24], suggesting that the IL-1 pathway is already activated in severe disease and that IL-1 activation may start before signs of severity appear.
- When severe disease develops, IL-1β is not detectable at high concentrations in the circulation by contrast to the other cytokines [16]. Since IL-1β and IL-6 are secreted in parallel from tissue macrophages, it may be hypothesized that the peak of IL-1β precedes the peak of the other cytokines.

3.4 How Can Early Activation of IL-1 Be Identified?

Not all patients with moderate-to-severe COVID-19 are at risk for progression into severe respiratory failure. This observation introduces the need for a biomarker that can identify activation of the IL-1 pathway early and that can prognosticate early which patients will deteriorate to develop severe respiratory failure. During March 2020, blood was drawn from 57 patients from three study sites in Greece on hospital admission for pneumonia. The concentrations of the biomarker suPAR (soluble urokinase plasminogen activator receptor) were measured. Despite the lack of signs of severe respiratory failure or respiratory distress at the time of admission, patients with concentrations of suPAR ≥6 ng/ml had 85.7% risk of progression into severe respiratory failure or death in the first 14 days of follow-up. This value was only

8.3% among patients with suPAR <6 ng/ml [25]. This finding was further validated in two later studies. The first study enrolled 352 patients and was multicenter in the United States, Denmark, Germany and Greece. Patients with suPAR ≥6.8 ng/ml on admission had 44.9% risk of progression into severe respiratory failure [26]. Finally, in the phase 2 study, SAVE (suPAR-guided anakinra treatment for validation of the risk and early management of severe respiratory failure by COVID-19), 59.2% of patients with suPAR ≥6 ng/ml receiving usual care progressed into severe respiratory failure or died the first 14 days contrary to only 3.7% of patients with suPAR <6 ng/ml [27]. Unpublished data from our group show that suPAR ≥6 ng/ml indicates increased circulating levels of the DAMP S100A8/A9 [28]. The above analysis on the role of DAMPs in priming tissue macrophages for pro-IL-1β led us to consider suPAR as an early biomarker of activation of the IL-1 pathway in patients which generates the risk for progression into severe respiratory failure.

3.5 SAVE Strategy: Early Blockade of IL-1 Guided by Biomarkers

The knowledge that suPAR may be an early biomarker for the risk of progression into severe respiratory failure led us to study its use to guide treatment with anakinra in one phase 2 and one phase 3 study. The therapeutic strategy targets hospitalized patients with COVID-19 pneumonia with a PaO_2:FiO_2 ratio ≥150 who do not need ICU treatment. If these patients have a plasma suPAR ≥6 ng/ml, early treatment with anakinra is started with one subcutaneous daily dose of 100 mg for 10 days.

The phase 2 study was given the acronym SAVE and was a single-arm, open-label trial (EudraCT number: 2020-001466-11; ClinicalTrials.gov Identifier: NCT04357366). Parallel comparators treated using standard-of-care in other departments of academic hospitals were recruited using the inclusion and exclusion criteria of the SAVE trial and were propensity-score matched for age, comorbidities, admission severity scores (Acute physiology and chronic health evaluation [APACHE] II, SOFA, pneumonia severity index, World Health Organization [WHO] scale) and for treatment with azithromycin, hydroxychloroquine, and dexamethasone. The incidence of severe respiratory failure or death after 14 days was 22.3% among anakinra-treated patients and 59.2% among comparators [27].

Following advice from the Emergency Task Force for COVID-19 of the European Medicine Agency, the pivotal, multicenter confirmatory phase III randomized controlled trial with the acronym SAVE-MORE was designed (EudraCT number: 2020-005828-11; ClinicalTrials.gov Identifier: NCT04680949). The study enrolled 594 patients who were subject to 1:2 stratified randomization into standard-of-care and placebo or standard-of-care and anakinra [29]. Stratified randomization was done taking into consideration, apart from allocation into placebo or anakinra, severity as defined by the need of oxygen therapy, intake of dexamethasone, body mass index, and geographic origin. On the day the study medication was started, 91.6% of participants were in need of supplemental oxygen. The primary study endpoint was comparison of the distribution of the scores from the 11-point WHO Clinical Progression ordinal Scale (CPS) on Day 28 as defined by ordinal multiple regression analysis. The adjusted proportional odds of having a worse score with anakinra than with placebo was 0.36 (95% confidence interval [CI] 0.26–0.50; p < 0.0001). Three supporting analyses of the primary endpoint were done. These were: (a) the distribution of the 11-point WHO-CPS on Day 14. The adjusted odds ratio was 0.58 (95% CI 0.42–0.79; p = 0.001); (b) proportion of patients with persistent disease at day 28 and with severe disease or death on day 28. Multivariate logistic regression analysis indicated that anakinra significantly reduced the risk of persistence (odds ratio 0.36; 95% CI 0.25–0.53; p < 0.0001) and of severe disease or death (odds ratio 0.46; 95% CI 0.26–0.83; p = 0.010); and (c) incidence of severe respiratory failure or death by day 14. This was 31.2% in the placebo arm and 20.7% in the anakinra arm (adjusted hazard ratio 0.67; p = 0.017). Secondary endpoints also favored anakinra treatment. More precisely: (1) the median absolute decrease in WHO-CPS by day 28 from baseline was 3 and 4 in the placebo and anakinra groups, respectively (odds ratio 0.40; p < 0.0001); (2) median absolute decrease in WHO-CPS by day 14 from baseline was 2 and 3 in the placebo and anakinra groups, respectively (odds ratio 0.64; p = 0.007); (3) median absolute decrease in SOFA score by day 7 from baseline was 0 and 1 in the placebo and anakinra groups, respectively (odds ratio 0.63; p = 0.004); (4) median time to hospital discharge was 12 and 11 days in the placebo and anakinra groups respectively (odds ratio 1.22; p = 0.033); and (5) median time for discharge from the ICU in case of ICU admission was 14 and 10 days in the placebo and anakinra groups, respectively (odds ratio 2.33; p = 0.026) [28]. It has to be noted that 11.1% of participants in the SAVE-MORE trial were not in need of supplemental oxygen at the time of screening for eligibility but had progressed into need for supplemental oxygen by mask or nasal prongs before the start of the study drug. As such, sudden need for oxygen may be considered a potential indication for anakinra treatment. The SAVE-MORE investigators also developed a prognostic score to help identify patients who may receive most benefit from anakinra treatment [29]. This score comprises aspartate aminotransferase >44 U/l; neutrophil to lymphocyte ratio > 5.5; C-reactive protein (CRP) >50 mg/l; and ferritin >700 ng/ml. Patients scoring positive for at least two of these elements had the greatest chance for improvement with anakinra treatment [29].

The CORIMUNO-ANA-1 study, which preceded the SAVE-MORE trial, did not give such favorable results. The patient population was similar to patients enrolled in the SAVE and SAVE-MORE trials, i.e., they were hospitalized and receiving nasal oxygen or oxygen by mask; 59 patients were randomized to treatment with anakinra and usual care and 55 patients to treatment with usual care alone [30]. The study was negative for the primary endpoint albeit showing a trend for anakinra benefit; 36% and 38% of patients respectively had a WHO-CPS score > 5 on day 4; and 47% and 51% respectively were receiving non-invasive ventilation or mechanical ventilation or had died by day 14 [30]. There are several possible explanations why the CORIMUNO-ANA-1 study was negative: (a) no biomarker was used for the selection of patients, so it is possible that some of the enrolled patients were not at a stage of early IL-1 activation; (b) no placebo was used; and (c) the duration of anakinra treatment was just 5 days.

In the CAN-COVID trial, 454 patients with hypoxic COVID-19 not requiring mechanical ventilation and with signs of hyperinflammation were randomized to a single injection of placebo or the anti-IL-1β monoclonal antibody, canakinumab

[31]. The primary endpoint was survival without need for non-invasive ventilation or mechanical ventilation by day 29. This endpoint was met in 88.8% of patients in the canakinumab arm and 85.7% of patients in the placebo arm. The superior efficacy of anakinra over canakinumab in a similar patient population may be explained by the activity of anakinra against IL-1α, which is not inhibited by canakinumab. An alternative explanation for this discrepancy is that suPAR was not used as a criterion for enrichment of the patient population.

3.6 Conclusion

The above analysis suggests there is great heterogeneity of patients at the time of hospital admission and that we need to understand early which patients are at risk for progression into severe respiratory failure so as to initiate early treatment aimed at preventing deterioration. This requires a personalized approach with the use of appropriate biomarkers (Fig. 3.1). In the case of anakinra, we suggest that the drug may be of benefit in patients admitted with COVID-19 pneumonia who do not

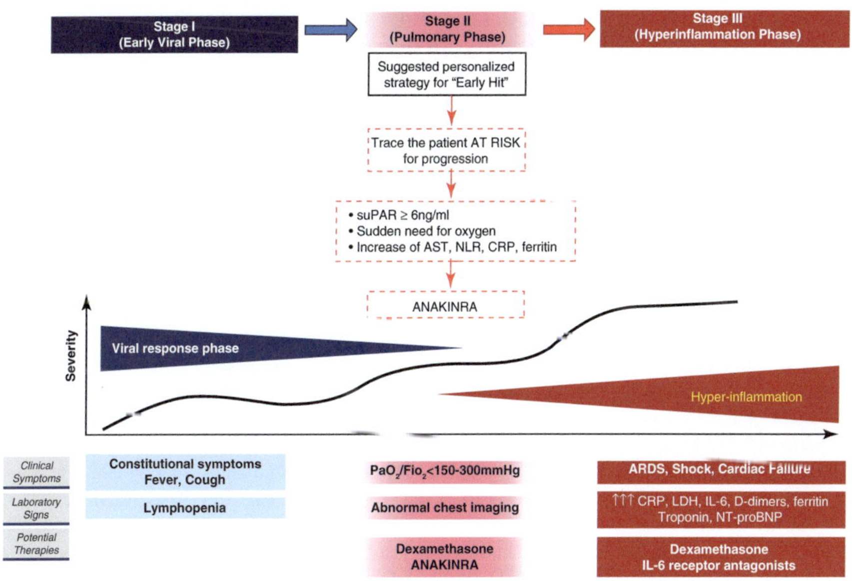

Fig. 3.1 Suggestion for early treatment with anakinra during the disease course of COVID-19 pneumonia. The results of the SAVE and SAVE-MORE trials [27, 29] suggest that anakinra could potentially be beneficial in patients who are at the pulmonary stage of the disease and at risk of progression to the hyperinflammatory stage. The patient at risk could be identified by at least one of following: soluble urokinase plasminogen activator receptor (suPAR) ≥6 ng/ml; sudden need for oxygen; increased circulating concentrations of at least two of aspartate aminotransferase (AST), neutrophil to lymphocyte ratio (NLR), C-reactive protein (CRP) and ferritin. *ARDS* acute respiratory distress syndrome, *BNP* brain natriuretic peptide, FiO_2 fraction of inspired oxygen, *IL* interleukin, *LDH* lactate dehydrogenase, PaO_2 partial oxygen pressure, ↑↑↑ extremely elevated

require ICU treatment. Existing evidence does not support the use of anakinra for patients already in severe respiratory failure.

Acknowledgements M. G. Netea is supported by an ERC Advanced Grant (#833247) and a Spinoza grant from the Netherlands Organization for Scientific Research.

References

1. Rhodes A, Evans LE, Alhazzani W, et al. Surviving sepsis campaign: international guidelines for management of sepsis and septic shock 2016. Crit Care Med. 2017;45:486–552.
2. Kumar A, Roberts D, Wood KE, et al. Duration of hypotension before initiation of effective antimicrobial therapy is the critical determinant of survival in human septic shock. Crit Care Med. 2006;34:1589–96.
3. Karakike E, Giamarellos-Bourboulis EJ, Kyprianou M, et al. Coronavirus disease 2019 as cause of viral sepsis: a systemic review and meta-analysis. Crit Care Med. 2021;49:2042–57.
4. Paranjape N, Husain M, Preistley J, Koonjah Y, Watts C, Havlik J. Early use of remdesivir in patients hospitalized with COVID-19 improves clinical outcomes: a retrospective observational study. Infect Dis Clin Pract. 2021;29:e282–6.
5. Laguna-Goyal R, Utrero-Rico A, Talayero P, et al. IL-6-based mortality risk model for hospitalized patients with COVID-19. J Allergy Clin Immunol. 2020;146:799–807.
6. Huntington KE, Louie DA, Lee CG, Elias JA, Ross EA, El-Deiry WS. Cytokine ranking via mutual information algorithm correlates cytokine profiles with presenting disease severity in patients infected with SARS-CoV-2. eLife. 2021;10:e64958.
7. Kerget B, Kerget F, Aksakal A, et al. Evaluation of alpha defensin, IL-1 receptor antagonist, and IL-18 levels in COVID-19 patients with macrophage activation syndrome and acute respiratory distress syndrome. J Med Virol. 2021;93:2090–8.
8. Wilson JG, Simpson LJ, Ferreira AM, et al. Cytokine profile in plasma of severe COVID-19 does not differ from ARDS and sepsis. JCI Insight. 2020;5:e140289.
9. McElvaney OJ, McEvoy NL, McElvaney OF, et al. Characterization of the inflammatory response to severe COVID-19 illness. Am J Resp Crit Care Med. 2020;202:812–21.
10. Wu J, Shen J, Han Y, et al. Upregulated IL-6 indicates a poor COVID-19 prognosis: a call for tocilizumab and convalescent plasma treatment. Front Immunol. 2021;12:598799.
11. Abers MS, Delmonte OM, Ricotta EE, et al. An immune-based biomarker signature is associated with mortality in COVID-19 patients. JCI Insight. 2021;6:e144455.
12. Santa-Cruz A, Mendes-Frias A, Oliveira AI, et al. Interleukin-6 as biomarker for the development of fatal severe acute respiratory syndrome coronavirus 2 pneumonia. Front Immunol. 2021;12:613422.
13. Li Q, Xu W, Li WX, Huang CL, Chen L. Dynamics of cytokines and lymphocyte subsets associated with poor prognosis of severe COVID-19. Eur Rev Med Pharmacol Sci. 2020;24:12536–44.
14. Saji R, Nishi M, Sakai K, et al. Combining IL-6 and SARS-CoV-2 RNAaemia-base risk stratification for fatal outcomes of COVID-19. PLoS One. 2021;16:e0256022.
15. Lavillegrand JR, Garnier M, Spaeth A, et al. Elevated plasma IL-6 and CRP levels are associated with adverse clinical outcomes and death in critically ill SARS-CoV-2 patients: inflammatory response of SARS-CoV-2 patients. Ann Intensive Care. 2021;11:9.
16. Del Valle DM, Kin-Schulze S, Huang HH, et al. An inflammatory cytokine signature predicts COVID-19 severity and survival. Nat Med. 2020;26:1636–43.
17. Saridaki M, Metallidis S, Grigoropoulou S, et al. Integration of heparin binding protein and interleukin-6 in the early prediction of respiratory failure and mortality in pneumonia by SARS-CoV-2 (COVID-19). Eur J Clin Microbiol Infect Dis. 2021;40:1405–12.
18. Karakike E, Giamarellos-Bourboulis EJ. Macrophage activation-like syndrome: a dinstict entity leading to early death in sepsis. Front Immunol. 2019;10:55.

19. Toldo S, Bussani R, Nuzzi V, et al. Inflammasome formation in the lungs of patients with fata COVID-19. Inflamm Res. 2021;70:7–10.
20. De Rivero VJ, Dietrich WD, Kean RW, de Rivero Vaccari JP. The inflammasomes in times of COVID-19. Front Immunol. 2020;11:583373.
21. Vora SM, Lieberman J, Wu H. Inflammasome activation at the crux of severe COVID-19. Nat Rev Immunol. 2021;21:694–703.
22. Rodrigues TS, de Sá KSG, Ishimoto AY, et al. Inflammasomes are activated in response to SARS-CoV-2 infection and are associated with COVID-19 severity in patients. J Exp Med. 2020;218:e20201707.
23. Cavalli G, Colafrancesco S, Emmi G, et al. Interleukin 1α: a comprehensive review on the role of IL-1α in the pathogenesis and treatment of autoimmune and inflammatory disorders. Autoimmun Rev. 2021;20:102763.
24. Kyriazopoulou E, Huet T, Cavalli G, et al. Effect of anakinra on mortality in patients with COVID-19: a systematic review and patient-level meta-analysis. Lancet Rheumatol. 2021;3:e690–7.
25. Rovina N, Akinosoglou K, Eugen-Olsen E, Hayek S, Reiser J, Giamarellos-Bourboulis EJ. Soluble urokinase plasminogen activator receptor (suPAR) as an early predictor of severe respiratory failure in patients with COVID-19 pneumonia. Crit Care. 2020;24:187.
26. Azam TU, Shadid HR, Blakely P, et al. Soluble urokinase receptor (suPAR) in COVID-19-related AKI. J Am Soc Nephrol. 2020;31:2725–35.
27. Kyriazopoulou E, Panagopoulos P, Metallidis S, et al. An open label trial of anakinra to prevent respiratory failure in COVID-19. eLife. 2021;10:e66125.
28. Renieris G, Karakike R, Gkavogianni T, et al. IL-1 mediates tissue specific inflammation and severe respiratory failure in Covid-19: clinical and experimental evidence. medRXiv 2021. https://doi.org/10.1101/2021.04.09.21255190
29. Kyriazopoulou E, Poulakou G, Milionis H, et al. Early treatment of COVID-19 with anakinra guided by soluble urokinase plasminogen activator receptor: a double-blind, randomized controlled phase 3 trial. Nat Med. 2021;27:1752–60.
30. CORIMUNO-19 Collaborative group. Effect of anakinra versus usual care in adults in hospital with COVID-19 and mild-to-moderate pneumonia (CORIMUNO-ANA-1): a randomised controlled trial. Lancet. Respir Med. 2021;9:295–304.
31. Carrichio R, Abbatte A, Gordeev I, et al. Effect of canakinumab vs placebo on survival without invasive mechanical ventilation in patients hospitalized with severe COVID-19. A randomized clinical trial. JAMA. 2021;326:230–9.

4 Hemoadsorption Therapy During ECMO: Emerging Evidence

A. Supady, T. Wengenmayer, and D. Brodie

4.1 Introduction

Over the past decade, venovenous extracorporeal membrane oxygenation (ECMO) has evolved to become a cornerstone for the treatment of patients with severe respiratory failure, and venoarterial ECMO has increasingly been used for cardiocirculatory support in patients with cardiogenic shock or cardiac arrest [1–3]. During the coronavirus disease 2019 (COVID-19) pandemic, there appears to be a continued role for ECMO in the treatment of patients with severe respiratory failure, although mortality remains high and appears to be worsening over the course of the pandemic [4, 5]. Therefore, it will be crucial to further refine the treatments and adjunctive therapies available to complement ECMO, with the potential to improve both survival and quality of life [6–8].

A. Supady (✉)
Department of Medicine III (Interdisciplinary Medical Intensive Care), Medical Center – University of Freiburg, Faculty of Medicine, University of Freiburg, Freiburg, Germany

Department of Cardiology and Angiology, Heart Center, University of Freiburg, Freiburg, Germany

Heidelberg Institute of Global Health, University of Heidelberg, Heidelberg, Germany
e-mail: alexander.supady@uniklinik-freiburg.de

T. Wengenmayer
Department of Medicine III (Interdisciplinary Medical Intensive Care), Medical Center – University of Freiburg, Faculty of Medicine, University of Freiburg, Freiburg, Germany

Department of Cardiology and Angiology, Heart Center, University of Freiburg, Freiburg, Germany

D. Brodie
Division of Pulmonary, Allergy and Critical Care Medicine, Columbia University College of Physicians and Surgeons, New York, NY, USA

Center for Acute Respiratory Failure, New York-Presbyterian Hospital, New York, NY, USA

J.-L. Vincent (ed.), *Annual Update in Intensive Care and Emergency Medicine 2022*, Annual Update in Intensive Care and Emergency Medicine,
https://doi.org/10.1007/978-3-030-93433-0_4

One adjunctive therapy that has received considerable attention is extracorporeal hemoadsorption. Hemoadsorption has been recommended for patients in severe inflammatory states [9]. The rationale for its use is the mitigation of a hyperactivated inflammatory response to a biologic insult through the removal of pathogen-associated molecular patterns (PAMPs) and damage-associated molecular patterns (DAMPs) [10, 11]. ECMO support itself has been suggested to activate or amplify host inflammation and may exacerbate the inflammatory milieu [12–14]. Current evidence for the use of extracorporeal hemoadsorption either with or without ECMO is limited and guidelines recommend its use only within clinical trials [15]. Nevertheless, hemoadsorption has been used and recommended frequently in this setting [16, 17]. In this chapter, we evaluate the available evidence for the use of hemoadsorption in combination with ECMO.

4.2 Devices and Implementation

There are several devices available with varying adsorption characteristics; however, the greatest clinical experience is with the CytoSorb adsorber, currently the most widely used hemoadsorption device [9, 18]. According to the manufacturer, the CytoSorb adsorber has been used for more than 140,000 treatments to date [19]. Some of the available devices, including the CytoSorb, may be incorporated as a stand-alone therapy in any kind of extracorporeal blood circuit, such as ECMO or continuous renal replacement therapy (CRRT), while others, such as the PentraSorb or the Oxiris, may only be used in combination with plasmapheresis or with hemofiltration in a renal replacement circuit (Fig. 4.1.) [20]. Data from preclinical and animal studies suggest that effective adsorption of various inflammatory mediators may be achieved, leading to reduced concentrations in the blood [11, 21–23].

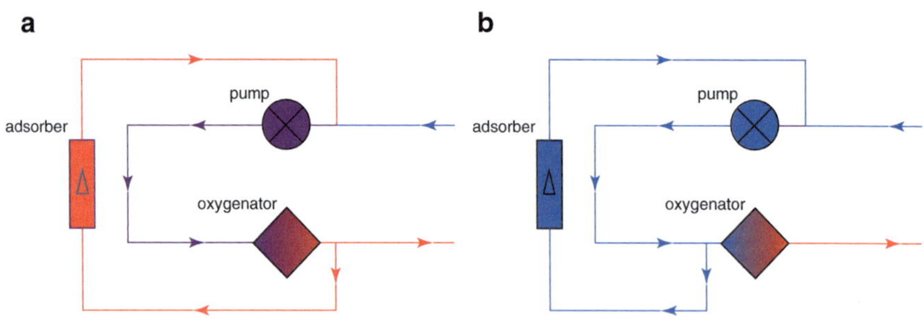

Fig. 4.1. Schematic structure of two options for the incorporation of the hemoadsorption device into an extracorporeal membrane oxygenation (ECMO) system. Blood flow is in the direction of the arrows. The bypass draining the blood from the ECMO circuit through the adsorber may start post-oxygenator (**a**) or pre-oxygenator (**b**) and then carry the blood to the adsorber that will be perfused from bottom to top before the blood is returned to the ECMO circuit pre-pump. The degree of oxygen content in the blood is represented by the color shown (blue = poorly oxygenated blood; purple = poorly oxygenated blood mixed with oxygenated blood from the bypass through the adsorber; red = oxygenated blood)

4.3 Hemoadsorption in Combination with ECMO

There is a growing, but still limited body of evidence regarding the use of hemoadsorption in combination with ECMO (Table 4.1) [16, 24]. Initial case reports suggested benefit from the use of hemoadsorption with ECMO in patients with the acute respiratory distress syndrome (ARDS) and in sepsis [25, 26]. Subsequent single-center case series also suggested that the use of hemoadsorption in severe respiratory failure, sepsis, and cardiocirculatory failure supported with ECMO may be beneficial [27, 28]. In these patients, following initiation of hemoadsorption, clinical improvement was observed, the need for vasopressors decreased as did lactate levels, the ratio of the partial pressure of arterial oxygen to the fraction of inspired oxygen (P/F ratio) improved, and positive end-expiratory pressure (PEEP) and peak pressure could be reduced. A reduction in inflammatory parameters and interleukins was suggested, but could not be supported by the data presented [29]. In severe rhabdomyolysis, hemoadsorption was associated with decreasing serum myoglobin concentrations and in liver failure it was associated with reduction of bilirubin levels [30, 31]. However, without control groups, it is not possible to confirm that these effects were due to hemoadsorption instead of overall management or tincture of time, as some cytokine levels would be expected to decay with time [32]. Further studies have so far failed to demonstrate any relevant benefit of treatment with hemoadsorption during ECMO compared to comparison groups without hemoadsorption [33–35]. Finally, a small retrospective observational study even suggested a negative effect of hemoadsorption on survival in patients after cardiac arrest [36].

4.4 Hemoadsorption in Severe COVID-19 Supported with ECMO

Early in the pandemic, severe presentations of COVID-19 were thought to be associated with an overwhelming inflammatory response, in what was termed "cytokine storm"; a contention that was later challenged [37, 38]. Based on these considerations, a potential role for hemoadsorption as an adjunctive treatment option was proposed and initial experience yielded promising results. In a single patient supported with ECMO, reported early during the pandemic, a significant reduction in inflammatory parameters and norepinephrine support was observed following initiation of hemoadsorption [39]. Subsequently, a comparison of four patients treated with ECMO and hemoadsorption with four patients treated with ECMO alone suggested a more pronounced and more sustained reduction of interleukin (IL)-6 levels in the patients treated with hemoadsorption [40]. Single-arm case series without comparison groups described a reduction in inflammatory parameters, reduced requirement for vasopressors, and improved ventilation parameters [41, 42].

In contrast to the initial hypothesis for the study, a randomized controlled trial (cytokine adsorption in patients with severe COVID-19 pneumonia requiring

Table 4.1 Overview of publications reporting data on patients treated with extracorporeal membrane oxygenation and hemoadsorption

Publication title	Publication type	Publication year	Hemoadsorption device	Number of patients on ECMO (with/without hemoadsorption)	Interpretation of the data by the authors of the original study	Reference
First successful combination of ECMO with cytokine removal therapy in cardiogenic septic shock: a case report	Case report	2015	CytoSorb	1 (1/0)	Favors hemoadsorption	[25]
Cytokine reduction in the setting of an ARDS-associated inflammatory response with multiple organ failure	Case report	2016	CytoSorb	1 (1/0)	Favors hemoadsorption	[26]
Cytokine adsorption in a patient with severe coronavirus disease 2019 related acute respiratory distress syndrome requiring extracorporeal membrane oxygenation therapy: A case report	Case report	2021	CytoSorb	1 (1/0)	Favors hemoadsorption	[39]
Acute respiratory distress syndrome caused by carbon monoxide poisoning and inhalation injury recovered after extracorporeal membrane oxygenation along with direct hemoperfusion with polymyxin B-immobilized fiber column: a case report	Case report	2021	Toraymyxin	1 (1/0)	Favors hemoadsorption	[46]
The Seraph®-100 Microbind Affinity blood filter does not affect vancomycin, tacrolimus, and mycophenolic acid plasma concentrations	Case report	2021	Seraph	1 (1/0)	Neutral with respect to hemoadsorption	[47]
A pilot study: a combined therapy using polymyxin-B hemoperfusion and extracorporeal membrane oxygenation for acute exacerbation of interstitial pneumonia	Case series	2015	Toraymyxin	3 (3/0)	Favors hemoadsorption	[48]
Blood purification with CytoSorb in critically ill patients: single-center preliminary experience	Case series	2018	CytoSorb	40 (40/0)	Favors hemoadsorption	[28]

Use of hemoadsorption in sepsis-associated ECMO-dependent severe ARDS: A case series	Case series	2020	CytoSorb	7 (7/0)	Favors hemoadsorption	[27]
Hemoadsorption treatment with CytoSorb® in patients with extracorporeal life support therapy: A case series	Case series	2019	CytoSorb	23 (23/0)	Favors hemoadsorption	[29]
Cytokine adsorption in patients with severe COVID-19 pneumonia requiring extracorporeal membrane oxygenation	Case series	2021	CytoSorb	8 (4/4)	Favors hemoadsorption	[40]
Continuous hemadsorption with cytokine adsorber for severe COVID-19: A case series of 15 patients	Case series	2021	CytoSorb	15 (11/4)	Favors hemoadsorption	[41]
Adjuvant hemoadsorption therapy in patients with severe COVID-19 and related organ failure requiring CRRT or ECMO therapy: A case series	Case series	2021	CytoSorb	8 (8/0)	Favors hemoadsorption	[42]
Hemoadsorption for management of patients on veno-venous ECMO support for severe COVID-19 acute respiratory distress syndrome	Case series	2021	CytoSorb	10(10/0)	Favors hemoadsorption	[49]
Longitudinal cytokine profiling in patients with severe COVID-19 on extracorporeal membrane oxygenation and hemoadsorption	Case series/ registry analysis	2021	CytoSorb	22 (11/11)	Neutral with respect to hemoadsortion	[44]
Blood purification with a cytokine adsorber for the elimination of myoglobin in critically ill patients with severe rhabdomyolysis	Registry analysis	2021	CytoSorb	14 (14/0)	Favors hemoadsorption	[30]
Successful elimination of bilirubin in critically ill patients with acute liver dysfunction using a cytokine adsorber and albumin dialysis: a pilot study	Registry analysis	2021	CytoSorb	33 (33/0)	Favors hemoadsorption	[31]
Can the cytokine adsorber CytoSorb® help to mitigate cytokine storm and reduce mortality in critically ill patients? A propensity score matching analysis	Registry analysis	2021	CytoSorb	27 (13/14)	Neutral with respect to hemoadsortion	[35]

(continued)

Table 4.1 (continued)

Publication title	Publication type	Publication year	Hemoadsorption device	Number of patients on ECMO (with/without hemoadsorption)	Interpretation of the data by the authors of the original study	Reference
Cytokine adsorption in severe acute respiratory failure requiring veno-venous extracorporeal membrane oxygenation	Registry analysis	2020	CytoSorb	18 (9/9)	Favors hemoadsorption	[33]
Effect of cytokine adsorption on survival and circulatory stabilization in patients receiving extracorporeal cardiopulmonary resuscitation	Registry analysis	2021	CytoSorb	46 (23/23)	Neutral with respect to hemoadsortion	[34]
Combined use of CytoSorb and ECMO in patients with severe pneumogenic sepsis	Registry analysis	2021	CytoSorb	20 (13/7)	Favors hemoadsorption	[50]
Early use of hemoadsorption in patients after out-of-hospital cardiac arrest—a matched pair analysis	Registry analysis	2020	CytoSorb	25 (7/17)	Discourages from the use of hemoadsorption	[36]
Cytokine adsorption in patients with severe COVID-19 pneumonia requiring extracorporeal membrane oxygenation (CYCOV): a single centre, open-label, randomized, controlled trial	Randomized controlled trial	2021	CytoSorb	34 (17/17)	Discourages from the use of hemoadsorption	[43]

The colors reflect the primary interpretation of the data as described in the publications (red: negative effect of hemoadsorption; orange: neutral effect of hemoadsorption; green: benefit of hemoadsorption). *ARDS* acute respiratory distress syndrome, *COVID-19* coronavirus disease 2019, *CRRT* continuous renal replacement therapy, *ECMO* extracorporeal membrane oxygenation extracorporeal membrane oxygenation, the CYCOV study), consisting of 17 patients supported with ECMO in combination with hemoadsorption over 72 h compared to 17 patients treated with ECMO alone, could not replicate these findings [43]. In this trial, IL-6 levels were not significantly affected by hemoadsorption and patients treated with hemoadsorption had a significantly higher risk of death. Another study, comparing COVID-19 patients receiving ECMO treated with hemoadsorption with a cohort without hemoadsorption, also failed to demonstrate a substantial effect on the concentrations of various cytokines [44]. Taken together, the available data do not support the use of hemoadsorption in COVID-19 patients supported with ECMO.

4.5 Discussion and Outlook

Extracorporeal hemoadsorption has been used in various settings. However, reliable proof of efficacy is lacking to date. Fundamental questions remain with regard to patient selection, indication, and dosage. So far, a clinically relevant reduction in pathophysiologically relevant inflammatory mediators as observed in *in vitro* settings has not been reliably confirmed in rigorous clinical trials.

The rationale for the use of hemoadsorption in combination with ECMO in severe inflammatory states, such as pneumonic sepsis, is clear, but available data are not sufficient to recommend its use in routine clinical practice. Pathophysiologic considerations and extrapolations from preclinical trials are likewise insufficient to justify its use. In fact, a degree of caution is warranted. Clinical data suggesting a potential benefit of extracorporeal hemoadsorption during ECMO come predominantly from case reports and small case series, mostly without comparison or control groups. The level of evidence for these recommendations is low, and they should therefore be interpreted with caution. In addition, the results of the randomized CYCOV trial and the results from retrospective analyses of patients after cardiopulmonary resuscitation or in septic shock, suggest the potential for increased mortality in patients treated with hemoadsorption [36, 43, 45]. Taken together, the use of hemoadsorption in the setting of ECMO should be confined to rigorous clinical trials.

4.6 Conclusion

The combination of hemoadsorption with ECMO has a seemingly sound basis in pathophysiology and is particularly appealing because the technical implementation of this dual-device strategy is not overly complex. However, the technical feasibility should not obscure the fact that its use is associated with potential risks. At this stage, further data from rigorously conducted clinical trials, including randomized controlled trials, are required. Until then, the uncritical use of extracorporeal hemoadsorption in patients receiving ECMO outside such trials should be avoided.

References

1. Becher PM, Gossling A, Schrage B, et al. Procedural volume and outcomes in patients undergoing VA-ECMO support. Crit Care. 2020;24:291.
2. Munshi L, Walkey A, Goligher E, Pham T, Uleryk EM, Fan E. Venovenous extracorporeal membrane oxygenation for acute respiratory distress syndrome: a systematic review and meta-analysis. Lancet Respir Med. 2019;7:163–72.
3. Bougouin W, Dumas F, Lamhaut L, et al. Extracorporeal cardiopulmonary resuscitation in out-of-hospital cardiac arrest: a registry study. Eur Heart J. 2020;41:1961–71.
4. Barbaro RP, MacLaren G, Boonstra PS, et al. Extracorporeal membrane oxygenation support in COVID-19: an international cohort study of the extracorporeal life support organization registry. Lancet. 2020;396:1071–8.
5. Barbaro RP, MacLaren G, Boonstra PS, et al. Extracorporeal membrane oxygenation for COVID-19: evolving outcomes from the international extracorporeal life support organization registry. Lancet. 2021;398:1230–8.
6. Abrams D, Ferguson ND, Brochard L, et al. ECMO for ARDS: from salvage to standard of care? Lancet Respir Med. 2019;7:108–10.
7. Petit M, Fetita C, Gaudemer A, Treluyer L, Lebreton G, Franchineau G, Hekimian G, Chommeloux J, Pineton de Chambrun M, Brechot N, et al. Prone-positioning for severe acute respiratory distress syndrome requiring extracorporeal membrane oxygenation. Crit Care Med. 2021; Jul 14. https://doi.org/10.1097/CCM.0000000000005145. Epub ahead of print.
8. Abrams D, Schmidt M, Pham T, Beitler JR, Fan E, Goligher EC, McNamee JJ, Patroniti N, Wilcox ME, Combes A, et al. Mechanical ventilation for acute respiratory distress syndrome during extracorporeal life support. Research and practice. Am J Respir Crit Care Med. 2020;201:514–25.
9. Bonavia A, Groff A, Karamchandani K, Singbartl K. Clinical utility of extracorporeal cytokine hemoadsorption therapy: a literature review. Blood Purif. 2018;46:337–49.
10. Honore PM, Hoste E, Molnar Z, et al. Cytokine removal in human septic shock: where are we and where are we going? Ann Intensive Care. 2019;9:56.
11. Gruda MC, Ruggeberg KG, O'Sullivan P, et al. Broad adsorption of sepsis-related PAMP and DAMP molecules, mycotoxins, and cytokines from whole blood using Consort(R) sorbent porous polymer beads. PLoS One. 2018;13:e0191676.
12. Cho HJ, Kayumov M, Kim D, et al. Acute immune response in venoarterial and venovenous extracorporeal membrane oxygenation models of rats. ASAIO J. 2021;67:546–53.
13. Millar JE, Fanning JP, McDonald CI, McAuley DF, Fraser JF. The inflammatory response to extracorporeal membrane oxygenation (ECMO): a review of the pathophysiology. Crit Care. 2016;20:387.
14. Henry BM. COVID-19, ECMO, and lymphopenia: a word of caution. Lancet Respir Med. 2020;8:e24.
15. Badulak J, Antonini MV, Stead CM, et al. Extracorporeal membrane oxygenation for COVID-19: updated 2021 guidelines from the extracorporeal life support organization. ASAIO J. 2021;67:485–95.
16. Napp LC, Ziegeler S, Kindgen-Milles D. Rationale of hemoadsorption during extracorporeal membrane oxygenation support. Blood Purif. 2019;48:203–14.
17. Ronco C, Bagshaw SM, Bellomo R, et al. Extracorporeal blood purification and organ support in the critically ill patient during COVID-19 pandemic: expert review and recommendation. Blood Purif. 2021;50:17–27.
18. Poli EC, Rimmele T, Schneider AG. Hemoadsorption with CytoSorb((R)). Intensive Care Med. 2019;45:236–9.
19. CytoSorb - The Therapy. Available at: https://cytosorb-therapy.com/en/the-therapy/. Accessed 3 Oct 2021.

20. Broman ME, Hansson F, Vincent JL, Bodelsson M. Endotoxin and cytokine reducing properties of the oXiris membrane in patients with septic shock: a randomized crossover double-blind study. PLoS One. 2019;14:e0220444.
21. Kellum JA, Song M, Venkataraman R. Hemoadsorption removes tumor necrosis factor, interleukin-6, and interleukin-10, reduces nuclear factor-kappaB DNA binding, and improves short-term survival in lethal endotoxemia. Crit Care Med. 2004;32:801–5.
22. Malard B, Lambert C, Kellum JA. In vitro comparison of the adsorption of inflammatory mediators by blood purification devices. Intensive Care Med Exp. 2018;6:12.
23. Song M, Winchester J, Albright RL, Capponi VJ, Choquette MD, Kellum JA. Cytokine removal with a novel adsorbent polymer. Blood Purif. 2004;22:428–34.
24. Napp LC, Lebreton G, De Somer F, Supady A, Pappalardo F. Opportunities, controversies and challenges of extracorporeal hemoadsorption with CytoSorb((R)) during ECMO. Artif Organs. 2021;45:1240–9.
25. Bruenger F, Kizner L, Weile J, Morshuis M, Gummert JF. First successful combination of ECMO with cytokine removal therapy in cardiogenic septic shock: a case report. Int J Artif Organs. 2015;38:113–6.
26. Träger K, Schütz C, Fischer G, et al. Cytokine reduction in the setting of an ARDS-associated inflammatory response with multiple organ failure. Case Rep Crit Care. 2016;2016:9852073.
27. Kogelmann K, Scheller M, Druner M, Jarczak D. Use of hemoadsorption in sepsis-associated ECMO-dependent severe ARDS: a case series. J Intensive Care Soc. 2020;21:183–90.
28. Calabro MG, Febres D, Recca G, et al. Blood purification with CytoSorb in critically ill patients: single-center preliminary experience. Artif Organs. 2019;43:189–94.
29. Trager K, Skrabal C, Fischer G, et al. Hemoadsorption treatment with CytoSorb((R)) in patients with extracorporeal life support therapy: a case series. Int J Artif Organs. 2020;43:422–9.
30. Scharf C, Liebchen U, Paal M, Irlbeck M, Zoller M, Schroeder I. Blood purification with a cytokine adsorber for the elimination of myoglobin in critically ill patients with severe rhabdomyolysis. Crit Care. 2021;25:41.
31. Scharf C, Liebchen U, Paal M, Becker-Pennrich A, Irlbeck M, Zoller M, Schroeder I. Successful elimination of bilirubin in critically ill patients with acute liver dysfunction using a cytokine adsorber and albumin dialysis: a pilot study. Sci Rep. 2021;11:10190.
32. Kellum JA, Kong L, Fink MP, et al. Understanding the inflammatory cytokine response in pneumonia and sepsis: results of the genetic and inflammatory markers of sepsis (GenIMS) study. Arch Intern Med. 2007;167:1655–63.
33. Rieder M, Duerschmied D, Zahn T, et al. Cytokine adsorption in severe acute respiratory failure requiring veno-venous extracorporeal membrane oxygenation. ASAIO J. 2021;67:332–8.
34. Supady A, Zahn T, Rieder M, et al. Effect of cytokine adsorption on survival and circulatory stabilization in patients receiving extracorporeal cardiopulmonary resuscitation. ASAIO J. 2021;68:64–72.
35. Scharf C, Schroeder I, Paal M, Winkels M, Irlbeck M, Zoller M, Liebchen U. Can the cytokine adsorber CytoSorb(®) help to mitigate cytokine storm and reduce mortality in critically ill patients? A propensity score matching analysis. Ann Intensive Care. 2021;11:115.
36. Akin M, Garcheva V, Sieweke JT, Flierl U, Daum HC, Bauersachs J, Schafer A. Early use of hemoadsorption in patients after out-of hospital cardiac arrest - a matched pair analysis. PLoS One. 2020;15:e0241709.
37. Sinha P, Matthay MA, Calfee CS. Is a “cytokine storm” relevant to COVID-19? JAMA Intern Med. 2020;180:1152–4.
38. Mehta P, McAuley DF, Brown M, et al. COVID-19: consider cytokine storm syndromes and immunosuppression. Lancet. 2020;395:1033–4.
39. Rieder M, Zahn T, Benk C, et al. Cytokine adsorption in a patient with severe coronavirus disease 2019 related acute respiratory distress syndrome requiring extracorporeal membrane oxygenation therapy: a case report. Artif Organs. 2021;45:191–4.
40. Rieder M, Wengenmayer T, Staudacher D, Duerschmied D, Supady A. Cytokine adsorption in patients with severe COVID-19 pneumonia requiring extracorporeal membrane oxygenation. Crit Care. 2020;24:435.

41. Paisey C, Patvardhan C, Mackay M, Vuylsteke A, Bhagra SK. Continuous hemadsorption with cytokine adsorber for severe COVID-19: a case series of 15 patients. Int J Artif Organs. 2021;44:664–74.
42. Wunderlich-Sperl F, Kautzky S, Pickem C, Hörmann C. Adjuvant hemoadsorption therapy in patients with severe COVID-19 and related organ failure requiring CRRT or ECMO therapy: a case series. Int J Artif Organs. 2021;44:694–702.
43. Supady A, Weber E, Rieder M, et al. Cytokine adsorption in patients with severe COVID-19 pneumonia requiring extracorporeal membrane oxygenation (CYCOV): a single Centre, open-label, randomised, controlled trial. Lancet Respir Med. 2021;9:755–62.
44. Lebreton G, Dorgham K, Quentric P, Combes A, Gorochov G, Schmidt M. Longitudinal cytokine profiling in patients with severe COVID-19 on extracorporeal membrane oxygenation and hemoadsorption. Am J Respir Crit Care Med. 2021;203:1433–5.
45. Wendel Garcia PD, Hilty MP, Held U, Kleinert EM, Maggiorini M. Cytokine adsorption in severe, refractory septic shock. Intensive Care Med. 2021;47:1334–6.
46. Jang JH, Jang HJ, Kim HK, et al. Acute respiratory distress syndrome caused by carbon monoxide poisoning and inhalation injury recovered after extracorporeal membrane oxygenation along with direct hemoperfusion with polymyxin B-immobilized fiber column: a case report. J Med Case Rep. 2021;15:456.
47. de Geus HRH, Smeets T, Hoek RAS, Endeman H, Hunfeld N. The seraph®-100 microbind affinity blood filter does not affect vancomycin, tacrolimus, and mycophenolic acid plasma concentrations. Blood Purif. 2021;50:971–5.
48. Itai J, Ohshimo S, Kida Y, et al. A pilot study: a combined therapy using polymyxin-B hemoperfusion and extracorporeal membrane oxygenation for acute exacerbation of interstitial pneumonia. Sarcoidosis Vasc Diffuse Lung Dis. 2015;31:343–9.
49. Geraci TC, Kon ZN, Moazami N, et al. Hemoadsorption for management of patients on venovenous ECMO support for severe COVID-19 acute respiratory distress syndrome. J Card Surg. 2021;36:4256–64.
50. Akil A, Ziegeler S, Reichelt J, Rehers S, Abdalla O, Semik M, Fischer S. Combined use of CytoSorb and ECMO in patients with severe pneumogenic sepsis. Thorac Cardiovasc Surg. 2021;69:246–51.

Part II

Respiratory Issues

The Forgotten Circulation and Transpulmonary Pressure Gradients

5

E. Bowcock, S. R. Orde, and A. S. McLean

5.1 Introduction

Pulmonary blood flow is as important as systemic flow yet is often forgotten, ignored, or misunderstood. Pulmonary blood flow carries the same blood load as the systemic circulation and can increase over five times during exercise without significant changes in pressure. The driving force of pulmonary blood flow is the pressure difference between the pulmonary artery and left atrium (known as the transpulmonary pressure gradient). This is the essential pressure that overcomes vascular resistance and is a cornerstone of hemodynamic resuscitation, enabling oxygenation and cardiac output. In this chapter, pulmonary blood flow and factors determining the transpulmonary pressure gradient will be considered with a focus on their relevance in the critically ill patient.

5.2 Pulmonary Vessel Anatomy

The pulmonary circulation comprises a pulmonary arterial tree, an extensive capillary bed, and a pulmonary venous tree (Fig. 5.1). These branching vessels create a low pressure, high capacitance system that provides a large surface area for gas exchange. Running alongside this are systemic bronchial arteries that are branches of the aortic arch. While a significant proportion of the systemic bronchial circulation drains directly back into the superior vena cava, blood that is distributed more peripherally passes through postcapillary anastomoses to join

E. Bowcock (✉) · S. R. Orde · A. S. McLean
Department of Intensive Care Medicine, Nepean Hospital, Kingswood, NSW, Australia
e-mail: Emma.Bowcock@health.nsw.gov.au

J.-L. Vincent (ed.), *Annual Update in Intensive Care and Emergency Medicine 2022*, Annual Update in Intensive Care and Emergency Medicine,
https://doi.org/10.1007/978-3-030-93433-0_5

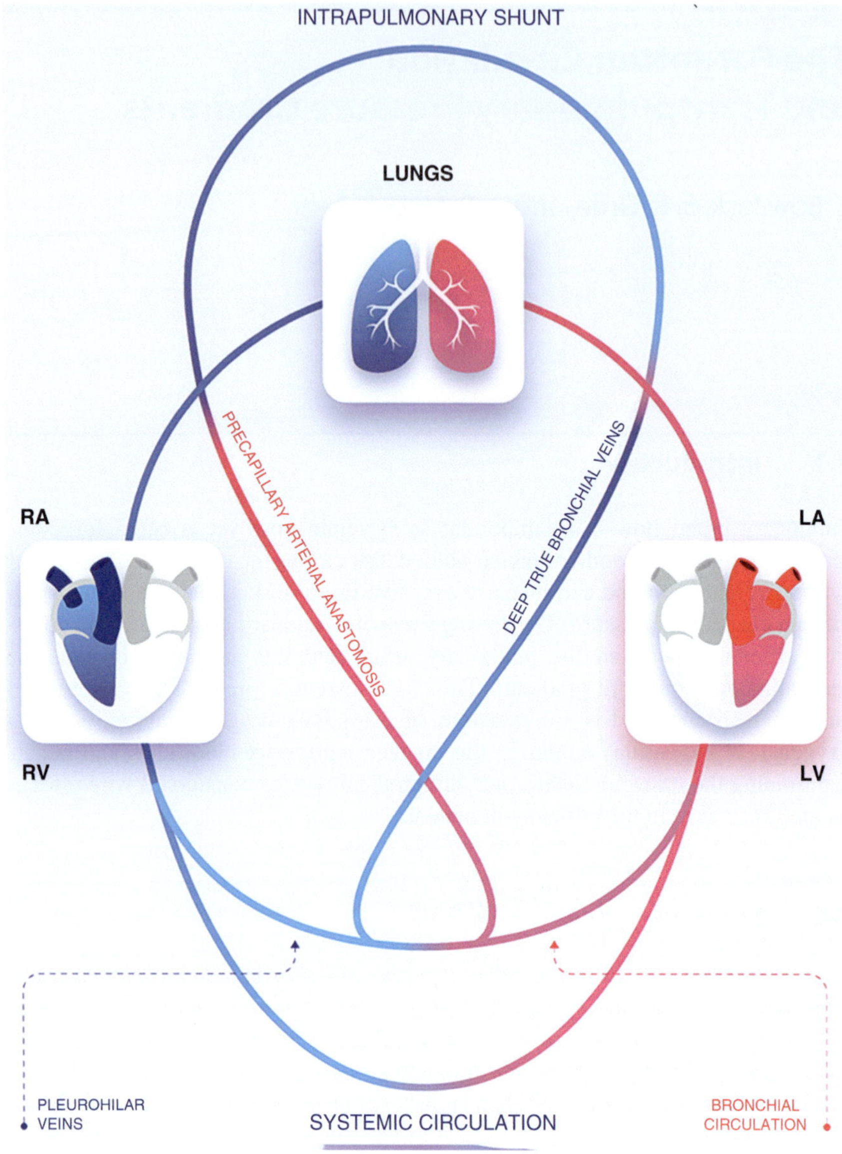

Fig. 5.1 Overview of the pulmonary circulation. LA left atrium, RA right atrium, LV left ventricle, RV right ventricle

the pulmonary veins, constituting venous admixture into the left atrium. There are also pre-capillary anastomoses from the bronchial arteries to the pulmonary arteries that are thought to act as sluice gates. In various lung injurious states, flow through these channels may be important but their precise function remains largely unknown [1].

5.3 Pulmonary Vascular Dysfunction

Unlike the systemic circulation where resistance is mainly determined by arterioles, pulmonary resistance is contributed to by arteries, capillaries and veins [2]. Pulmonary vascular dysfunction can be thought of as a process that brings about increases in the transpulmonary pressure gradient and pulmonary vascular resistance (PVR) [3]. It is central to many disease processes in the critically ill and has been investigated in acute respiratory distress syndrome (ARDS) and sepsis where it is associated with worse outcomes [4, 5]. In brief, pulmonary vascular dysfunction includes pulmonary endothelial dysfunction, microthrombosis, altered vascular permeability, vasoactive mediator imbalance, hypoxic pulmonary vasoconstriction, and vascular remodeling [6–8]. In comparison to pulmonary arteries and capillary endothelium, the pulmonary veins receive little attention and their exact role in different disease states is unknown, though studies have shown that they may contribute significantly to increased PVR [9, 10]. Studies evaluating kinetics of endothelium-bound angiotensin converting enzymes (ACE) provide insights into pulmonary capillary function [11]. The severe acute respiratory syndrome coronavirus 2 (SARS-CoV-2) pandemic has brought attention back to the pulmonary microcirculation where 'endotheliitis' and microthrombosis are predominant features [12]. Despite decades of interest in the pathobiology of pulmonary vascular dysfunction in critical illness, much remains unproven with regards to specific targeted treatment [8]. As we focus our attention at the bedside on the tenants of hemodynamic resuscitation—pressure, flow and resistance—other important cellular factors are likely to be at play within the 'forgotten microcirculation'. Molecular biology research brings the hope of therapies targeted at the molecular level that will alter patient outcome or offer pathways to individualized resuscitation.

5.4 Pulmonary Circulation and Its Components

5.4.1 The Transpulmonary Driving Pressure: A Small Gradient with Big Importance

Pulmonary blood flow is around 6 l/min at rest and approximates cardiac output. In contrast to the systemic circulation, the pressure drop from pulmonary arterioles to veins is very small and capillary flow remains highly pulsatile. The transpulmonary driving pressure gradient equals MPAP (15 mmHg) – LAP (8 mmHg) = 7 mmHg, where MPAP is the mean pulmonary artery pressure and LAP the left atrial pressure (Fig. 5.2). In comparison, the systemic driving pressure gradient equals MAP (90 mmHg) – RAP (5 mm Hg) = 85 mmHg, where MAP is the mean arterial pressure and RAP the right atrial pressure. If the transpulmonary pressure gradient is elevated, it leads to right ventricular (RV) pressure overload. In the acute setting, the right ventricle adapts poorly to increased pressure loading leading to RV dysfunction [13]. Careful attention to the transpulmonary pressure gradient is important if we are to minimize insults to the pressure sensitive right ventricle.

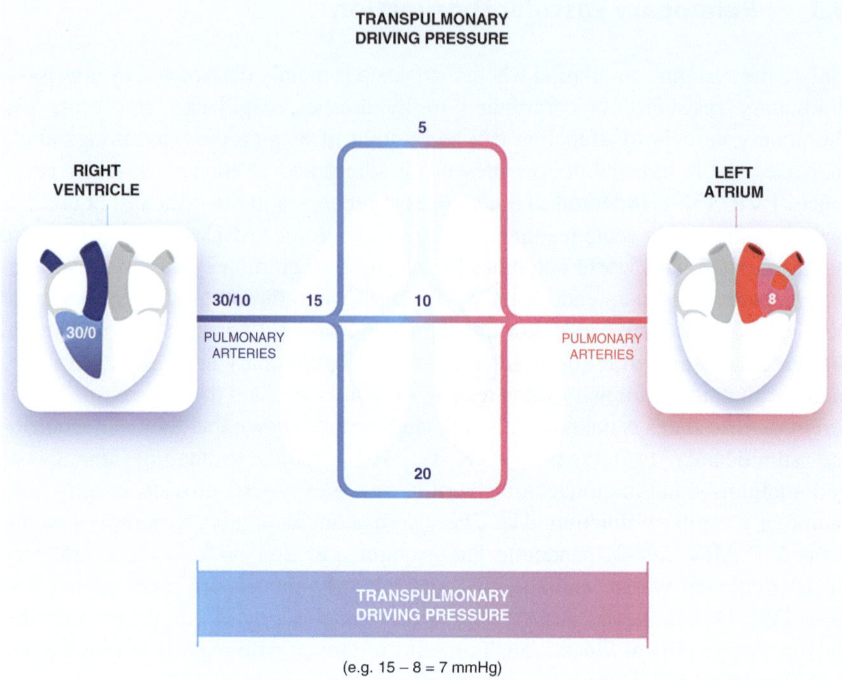

Fig. 5.2 Conceptual diagram of the transpulmonary driving pressure gradient (TPG). TPG = MPAP (15 mmHg) – LAP (8 mmHg) = 7 mmHg, where MPAP = mean pulmonary artery pressure, LAP = left atrial pressure. All values have mmHg as units. Note the pressures from apex to base are to illustrate intravascular pressure gradients from apex to base and are not true values

5.4.2 Pulmonary Vascular Resistance and 'Closing Pressures'

Simplifying the pulsatile cardiopulmonary unit to a model of static Newtonian flow, the relationship between pulmonary pressure, resistance, and flow can be estimated using Ohm's law:

$$\mathrm{PVR} = 80 \times \mathrm{MPAP} - \mathrm{PAOP/CO} \tag{5.1}$$

where PAOP is the pulmonary artery occlusion pressure and CO the cardiac output. The normal PVR range is 0.6–1.7 mmHg/l/min or 37–250 dynes/s/cm^5.

However, unlike the systemic circulation for which Ohm's law provides a reasonable approximation of the linearity between flow and pressure, there are a number of complexities to consider in the pulmonary circulation. First, we must consider the inherent flaw of Poiseuille's resistance equation assuming blood behaves as a Newtonian non-viscous fluid and that pulmonary vessels behave as circular, non-branching, rigid pipes. Blood viscosity is not of purely academic interest. An increased hematocrit is associated with increased pulmonary artery pressure for a

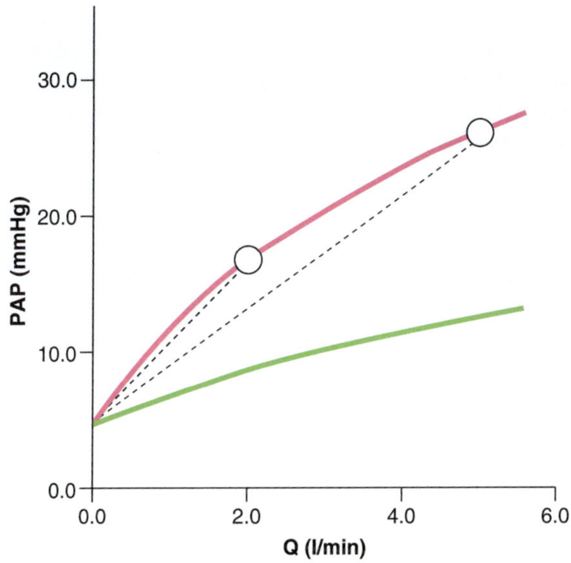

Fig. 5.3 A plot of pulmonary arterial pressure (PAP) against flow or cardiac output (Q) is curvilinear with an intercept on the pressure axis that is equal to left atrial pressure or the closing pressure (Pc). The green curve represents a normal pressure–flow curve while the pink curve represents the pressure–flow curve in the presence of disease such as ARDS. The two circles show a normal cardiac output and a reduced cardiac output. At each cardiac output the pulmonary vascular resistance (PVR) is illustrated as the slope of the straight gray dashed line. Even though the two points are each on the same pressure–flow curve, the calculated PVR is different at the different cardiac outputs. PVR and cardiac output have an inverse relation that holds true in ARDS

given flow. This response is exaggerated in those with less distensible vessels, the elderly for example [14].

Pulmonary vessels are highly distensible and pulmonary capillary flow is dynamic, such that at low flows distension is dominant and at higher flows recruitment is dominant [15]. With this in mind, a complex multipoint curvilinear fit of the pressure–flow relationship may be more accurate [16], as depicted in Fig. 5.3. The importance of distensibility of the pulmonary circulation is increasingly recognized and there are mathematical models that take into account the distensibility coefficient ($\propto$) given by Eq. (5.2) [17]:

$$\mathrm{MPAP} = \left(\left[\left(1 + \propto \mathrm{LAP}\right)^5 + 5 \propto \mathrm{R}_0 \left(\mathrm{CO}\right) \right]^{1/5} - 1 \right) / \propto \tag{5.2}$$

where R_0 is the total PVR at rest. The notion that pulmonary blood flow is largely governed by the pressure difference between MPAP and LAP is not the complete picture. Seminal works by West et al. [18] using a Starling resistor analogy, Permutt et al. [19] using a waterfall analogy, and insightful interpretation by others afford an integrated understanding of the complexities [20].

Central to these is the role of a ‘closing pressure’ (Pc), shown as the positive intercept in Fig. 5.3 [20, 21]. Pc is greater than LAP in any disease state with high alveolar pressure and /or increased pulmonary vessel tone. This scenario would be fairly common in the critically ill patient with ARDS, sepsis, pulmonary hypertension, high positive end-expiratory pressure (PEEP), or West zone 1–2 conditions with low cardiac output. LAP then becomes irrelevant to flow and is said to become the ‘apparent outflow pressure’ and the Pc the ‘effective outflow pressure’. An animal model of ARDS can be used to demonstrate these concepts (Fig. 5.4) [21, 22].

The clinical implication is that in disease states like ARDS where Pc > LAP, the downstream pressure may not be transmitted to the upstream pulmonary vasculature and MPAP becomes less or insensitive to changes in flow or LAP [20]. In addition, the calculated PVR rapidly decreases with increased cardiac output [4]. PVR calculations remain applicable to evaluate the functional state of the pulmonary circulation, provided that the apparent downstream pressure (LAP) is replaced by the effective one (Pc). Uncertainty exists however, because this effective pressure is largely unknown in individual patients [20].

Relying solely on pulmonary pressures or uncorrected PVR measurement may lead to erroneous conclusions. Overcoming these inherent challenges at the bedside

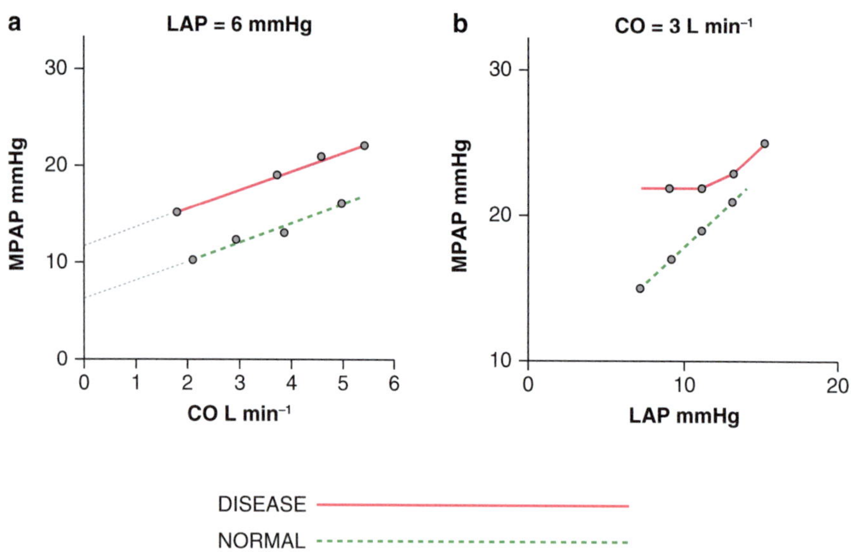

Fig. 5.4 (**a**) Mean pulmonary artery pressure (MPAP) as a function of cardiac output (CO) at constant left atrial pressure (LAP) and (**b**) MPAP as a function of LAP at constant CO in an animal before (normal) and after (disease) induction of lung injury by the injection of oleic acid (OA). Normal (green): (**a**) MPAP–CO plots presented with an extrapolated pressure intercept equal to LAP and (**b**) any increase in LAP was transmitted upstream to MPAP. ARDS model (pink): (**a**) MPAP–CO plots presented with an extrapolated pressure intercept higher than LAP and in (**b**) LAP was not transmitted upstream to MPAP below a pressure equal to that value. These observations suggest that OA-induced pulmonary hypertension is caused by an increase in the closing pressure of the pulmonary circulation. Data from [22]

is not easy. The evolution of contemporary pulmonary artery catheters using advanced thermodilution techniques with pulmonary vascular and RV measurements alongside echocardiography may provide useful insight for further validation studies.

5.5 Measuring the Transpulmonary Pressure Gradient

The transpulmonary pressure gradient is measured using a surrogate of LAP, the PAOP, and is equal to MPAP–PAOP. It is an assumption that PAOP = LAP = effective closing pressure at zero flow state and though important it will not be further discussed in this article. The transpulmonary pressure gradient had previously been incorporated into pulmonary hypertension guidelines and a cut off value of ≥12 mmHg was used to help differentiate 'isolated' post-capillary from 'mixed' pulmonary hypertension as discussed further later [23]. This value is now considered somewhat arbitrary given the transpulmonary pressure gradient is so sensitive to all factors that alter MPAP: cardiac ouput, PVR, and left sided filling pressures. In addition, the pulsatile nature of pulmonary blood flow and thus MPAP is affected by arterial compliance [21]. To overcome these issues, various authors and most recent pulmonary hypertension guidelines have suggested the integrated use of a diastolic pulmonary gradient [21, 24]. The diastolic pulmonary gradient is calculated by subtracting the mean PAOP from the diastolic pulmonary artery pressure (DPAP). A normal diastolic pulmonary gradient is between 1–3 mmHg owing to the large capillary reserve, which offers such low resistance to run off during diastole. A value of ≥7 mmHg is suggested as discriminating between whether pulmonary pressures are elevated due to passive upstream transmission of LAP (isolated post-capillary pulmonary hypertension) or from increased PVR due to pulmonary vasoconstriction and/or pulmonary vascular remodeling (mixed pre- and post-capillary pulmonary hypertension) [25].

The use of the diastolic pulmonary gradient has been scrutinized as studies have found physiologically impossible negative values, mostly related to improper wedging of the catheter tip or due to the mean PAOP overestimating the LAP [26, 27]. Further work evaluating the impact of pressure pulsatility on diastolic pulmonary gradient measurement in those with left heart-induced pulmonary hypertension, has shown that using the 'Y' descent of the PAOP trace rather than the mean PAOP might yield a more reliable assessment, possibly due to the reduced oscillatory effect of V-waves [26].

In 1978, Sibbald et al. explored the diastolic pulmonary gradient in 37 patients with sepsis and showed that a higher gradient was associated with increased mortality [5]. Similarly in 1988, measurement of the diastolic pulmonary gradient in 128 critically patients showed a higher mortality in those with a gradient >6 mmHg. Of 1922 measurements, 18.5% of readings were erroneous and were fixed by changing catheter tip position [27]. In recent times, use of the diastolic pulmonary gradient in critical illness has received relatively little attention, this possibly correlates to the decreasing use of pulmonary artery catheters and possibly that it is a forgotten number in critical care.

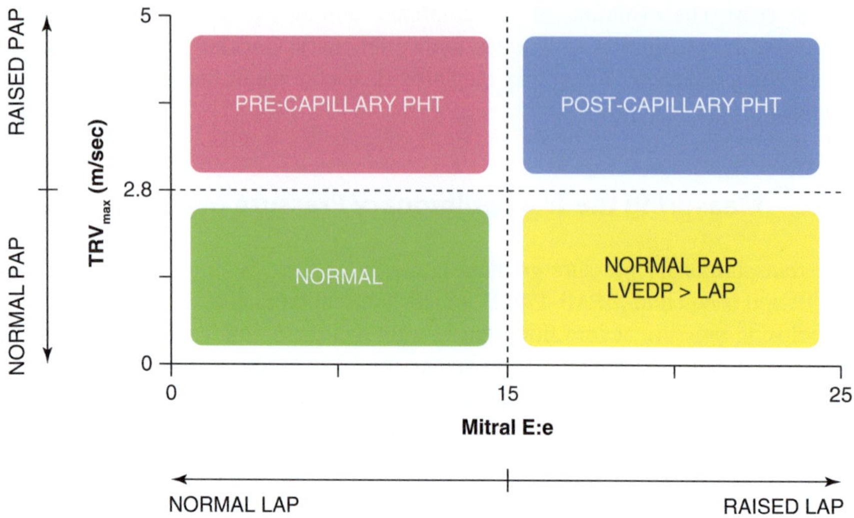

Fig. 5.5 ePLAR (echocardiographic pulmonary to left atrial pressure ratio). Post-capillary pulmonary hypertension (PHT) is likely if E/e' is >15 and tricuspid regurgitant maximal velocity (TRVmax) >2.8 m/s. LVEDP = left ventricular end-diastolic pressure in mmHg, LAP = left atrial pressure in mmHg, mitral E velocity = early mitral inflow velocity in m/s, mitral e' = mitral annular early diastolic velocity in m/s, measured with tissue Doppler imaging (TDI). Normal PAP, LVEDP>LAP = left heart failure with normal pulmonary pressures

Non-invasively, an echo Doppler ratio known as ePLAR (echocardiographic pulmonary to left atrial ratio) is calculated by the maximum tricuspid regurgitant velocity (TRVmax, m/s) divided by the E/e' (Fig. 5.5). It has been used to help differentiate pre-capillary and post-capillary pulmonary hypertension and has shown reasonable performance in this population: sensitivity of 94% and specificity of 65% for a cut-off ratio of ≤0.2 for post-capillary pulmonary hypertension with an area under the receiver operating characteristic (ROC) curve of 0.87 [28].

If the diastolic pulmonary gradient or ePLAR is to be incorporated into bedside assessment of pulmonary hypertension in critical illness, further prospective work is needed to assess their feasibility and utility.

5.6 The Evolving Role of Pulmonary Arterial Compliance

The key elements of total pulmonary vascular load are the resistive and pulsatile forces from PVR and pulmonary arterial compliance, respectively. PVR and pulmonary arterial compliance are inversely related, and their product (arterial time constant of the pulmonary circulation [RC]) is thought to be constant in health and disease (RC = PVR x pulmonary arterial compliance) [29, 30].

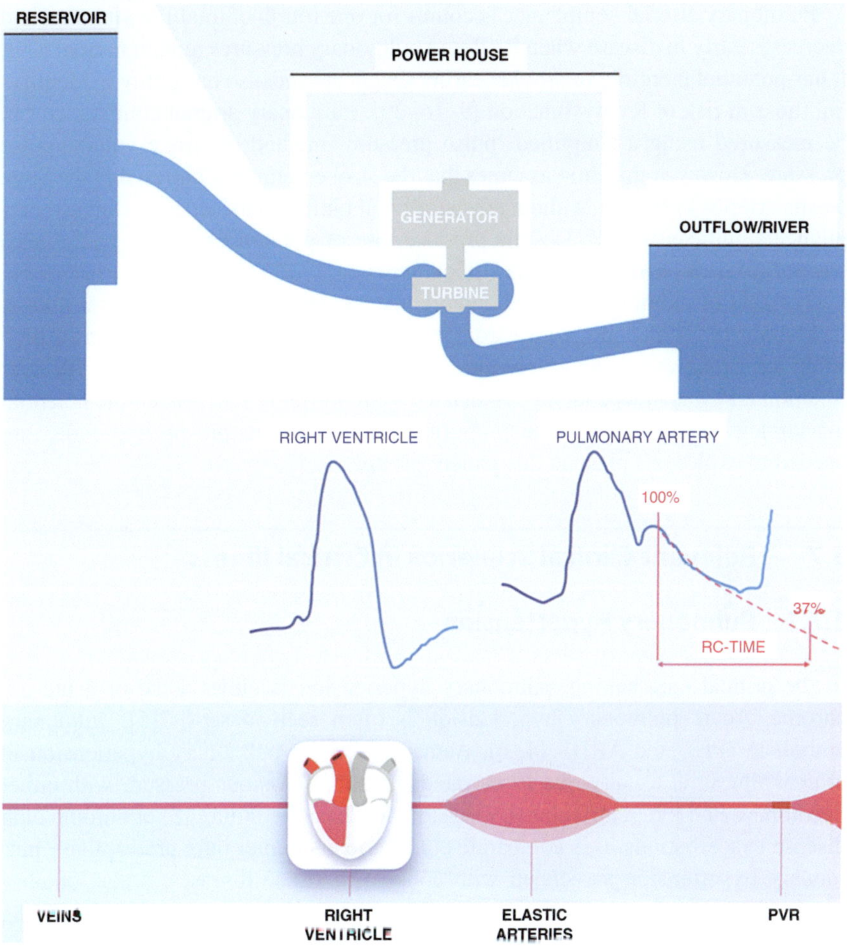

Fig. 5.6 Comparison of the right ventricle–pulmonary circulatory unit with a hydroelectric dam demonstrating the key elements linked with the RC-time (arterial time constant of the pulmonary circulation). RC time, seconds = compliance x resistance

The decrease of pressure in diastole depends on PVR and pulmonary arterial compliance. A high PVR means a small run-off and a high pulmonary arterial compliance implies a large storage volume, both of which result in a small pulmonary pressure decrease in diastole. Practically we can characterize this decrease in pressure in diastole by measuring the exponential decrease with RC time as illustrated in Fig. 5.6 [31].

This mathematical assumption has practical benefit in that if their product is constant, knowledge of one is sufficient to derive the value of the other. However, recent works have shown that this may be inaccurate, with shorter RC-times found in post-capillary than in pre-capillary pulmonary hypertension [32].

Pulmonary arterial compliance accounts for one fourth of total RV afterload and decreases early in disease when PVR and pulmonary pressures remain normal [29]. It has potential therefore to provide earlier diagnosis and also has utility in identifying those at risk of RV dysfunction [9, 16, 29]. Pulmonary arterial compliance can be measured using a simplified 'pulse pressure' method of stroke volume/pulse pressure. However, this ratio assumes that the stroke volume is buffered in the large elastic arteries in systole, without any peripheral outflow and can overestimate compliance significantly [33]. Despite promise, use of pulmonary arterial compliance has not yet translated into routine clinical practice.

The role of pulmonary arterial compliance has been explored in critical illness. In a study of 91 patients with cardiogenic shock, a lower compliance measured using the stroke volume/pulse pressure method was associated with severe RV dysfunction and was independently associated with mortality [34]. Given the potential inaccuracies and the heterogeneity of critical illness, further prospective studies are needed to explore its place in this patient group.

5.7 Relevant Clinical Scenarios in Critical Illness

5.7.1 Pulmonary Hypertension

In the critical care setting, pulmonary hypertension is either acute or acute-on-chronic. Acute pulmonary hypertension is often seen in sepsis [5], pulmonary embolism (PE), and ARDS [4, 6]. Acute-on-chronic pulmonary hypertension in critical illness is usually due to elevated pulmonary venous pressure with either decompensated left ventricular (LV) systolic or diastolic failure [8] or chronic lung disease exacerbations. It is comparatively rare to encounter pure pre-capillary pulmonary hypertension associated with connective tissue diseases, drugs, or idiopathic, for example. Although there is a lot of importance placed upon classifying pulmonary hypertension in the non-critical care setting [24], pulmonary hypertension associated with critical illness is often placed under an 'umbrella' of pulmonary vascular dysfunction. Rarely is there a quest to differentiate the dominant factors at play; doing so may have benefit in guiding individualized treatments as discussed below.

Patients are characterized as pre-capillary pulmonary hypertension when MPAP ≥25 mm Hg, PAOP ≤15 mm Hg, and PVR ≥3 Wood units (WU). In contrast, post-capillary pulmonary hypertension is diagnosed when PAOP is >15 mmHg. Post-capillary cases are then divided into two groups. Isolated post-capillary pulmonary hypertension, with no secondary reactive pulmonary arteriolar disease, has a low diastolic pressure gradient (≤7 mmHg) and PVR (≤3 WU). However, many patients with elevated LAP develop secondary perivascular pulmonary arteriolar sclerosis resulting in increased diastolic pulmonary gradient (≥7 mmHg) and/or PVR (≥3 WU) [25].

Right heart catheterization using a pulmonary artery catheter is the gold standard diagnostic tool to invasively measure the pulmonary arterial systolic (PASP), mean

(MPAP), and diastolic (PADP) pressures and to calculate cardiac output and PVR [24]. In critical care, non-invasive echocardiographic measurement of PASP is often more practical. PASP is calculated by applying the simplified Bernoulli's principle to TRVmax where PASP = 4 × TRVmax^2 + RAP, assuming no RV outflow tract (RVOT) obstruction. If present, the pulmonary regurgitant jet can be used to estimate MPAP and PADP using the same Doppler principles by adding RAP to pulmonary regurgitation peak velocity and pulmonary regurgitation end velocity, respectively (Fig. 5.7). Although enticing, these measurements are technically challenging in the critically ill population [35]. Non-invasive assessment of PVR is made using the pulmonary arterial acceleration time with values less than 90 ms correlating with raised PVR >3 WU [36]. The pulmonary arterial acceleration time can be often used to suggest pulmonary hypertension in those where estimates of PASP cannot be made or is underestimated, with lack of a tricuspid regurgitation jet, acute RV dysfunction or free flowing tricuspid regurgitation, for example. Interesting work in the pulmonary hypertension population interrogating the RVOT pulsed wave Doppler trace, found that the presence of notching and mid-systolic deceleration times of <120 ms was associated with reduced survival [37]. Investigation into the feasibility and utility of such detailed analysis in the critically ill is needed. The severity of pulmonary hypertension will also depend on chronicity given that a 'trained', hypertrophied right ventricle can generate much higher pressures. The

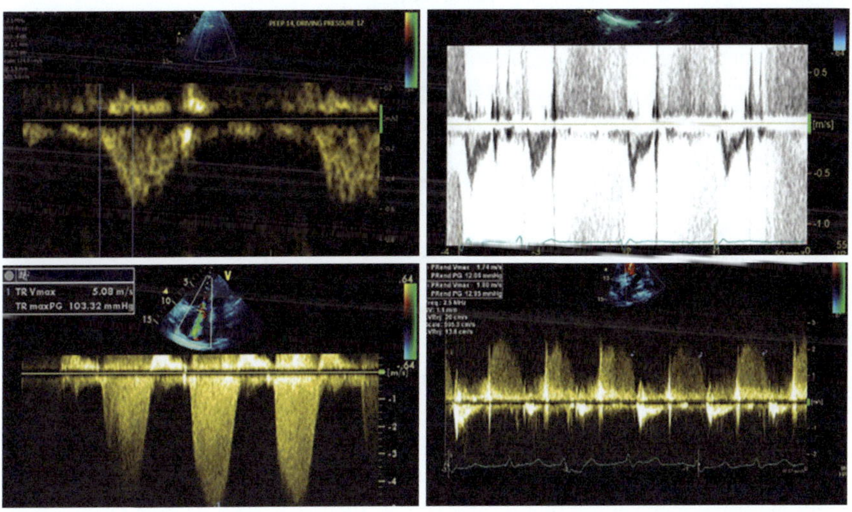

Fig. 5.7 Upper left—pulsed wave Doppler (PWD) of right ventricular outflow tract (RVOT) and measurement of pulmonary valve acceleration time (PAT); upper right—notching of the RVOT PWD trace signifying significantly raised PVR; lower left—continuous wave Doppler (CWD) of tricuspid regurgitation jet maximum velocity (TRVmax) and pressure gradient (TRmaxPG) calculated from modified Bernoulli using 4V^2. Adding RAP to the TRmaxPG gives pulmonary artery systolic pressure (PASP); lower right—CWD of pulmonary regurgitant jet and measurement of end-diastolic velocity and pressure gradient (PRendPG) calculated from modified Bernoulli using 4V^2. Adding RAP to the PRendPG gives pulmonary artery diastolic pressure (PADP)

presence of RV dysfunction in pulmonary hypertension is a poor prognostic marker [38] and this serves to highlight the important role of echocardiography in this cohort.

Differentiating types of pulmonary hypertension in critical illness seems important as treatment strategies for one can be at the cost of the other. For example, the use of pulmonary vasodilators, such as nitric oxide (NO), in patients with pure post-capillary pulmonary hypertension may cause harm with worsening pulmonary edema [39]. Yet in RV dysfunction secondary to ARDS with pulmonary hypertension, for example, the use of a pulmonary vasodilator would have physiological plausibility and may have beneficial effect [40].

Incorporating clinical, pulmonary artery catheter, and echocardiographic assessment may be helpful in differentiating pre- from post-capillary pulmonary hypertension and may help guide hemodynamic resuscitation, particularly in those with concomitant RV dysfunction. As always, acute changes to loading conditions and measurement pitfalls must be remembered [35]. In addition, identifying and characterizing the 'RV–pulmonary circuit phenotype' may have longer term benefit. For example, discerning the higher risk phenotypes and organizing post-ICU follow up in specialized pulmonary hypertension clinics could potentially lead to improvements in long-term patient outcomes. Prospective longitudinal studies are desperately needed in this critical care cohort.

5.7.2 Right Ventricular Dysfunction

RV dysfunction, admittedly a loose term, is well recognized in the critically ill, manifesting as acute or acute-on-chronic phenotypes. Echocardiography is the reference standard for analysis of RV size and function in the critically ill. It has an important role in acute hemodynamic resuscitation and in determining chronicity through assessment of features including RV wall thickness, chamber size, pulmonary artery dimensions, and evaluation of contributing left heart pathology. As the RV begins to fail from increased afterload, decreases in stroke volume will manifest as decreases in pulmonary arterial pressures, although PVR is likely to remain elevated. Therefore, contextualization of pressure and resistance measures with concomitant echocardiographic assessment of RV and LV systolic, diastolic, and valvular function is crucial to guide treatment decisions. Frequent studies have indicated the prognostic significance of RV dysfunction, particularly when severe [41]. However, from a clinical perspective it is often more relevant to recognize the 'at risk' right ventricle in order to hone therapeutic methods. Perhaps this is where more sensitive echocardiographic assessment methods, such as speckle tracking echocardiography, may be helpful. This relatively novel echocardiographic technique has been found to be feasible in the critically ill and has been used in studies assessing optimal PEEP assessment for example [42].

There is emerging interest in the pathobiology of RV dysfunction. Very briefly, there are a number of *ex vivo* models (pulmonary artery banding, chronic hypoxia, Sugen-hypoxia, monocrotaline) that are leading to a number of discoveries: the role of estrogen and sex, cytoskeleton and myocardial fibrosis, sarcomere dysfunction in scleroderma induced pulmonary hypertension, BMPR2 gene dysfunction in hereditary pulmonary hypertension as well as downregulation of micro-RNAs, among others [16, 43]. Where this lies in the critical care landscape remains uncertain.

We are increasingly aware that RV dysfunction is not a single physiological entity, but rather part of a broader 'RV–pulmonary circuit' dysfunction. RV dysfunction requires correction of the underlying pathology and careful assessment of loading factors. RV dysfunction from PE, myocardial infarction, septic cardiomyopathy or raised RV afterload from ARDS or sepsis all require a different approach, particularly from a fluid management perspective. For example, if RV dysfunction occurs in the setting of increased RV afterload, as occurs in a patient with ARDS, volume loading can result in displacement of the septum toward the left ventricle impairing LV diastolic filling [44]. Precisely how early RV remodeling in response to the complex microcirculation alterations in various disease states impacts acute critical care management remains unanswered for now.

5.8 Can Right Ventricular–Pulmonary Arterial (RV–PA) Coupling Shed more Light on the RV–Pulmonary Circuit in Critical Illness?

Put simply, RV–PA coupling is the linking of RV contractility to RV afterload to maintain an adequate cardiac output at the lowest possible energy cost. If the RV contractile load cannot match the pulmonary afterload it is said to be 'uncoupled' [45]. There is emerging interest in regard to uncoupling of the right ventricle and its role in therapeutics and prognostication in critical illness. The gold standard ratio in assessing RV–PA coupling is ventricular end-systolic (Ees) to arterial elastance (Ea) and a Ees/Ea ratio between 1-2 is considered normal [16]. In the chronic pulmonary hypertension cohort, Es/Ea ratios of <0.8 were associated with RV dysfunction, defined as a RV ejection fraction of <35% in one study of 42 patients [46]. This approach however requires invasive and impractical measurement of pressure volume loops and pragmatic surrogates have been explored. Studies using surrogates in critical illness have included: RV fractional area change (FAC)/PASP, tricuspid annular plane systolic excursion (TAPSE)/PASP and tricuspid annular systolic velocity (TASV)/PASP ratios [47–49]. In these studies, the indices have been shown to have prognostic utility in critical illness. Further prospective work on RV–PA coupling is needed, not only to assess its prognostic benefit, but also its utility as a novel hemodynamic tool, possibly as part of an elastance-based resuscitation strategy.

5.9 Conclusion

It is reasonable to conclude that pulmonary pressures and PVR cannot be used interchangeably when considering pulmonary hemodynamics in critically ill patients. Consideration of the whole 'RV–pulmonary circulatory unit' is key. Understanding the driving processes of acute or acute-on-chronic pulmonary hypertension and/or RV dysfunction may enable targeted hemodynamic resuscitation strategies. Future work exploring the feasibility and utility of bedside measures of PVR, total arterial compliance, and transpulmonary pressure gradients in disease states such as ARDS and sepsis is needed. With an increasing skill set in advanced echocardiography and possible resurgence in the use of the contemporary pulmonary artery catheter, intensivists can lead the way in bedside research. This may parallel bench side investigation into the anatomical and molecular basis of RV–pulmonary vascular dysfunction. Arguably then, the most important pathway for the intensive care physician at the bedside is the route linking the right and left atria across the pulmonary circulation and perhaps this 'forgotten circulation' is where we should focus our attention if we are to make headway with individualized, targeted resuscitation.

References

1. Tobin CE. Arteriovenous shunts in the peripheral pulmonary circulation in the human lung. Thorax. 1966;21:197–204.
2. Lumb A. The Pulmonary Circulation. In: Lumb AB, editor. Nunn's applied respiratory physiology. 7th ed. Philadelphia: Lippincott Williams and WIlkins; 2010. p. 3782–4524.
3. Bull TM, Clark B, McFann K, Moss M. Pulmonary vascular dysfunction is associated with poor outcomes in patients with acute lung injury. Am J Respir Crit Care Med. 2010;182:1123–8.
4. Zapol WM, Snider MT. Pulmonary hypertension in severe acute respiratory failure. N Engl J Med. 1977;296:476–80.
5. Sibbald W, Paterson NAM, Holliday RL, Anderson RA, Lobb TR, Duff JH. Pulmonary hypertension in sepsis. Measurement by the pulmonary arterial diastolic-pulmonary wedge pressure gradient and the influence of passive and active factors. Chest. 1978;73:583–91.
6. Price LC, McAuley DF, Marino PS, Finney SJ, Griffiths MJ, Wort SJ. Pathophysiology of pulmonary hypertension in acute lung injury. Am J Physiol Lung Cell Mol Physiol. 2012;302:L803–15.
7. Pandol R, Barreira B, Moreno E, et al. Role of acid sphingomyelinase and IL-6 as mediators of endotoxin-induced pulmonary vascular dysfunction. Thorax. 2017;72:460–71.
8. Price LC, Wort SJ, Finney SJ, Marino PS, Brett SJ. Pulmonary vascular and right ventricular dysfunction in adult critical care: current and emerging options for management: a systematic literature review. Crit Care. 2010;14:R169.
9. Vonk Noordegraaf A, Westerhof BE, Westerhof N. The relationship between the right ventricle and its load in pulmonary hypertension. J Am Coll Cardiol. 2017;69:236–43.
10. Chazova I, Loyd JE, Zhdanov VS, Newman JH, Belenkov Y, Meyrickt B. Pulmonary artery adventitial changes and venous involvement in primary pulmonary hypertension. Am J Pathol. 1995;146:389–97.
11. Toivonen HJ, Catravas JD. Effects of blood flow on lung ACE kinetics: evidence for microvascular recruitment. J Appl Physiol. 1991;71:2244–54.
12. Huertas A, Montani D, Savale L, et al. Endothelial cell dysfunction: a major player in SARS-CoV-2 infection (COVID-19)? Eur Respir J. 2020;56:2001634.
13. Piazza G, Goldhaber SZ. The acutely decompensated right ventricle: pathways for diagnosis and management. Chest. 2005;128:1836–52.
14. Vanderpool RR, Naeije R. Hematocrit-corrected pulmonary vascular resistance. Am J Respir Crit Care Med. 2018;198:305–9.
15. Reeves JT, Linehan JH, Stenmark KR. Distensibility of the normal human lung circulation during exercise. Am J Physiol Lung Cell Mol Physiol. 2005;288:419–25.

16. Vonk Noordegraaf A, Chin KM, Haddad F, et al. Pathophysiology of the right ventricle and of the pulmonary circulation in pulmonary hypertension: an update. Eur Respir J. 2019;53:1801900.
17. Linehan JH, Haworth S, Nelin L, Krenz G. A simple distensible model for interpreting pulmonary vascular pressure-flow curves. J Appl Physiol. 1992;73:987–94.
18. West JB, Dollery CT, Naimark A. Distribution of blood flow in isolated lung; relation to vascular and alveolar pressures. J Appl Physiol. 1964;19:713–24.
19. Permutt S, Bromberger-Barnea B, Bane H. Alveolar pressure, pulmonary venous pressure, and the vascular waterfall. Med Thorac. 1962;19:239–60.
20. Naeije R. Pulmonary vascular resistance. A meaningless variable? In: Pinsky MR, Brochard L, Hedenstierna G, Antonelli M, editors. Applied physiology in intensive care medicine. 2nd ed. Berlin: Springer; 2009. p. 65–7.
21. Naeije R, Vachiery JL, Yerly P, Vanderpool R. The transpulmonary pressure gradient for the diagnosis of pulmonary vascular disease. Eur Respir J. 2013;41:217–23.
22. Leeman M, Lejeune P, Closset J, Vachiery JL, Melot C, Naeije R. Nature of pulmonary hypertension in canine oleic acid pulmonary edema. J Appl Physiol. 1990;69:293–8.
23. Galiè N, Hoeper MM, Humbert M, et al. Guidelines for the diagnosis and treatment of pulmonary hypertension. Eur Heart J. 2009;30:2493–537.
24. Galiè N, Humbert M, Vachiery JL, et al. 2015 ESC/ERS guidelines for the diagnosis and treatment of pulmonary hypertension. Eur Respir J. 2015;46:903–75.
25. Gerges C, Gerges M, Lang MB, et al. Diastolic pulmonary vascular pressure gradient: a predictor of prognosis in "out-of-proportion" pulmonary hypertension. Chest. 2013;143:758–66.
26. Manouras A, Johnson J, Lund LH, Nagy AI. Optimizing diastolic pressure gradient assessment. Clin Res Cardiol. 2020;109:1411–22.
27. Wilson RF, Beckman SB, Tyburski JG, Scholten DJ. Pulmonary artery diastolic and wedge pressure relationships in critically ill and injured patients. Arch Surg. 1988;123:933–6.
28. Scalia GM, Scalia IG, Kierle R, et al. ePLAR - the echocardiographic pulmonary to left atrial ratio - a novel non-invasive parameter to differentiate pre-capillary and post-capillary pulmonary hypertension. Int J Cardiol. 2016;212:379–86.
29. Thenappan T, Prins KW, Pritzker MR, Scandurra J, Volmers K, Weir EK. The critical role of pulmonary arterial compliance in pulmonary hypertension. Ann Am Thorac Soc. 2016;13:276–84.
30. Lankhaar JW, Westerhof N, Faes TJC, et al. Pulmonary vascular resistance and compliance relationship instay inversely related during treatment of pulmonary hypertension. Eur Heart J. 2008;29:1688–95.
31. Saouti N, Westerhof N, Postmus PE, Vonk-Noordegraaf A. The arterial load in pulmonary hypertension. Eur Respir Rev. 2010;19:197–203.
32. Chemla D, Lau EMT, Papelier Y, Attal P, Hervé P. Pulmonary vascular resistance and compliance relationship in pulmonary hypertension. Eur Respir J. 2015;46:1178–89.
33. Souza R. Assessment of compliance in pulmonary arterial hypertension. Eur Heart J. 2008;29:1603–4.
34. Zorzi MF, Cancelli E, Rusca M, Kirsch M, Yerly P, Liaudet L. The prognostic value of pulmonary artery compliance in cardiogenic shock. Pulm Circ. 2019;9:2045894019877161.
35. Orde S, Slama M, Hilton A, Yastrebov K, McLean A. Pearls and pitfalls in comprehensive critical care echocardiography. Crit Care. 2017;21:1–10.
36. Tossavainen E, Söderberg S, Grönlund C, Gonzalez M, Henein MY, Lindqvist P. Pulmonary artery acceleration time in identifying pulmonary hypertension patients with raised pulmonary vascular resistance. Eur Heart J Cardiovasc Imaging. 2013;14:890–7.
37. Takahama H, McCully RB, Frantz RP, Kane GC. Unraveling the RV ejection Doppler envelope: insight into pulmonary artery hemodynamics and disease severity. JACC Cardiovasc Imaging. 2017;10:1268–77.
38. Prins KW, Rose L, Archer SL, et al. Clinical determinants and prognostic implications of right ventricular dysfunction in pulmonary hypertension caused by chronic lung disease. J Am Heart Assoc. 2019;8:1–15.

39. Hayward CS, Macdonald PS, Keogh AM. Inhaled nitric oxide in cardiology practice. Cardiovasc Res. 1999;43:628–38.
40. Feng WX, Yang Y, Wen J, Liu YX, Liu L, Feng C. Implication of inhaled nitric oxide for the treatment of critically ill COVID-19 patients with pulmonary hypertension. ESC Heart Fail. 2021;8:714–8.
41. Harjola VP, Mebazaa A, Čelutkiene J, et al. Contemporary management of acute right ventricular failure: a statement from the heart failure association and the working group on pulmonary circulation and right ventricular function of the European Society of Cardiology. Eur J Heart Fail. 2016;18:226–41.
42. Mercado P, Maizel J, Kontar L, et al. Moderate and severe acute respiratory distress syndrome: hemodynamic and cardiac effects of an open lung strategy with recruitment maneuver analyzed using echocardiography. Crit Care Med. 2018;46:1608–16.
43. Prisco SZ, Thenappan T, Prins KW. Treatment targets for right ventricular dysfunction in pulmonary arterial hypertension. JACC Bas Transl Sci. 2020;5:1244–60.
44. Chan C, Klinger JR. Sepsis and pulmonary arterial hypertension in the ICU. Adv Pulm Hypertens. 2015;13:188–96.
45. Pinsky MR. The right ventricle: interaction with the pulmonary circulation. Crit Care. 2016;20:1–9.
46. Tello K, Dalmer A, Axmann J, Naeije R, et al. Reserve of right ventricular-arterial coupling in the setting of chronic overload. Circ Heart Fail. 2019;12:e005512.
47. Jentzer JC, Anavekar NS, Reddy YNV, et al. Right ventricular pulmonary artery coupling and mortality in cardiac intensive care unit patients. J Am Heart Assoc. 2021;10:e019015.
48. D'Alto M, Marra AM, Severino S, et al. Right ventricular-arterial uncoupling independently predicts survival in COVID-19 ARDS. Crit Care. 2020;24:670.
49. Bleakley C, Singh S, Garfield B, Al E. Right ventricular dysfunction in critically ill COVID-19 ARDS. Int J Cardiol. 2021;327:251–9.

Oxygen: Origin, Physiology, Pathophysiology, and Use in the Critically Ill

6

H. P. M. M. Gelissen, H. J. de Grooth, and A. M. E. de Man

6.1 Introduction

Oxygen is crucial for the critically ill. These patients have a high risk of hypoxemic harm, which can lead to compensatory hyperoxemia by superfluous oxygen administration. Hyperoxia can cause direct toxic effects on the lungs, whereas hyperoxemia can exert vasoconstrictive effects on the circulation, and lead to cellular and organ injury by increased production of reactive oxygen species (ROS). In the last 5 years, an increasing number of large randomized, controlled trials (RCTs) have been performed to determine optimal oxygenation targets, but the discussion is ongoing. In this chapter, we will elaborate on the physiological and pathophysiological background of oxygen, and subsequently discuss the current status of clinical evidence.

6.2 Origin of Oxygen in the Earth's Atmosphere

Over a period of approximately 4.5 billion years, the oxygen fraction (FO_2) of the atmosphere of the earth changed from 0 to 0.21. A complex interaction between biological evolution and geology led to the present FO_2 and the diversity of life forms on earth [1, 2]. Based on the distance to the sun and the position in the solar

H. P. M. M. Gelissen · H. J. de Grooth · A. M. E. de Man (✉)
Department of Intensive Care, Amsterdam UMC, Location VUmc, Amsterdam, The Netherlands

Amsterdam Cardiovascular Science, Amsterdam, The Netherlands

Amsterdam Infection and Immunity Institute, Amsterdam, The Netherlands

Amsterdam Medical Data Science, Amsterdam, The Netherlands
e-mail: ame.deman@amsterdamumc.nl

J.-L. Vincent (ed.), *Annual Update in Intensive Care and Emergency Medicine 2022*, Annual Update in Intensive Care and Emergency Medicine,
https://doi.org/10.1007/978-3-030-93433-0_6

system, the earth is within the 'habitable zone'. Oxygen is an extremely reactive element produced by photosynthesis in cyanobacteria or plants' chloroplasts. Contemporary plants still use symbiosis with cyanobacteria for photosynthesis. Before the appearance of cyanobacteria, anaerobic microbes used sulfate instead of oxygen for their energetic needs. Approximately 2.45 billion years ago, cyanobacteria took over from anaerobes, producing the extremely reactive element oxygen in the period known as the Great Oxidation Event. After another billion years, during which there were very few new developments (the boring billion), the O_2 concentration became high enough for the development and further evolution of animal life. During the history of the earth's atmosphere, a maximum FO_2 of approximately 0.30 has been reached, now stabilizing at 0.21. Its high electronegativity and abundance made oxygen uniquely suitable as the final electron acceptor in a series of transfers from high-energy to low-energy molecular states: the electron transport chain. In this way, the increasing oxygen levels were a prerequisite for the development of many new organisms, including human beings. However, the same levels were toxic for others. Oxygen's propensity to acquire electrons meant that organisms had to develop antioxidant defenses to prevent inadvertent molecular oxidation and dysfunction. As Paracelsus stated "the dose makes the poison".

6.3 Measurements and Estimations of Oxygenation

To estimate the oxygenation status of critically ill patients, several different methods and parameters can be used: oxygen saturation of the blood (SO_2) by pulse oximetry (SpO_2) or by arterial blood gas analysis (SaO_2), oxygen pressure (PO_2) by arterial blood gas analysis, oxygen extraction by adding central or mixed venous blood gas analysis ($ScvO_2$ or SvO_2), lactate concentration and oxygen delivery (DO_2). A pulse oximeter measures SpO_2 with use of two near infrared wavelengths combined with the circulatory pulsations. The two wavelengths are differently absorbed by oxygenated (O_2-Hb) versus de-oxygenated (H-Hb) hemoglobin. Carbon monoxide bonded to hemoglobin (CO-Hb) is not differentiated from O_2-Hb by the two wavelength pulse oximeter and will thus cause a falsely high SpO_2 reading. The main advantages of SpO_2 measurement are that it can be measured easily, continuously, and non-invasively. Disadvantages are the relative unreliable results in patients with dark skin color [3] and the impossibility to detect hyperoxemia. The method using near infrared wavelengths can also be used directly on blood and with up to four different wavelengths instead of the two used in pulse oximetry, enabling determination of concentrations of methemoglobin and CO-Hb [4]. PO_2 can be measured in blood samples with a polarographic electrode that has an electrical resistance varying with PO_2, and tissue PO_2 can be measured by small polarographic electrodes on the skin or on organs. The major limitation of this application is the restricted depth of the measurements. The advantage of PO_2 measurements in arterial blood (PaO_2) is its accuracy. In addition, pressure is the driving force of O_2 diffusion, making pressure a more relevant parameter than saturation, which is not directly related to O_2 diffusion. Disadvantages are the discontinuous and invasive nature of this method. There are equations to calculate PO_2 from SO_2, and *vice versa*, for oxygen levels within normal ranges [5, 6]. However, these equations do not completely take into account the effects of temperature, 2,3-diphosphoglycerate, pH and PCO_2 (the Bohr effect) on the lateral position (right or left shift) of the oxyhemoglobin dissociation curve and are thus only of limited clinical value. Furthermore, in the high oxygen range with high arterial O_2 saturations (SaO_2 > 97%) large changes of PO_2 are related to extremely small changes of SO_2 that cannot be accurately measured. Thus in the SpO_2 range > 97% hyperoxemia can go undetected unless PO_2 is simultaneously measured. Adequate oxygenation can be estimated by calculating oxygen extraction between arterial and venous blood or by measuring lactate production [7]. Extraction of oxygen and production of lactate depends on severity of hypoxemia, but also on the conservation of tissue perfusion and adequate supply of glucose or other metabolic substrates. Calculating oxygen extraction of the whole body can be done by simultaneous sampling of arterial and central or preferably mixed venous blood. $ScvO_2$ can be sampled relative easily and is a well-documented parameter for assessing the circulation of patients in shock. The problem of SvO_2 measurement is the requirement of a pulmonary artery catheter. Lactate is a simple measurement, but its level can be affected by many other variables [8]. Tissue DO_2 can be calculated using Hb, SaO_2, and PaO_2 [(1.34 x Hb x SpO_2 x 0.01) + (0.023 x PaO_2)] and cardiac output and is about 1000 ml of O_2 per minute under normal conditions. DO_2 is related to oxygen extraction and to oxygen uptake (VO_2), but dependent on many circulatory and metabolic variables.

6.4 Definition of Hypoxemia, Normoxemia, and Hyperoxemia

Administration of extra oxygen can lead to hyperoxia, which is generally defined as any FO_2 >0.21. Supranormal FO_2 in normal physiological conditions will lead to hyperoxemia or higher than normal PaO_2. The normal range of PaO_2 is 10–13.3 kPa. Thus any PaO_2 >13.3 kPa can be considered as hyperoxemia and any PaO_2 value <10 kPa as hypoxemia. Many different definitions and cut-off values for hypoxemia, normoxemia, and (mild, moderate, or severe) hyperoxemia are used in the O_2-literature, which makes comparison of study results very difficult. Due to the shape of the oxyhemoglobin dissociation curve and the weak correlation, especially at the high extreme of the SO_2 range, between PaO_2 and SO_2, the measurement of SO_2 is an unreliable method to distinguish mild, moderate, and severe hyperoxemia.

6.5 Physiology of Oxygen in Humans

The transport and the levels of oxygen (expressed as PO_2) from the inspired gas (air and/or O_2) to the mitochondria are described in the oxygen cascade (Fig. 6.1). Oxygen transport along the cascade is facilitated by ventilation and circulation on the one hand

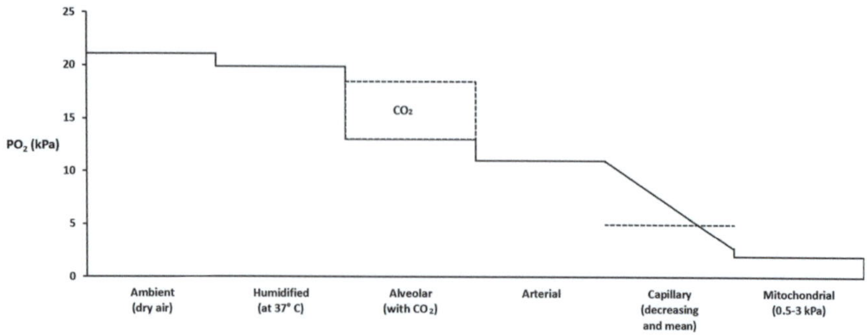

Fig. 6.1 The oxygen cascade: steps from dry ambient air to the mitochondria

and by diffusion on the other. The PO_2 of dry atmospheric air is 21.1 kPa. In the airways, the air is saturated with H_2O at 37 ° C and the inspiratory PO_2 (PIO_2) drops from 21.1 kPa to 19.9 kPa. The next decrease is caused by the exhalation of carbon dioxide (CO_2) in the alveoli. The alveolar carbon dioxide pressure ($PACO_2$) is determined by the alveolar ventilation. Using a simplified alveolar air equation and the respiratory exchange ratio (RQ), the alveolar PAO_2 can be calculated to be approximately 13 kPa under normal conditions and when breathing air. Hypoventilation when breathing air may cause a significant decrease in PAO_2; hyperventilation on the contrary causes only a relatively small increase of PAO_2. This can also be explained by using the alveolar air equation and the PIO_2 (19.9 kPa) in H_2O saturated air in the airways. The highest PAO_2 will be (19.9-$PACO_2$) kPa when breathing air.

Before the circulation takes over the oxygen transport, diffusion of oxygen from the alveoli to the arterial blood is necessary. In normal subjects the alveolar/arterial PO_2 gradient ($\Delta PA\text{-}aO_2$) is limited to less than 2 kPa and is mainly caused by resistance to diffusion. Venous admixture, decreased ventilation/perfusion ratios within the lung, and decreased PAO_2 are the most common causes of an increased $\Delta PA\text{-}aO_2$. The normal arterial O_2 pressure (PaO_2) is therefore slightly higher than 11 kPa. This is the pressure available for diffusion and is directly related to the small amount of oxygen dissolved in blood (0.0232 ml O_2 per 100 ml blood per kPa PO_2).

Most oxygen carried by the blood is bound to hemoglobin (maximum 1.39 ml oxygen per gram of hemoglobin at an SO_2 of 100%). There is a direct equilibrium between dissolved oxygen in blood and oxygen bound to hemoglobin, determined by the oxyhemoglobin dissociation curve and its lateral position. The next stop in the oxygen cascade is the capillary. Over its length in the tissues, more and more O_2 is extracted from the blood by diffusion along a pressure gradient to the tissues. The mean value of PO_2 in capillary blood is slightly >5 kPa. Further steps in the cascade are from capillary to tissue and within the cell. Finally, oxygen reaches the mitochondria. Physiological mitochondrial PO_2 is estimated to be between 3 and 0.5 kPa. In the cells and the mitochondria, O_2 is used by enzymes (oxidases), such as the cytochrome c oxidase system and cytochrome P450. In the mitochondria, O_2 is utilized for aerobic metabolism by oxidation of mainly carbohydrates (glucose). The first step of this process is anaerobic glycolysis taking place in the cells and converting glucose into pyruvate while producing only two ATP per glucose molecule. In anaerobic conditions, the next step will be the conversion of pyruvate to lactate. Lactate levels in metabolic acidosis can be used to estimate the severity of disease and to a lesser extent of hypoxia [8, 9]. In aerobic circumstances, pyruvate will enter the tricarboxylic acid (TCA) cycle in the mitochondria allowing oxidative phosphorylation, thus producing as much as 36 ATP for each glucose molecule. Further products of this metabolic pathway are CO_2, NADH, $FADH_2$ and H_2O.

6.6 Pathophysiology of Oxygen in Humans: Hypoxemia and Effects of Lack of O_2

When critically ill patients become hypoxemic, aerobic glycolysis will be hampered, causing energy depletion, cellular dysfunction, and progressive metabolic lactic acidosis. Longer lasting (chronic) hypoxemia activates intracellular hypoxia-inducible factor, which can activate gene transcription leading to pathophysiological effects opposing hypoxia. These effects include: increased production of hemoglobin through erythropoietin, an increase in vascular growth factors improving tissue perfusion, and sympathetic activation.

6.7 Pathophysiology of Oxygen in Humans: Hyperoxia, Hyperoxemia, and O_2 Toxicity

At a normal atmospheric pressure of 101 kPa, changing FO_2 from 0.21 to 1.0 has negligible effects on SaO_2 and thus on O_2 content ($C\text{-}O_2$) of the blood. However, PaO_2 will largely increase with an increase in FO_2. Hyperoxia therefore will increase the risks of O_2 toxicity without significantly increasing tissue DO_2. Increasing FO_2 is used in clinical medicine to improve oxygenation in cases of hypoventilation, venous admixture or pulmonary pathology with a diffusion disorder. In anemic patients, the factor limiting $C\text{-}O_2$ is hemoglobin and administration of red blood cells (RBCs) is far more efficient than an increase in FO_2; in patients in shock, tissue DO_2 can best be improved by optimizing the circulation. The increase in FO_2 results in hyperoxia, which has a direct effect on the airways and lungs [10]. Signs and symptoms of toxicity are tracheobronchial inflammation, retrosternal pain, cough, resorption atelectasis, and finally hyperoxic acute lung injury (HALI) at the alveolar level. Alveolar damage is related to nitric oxide (NO) production increased by inflammation.

Hyperoxemia leads to higher than normal levels of O_2 in the cells and mitochondria. At these high levels, mitochondrial O_2 can be transformed to ROS, which have unpaired electrons in the outer shell. *In vitro* experiments showed a strong, exponential correlation between increasing oxygen levels and ROS production in porcine lung mitochondria [11] and capillary endothelial cells from rat lungs [12]. In a reperfusion/re-oxygenation model of cultured hepatocytes, increasing oxygen from 0 to 2% led to a sharp increase in ROS production, whereas further increase in the oxygen content up to 95% induced a steady rise in the formation of ROS [13].

ROS are highly reactive and harmful because they react with intracellular molecules damaging proteins and DNA [14–16]. Thus, unopposed ROS react with fatty acids of lipid membranes causing damage to these membranes and lipid peroxidase reactions leading to further cell damage. The effects of ROS may be increased by systemic inflammation, frequently present in critically ill patients. ROS are physiologically inactivated by superoxide dismutase and catalase, enzymes which support the conversion of ROS into H_2O and normal O_2. ROS can also be inactivated by for example vitamin C, vitamin E, and glutathione in the cells. Antioxidant drugs are pharmacological options to influence ROS formation and deformation. Hyperoxemia not only increases serum ROS but also inflammatory cytokines and is linked to progressive inflammation and organ dysfunction. Oxidative stress in hyperoxemia lowers NO levels and causes vasoconstriction in the microcirculation. Depending on circulatory pathology (the type of shock), vasoconstriction may have different effects on the circulation.

6.8 Effects of Normoxia, Hypoxia and Hyperoxia in Critically Ill Patients

Based on the effects of hypoxemia and hyperoxemia described above, large numbers of observational and interventional studies have been performed over the last decade in critically ill patients. In 2008, a retrospective observational landmark study described the oxygenation targets in 36,307 ICU patients in 50 ICUs in the Netherlands and the relationships between used FiO_2 or achieved PaO_2 and clinical outcome [17]. A U-shaped relationship between PaO_2 and mortality (corrected for several variables) was found, with the lowest mortality in the PaO_2 range from 8.9 to 10.6 kPa. Recently [18], a higher nadir for the relationship between PaO_2 and hospital mortality (13.2 kPa) and ICU mortality (13.5 kPa) was reported in ARDS patients. Since 2008, several RCTs have studied the effects of lower versus higher FiO_2, PaO_2, SaO_2 and/or SpO_2 in critically ill patients [19–25]. These RCTs differed in patient selection, target oxygenation in the low and high oxygen groups, and in primary and secondary endpoints. Table 6.1 gives an overview of the characteristics of the RCTs and of two ongoing RCTs.

The first study [19] was a small feasibility study with 103 participants. There were significant differences between PaO_2, SaO_2, and SpO_2 in the experimental and control groups. The authors concluded that conservative oxygenation targets were feasible even though there were significantly more hypoxemic ($SpO_2 < 88\%$) and hyperoxemic ($SpO_2 > 98\%$) saturations found in the conservative versus the liberal oxygenation groups, respectively. The secondary endpoints (new organ dysfunction, mortality in the ICU and at 90 days) were not significantly different in the two groups in this small study.

The Oxygen-ICU study [20] planned to include 660 patients randomized to normoxic PaO_2 and SpO_2 targets versus 'standard practice' of allowing hyperoxic PaO_2 and SpO_2 values. The study was stopped prematurely after inclusion of 480 patients of whom 434 were analyzed. The primary endpoint (ICU mortality) was

Table 6.1 RCTs comparing conventional (high) and conservative (low) oxygenation targets in critically ill patients ventilated in the intensive care unit (ICU)

Study	Year of publication	Type of patients	Number of participants Conservative/ Conventional	Oxygenation targets		Endpoints		
				Conservative (low) O_2	Conventional (high) O_2	Primary	Secondary	Primary endpoint conclusion
Panwar [19]	2016	Mechanically ventilated in ICU	52/51	SpO_2 88–92%	$SpO_2 \geq 96\%$	Feasibility	New organ dysfunction Mortality	Feasible No difference
Oxygen-ICU Girardis [20]	2016	ICU ≥ 72 h	216/218 (prematurely stopped)	SpO_2 94–88% or PaO_2 70–100 mmHg	$PaO_2 \leq 150$ mmHg SpO_2 97–100% ($FiO_2 \geq 0.4$)	ICU mortality	New organ failure New infection	Primary and many secondary end points: Conservative favorable
HYPERS2S Asfar [21]	2017	Septic shock with mechanical ventilation	223/219 (prematurely stopped)	SpO_2 88–95%	FiO_2 1.0 (24 h)	Mortality 28 d	SAEs	No difference more SAEs in hyperoxia
ICU-ROX Mackle [22]	2020	Mechanically ventilated in ICU	501/499	SpO_2 90–97%	No limit FiO_2 or SpO_2	Ventilator-free days 28 d	Mortality 180 d	No difference
LOCO$_2$ Barrot [23]	2020	ARDS	99/102 (prematurely stopped)	PaO_2 55–70 mmHg SpO_2 88–92%	PaO_2 90–105 mmHg $SpO_2 \geq 96\%$	Mortality 28 d	Mesenteric ischemia	No difference More mesenteric ischemia in conservative group
ICU-ROX post-hoc Young [27]	2020	Sepsis	130/120	SpO_2 90–97%	No limit FiO_2 or SpO_2	Mortality 90 d	ICU/hospital length of stay Ventilator-free days	No difference

(continued)

Table 6.1 (continued)

Study	Year of publication	Type of patients	Number of participants Conservative/ Conventional	Oxygenation targets		Endpoints		
				Conservative (low) O_2	Conventional (high) O_2	Primary	Secondary	Primary endpoint conclusion
HOT-ICU Schjørring [24]	2021	ICU and hypoxia	1441/1447	PaO_2 60 mmHg	PaO_2 90 mmHg	Mortality 90 d	Shock, myocardial ischemia, ischemic stroke, intestinal ischemia	No difference
Gelissen [25]	2021	SIRS in ICU	205/195	PaO_2 8–12 kPa	$FiO_2 \leq 0.6$ PaO_2 14–18 kPa	$SOFA_{RANK}$	Mortality	No difference
Study	*Inclusion period*		*Total planned*					
UK-ROX [33]	2020–2023	Invasive ventilation in ICU	16,500	SpO_2 88-92%	No limit	Mortality 90 d costs/ QALY	Mortality (ICU, hospital, 1 year) Stay (ICU, hospital) Economic	
Mega-ROX [32]	2020–2025	Invasive ventilation in ICU	40,000	$SpO_2 < 94\%$ and FiO_2 0.21 with SpO_2 target 90%	$FiO_2 > 0.3$	Mortality in hospital	Duration of survival, length of stay (ICU, hospital)	

SpO_2 oxygen saturation by pulse oximetry, *FiO_2* inspired oxygen fraction, *QALY* quality-adjusted life year, *$SOFA_{RANK}$* ranked sequential organ failure assessment, *SIRS* systemic inflammatory response syndrome, *ARDS* acute respiratory distress syndrome, *SAE* serious adverse event

significantly lower in the conservative group (12% vs. 20%). Among the secondary endpoints, new shock, new liver failure, and bloodstream infections occurred less frequently in the conservative group. The authors considered their conclusions to be preliminary due to the smaller than planned size of the analyzed groups.

The HYPERS2S study [21] combined a study of oxygenation targets (hyperoxia at FiO_2 of 1.00 compared to SO_2 of 88 to 95%) with a study of isotonic versus hypertonic saline infusion in a two-by-two factorial, multicenter RCT in mechanically ventilated patients with septic shock. The primary endpoint of 28-day mortality was not significantly different in the two oxygenation groups. However, the trial was stopped prematurely due to a high number of serious adverse events (SAEs) in the hyperoxia group. Atelectasis occurred significantly more frequent with an FiO_2 of 1.00 and there was a potentially important but statistically not significant difference in the incidence of ICU-acquired weakness. The authors concluded that in patients with septic shock an FiO_2 of 1.00 might increase the risk of mortality, although at the moment of discontinuation, mortality was not significantly higher in the hyperoxic group.

The ICU-ROX trial [22] included 1000 patients with at least 1 day of mechanical ventilation. Hypoxemia was prevented by setting the lower limit of SpO_2 to 90%. In the conservative group, the upper limit of SpO_2 was 97% and the FiO_2 was lowered to a minimal value of 0.21 as long as SpO_2 was >90%. In the usual (conventional) oxygen group, there were no limits to FiO_2 or SpO_2. The primary endpoint (ventilator-free days at day 28) was not different between the usual and experimental oxygenation groups. Mortality up to 180 days after inclusion was also not different.

In the $LOCO_2$ trial [23], patients with acute respiratory distress syndrome (ARDS) were exposed to either conservative oxygenation targets (PaO_2 55–80 mmHg and SpO_2 88–92%) or liberal oxygenation targets (PaO_2 90 to 105 mmHg and SpO_2 ≥96%) for 7 days. Mechanical ventilation strategies were identical in both groups. The primary endpoint of mortality at 28 days was not significantly different between the groups. However, the trial was stopped prematurely because five cases of mesenteric ischemia occurred in the conservative oxygenation group versus none in the liberal oxygenation group and because the mortality at 90 days was higher (44 vs. 30%) in the conservative oxygenation group.

The HOT-ICU [24] is the largest RCT of lower-oxygenation versus higher-oxygenation in critically ill patients up to now, in which 2888 patients admitted to the ICU for hypoxemic respiratory failure were randomized for target PaO_2 of either 60 mmHg or 90 mmHg. The primary outcome of mortality after 90 days was not significantly different, at 42.9% and 42.2% in the lower-oxygenation and the higher oxygenation groups, respectively. Secondary endpoints were similar in the two groups.

Recently we published results from an RCT in 400 patients with at least two positive systemic inflammatory response syndrome (SIRS) criteria [25]. Target oxygenation was chosen within the range of clinical practice for both the control and the experimental groups. The control group (high-normal) was targeted for a PaO_2 of 14 to 18 kPa and the risk of hyperoxic pulmonary damage was limited by restricting the FiO_2 to a maximum of 0.60 in this group as much as clinically possible. The experimental group (low-normal) had a target PaO_2 of 8 to 12 kPa. A novel substitute endpoint for organ failure (ranked sequential organ failure assessment [$SOFA_{RANK}$]) was developed based on a previous study [26]. $SOFA_{RANK}$ is a ranked outcome of SOFA scores over the first 14 days after randomization and excluding the respiratory component of the SOFA score since that is being influenced by the targeted oxygenation. Organ failure ranking in the two groups was not significantly different ($p = 0.06$), but tended to favor the high-normal oxygenation target (i.e., the confidence interval was not consistent with clinically important harm from high-normal oxygen target). Mild hypoxemia occurred more often in the low-normal oxygenation group, but severe hypoxemia (PaO_2 <5 kPa) was similar in both the oxygenation groups. Other secondary endpoints (duration of mechanical ventilation and mortality) were similar in the two groups.

In a *post hoc* subgroup analysis of ventilated patients with sepsis from the ICU-ROX study [27], no differences were found between conservative and usual oxygen therapy for the primary endpoint (mortality at day 90) or for any of the secondary endpoints. Point estimates of treatment effects favored usual (conventional) oxygen therapy, in line with our recent results [25].

Since 2014, a number of systematic reviews and meta-analyses [28–31] including the above mentioned RCTs and other studies in critically ill patients have been published.

In 2014, a meta-analysis was published [28] including 17 observational studies and 1 prospective before-after study. Only four of the included studies specifically addressed critical care patients. Due to the heterogeneity of these four studies, data could not be pooled. Mortality was increased in the hyperoxic groups in the pooled studies of post-cardiac arrest, stroke, and traumatic brain injury patients.

In the IOTA systematic review and meta-analysis [29], 27 RCTs with 16,037 acutely ill patients from several subgroups were included. In-hospital, 30 day, and longest follow-up mortality were significantly increased in the overall liberal oxygen versus the overall conservative oxygenation groups.

In 2021, a meta-analysis including seven RCTs with 5265 patients was published [30]. Longest follow-up mortality was identical in the conservative and conventional oxygenation groups overall. However, in a subgroup analysis of three studies that only included patients with mild to moderate hypoxemia (PaO_2/FiO_2 >100 mmHg), mortality was significantly lower when using conservative oxygen therapy.

Also in 2021, a network meta-analysis of eight RCTs in mechanically ventilated critically ill patients was performed [31]. Surface under the cumulative ranking (SUCRA) scores and survival curves suggested superiority of the moderate (90–150 mmHg) PaO_2 target in the trinary and quadruple classification and also the conservative (70–90 mmHg) PaO_2 in the quadruple classification when compared to liberal (>150 mmHg) and far-conservative targets (55–70 mmHg).

6.9 Future Studies

Two large ongoing RCTs comparing conservative versus conventional oxygenation targets in ICU patients have been registered and are currently recruiting [32, 33]. The Mega-ROX trial [32] aims to include 40,000 adults admitted to the ICU for invasive mechanical ventilation or starting invasive mechanical ventilation after admission. For the control group (liberal oxygen or usual care) the only condition is $FiO_2 \geq 0.30$. In the treatment group (conservative oxygen therapy), FiO_2 will be decreased to 0.21 if possible, but limited to a minimum acceptable SpO_2 of 90% and aiming for a maximum SpO_2 of 94 or 95%. The primary endpoint is in-hospital mortality up to 90 days after randomization. Using a response-adaptive randomization procedure, more subjects will be assigned to the group with the lowest mortality during the ongoing period of recruitment, stratified by subgroup. Power calculations were made based on data from the IOTA systematic review and meta-analysis [29] and from the ICU-ROX trial [22]. Heterogeneity of treatment effect in diagnostic subgroups (hypoxic ischemic encephalopathy, acute brain injury, and sepsis) of critically ill patients will be explored.

The UK-ROX trial [33] aims to include 16,500 adult patients admitted to the critical care unit for mechanical ventilation or receiving mechanical ventilation after being admitted for another reason. For the control group (usual oxygen therapy), there are no conditions other than usual care as per local practice. For the intervention group (conservative oxygen therapy), SpO_2 values of 88 to 92% are the target. The primary endpoints are mortality at day 90 and economic outcome (incremental costs, quality-adjusted life year (QALY) and net monetary benefit at 90 days). Economic outcome has not been studied previously in this setting.

6.10 Conclusion

In heterogeneous critically ill patients, the potentially deleterious effects of hyperoxemia found in preclinical research and large observational studies have not been confirmed in well-sized RCTs. In view of the current body of literature, it seems reasonable and prudent to avoid far-conservative and far-liberal oxygenation values. It is presently unknown whether there are specific subgroups or conditions within the critically ill population that might benefit from oxygenation targets outside the normoxemia range. As far as oxygen is concerned half a millennium after the Paracelsus statement "the dose makes the poison", it is still not completely clear at what dose the transition from useful drug to dangerous poison takes place.

References

1. Canfield DE. Oxygen: a four billion year history. Princeton: Princeton University Press; 2014.
2. Kump LR. The rise of atmospheric oxygen. Nature. 2008;451:277–8.

3. Sjoding MW, Dickson RP, Iwashyna TJ, Gay SE, Valley TS. Racial bias in pulse oximetry measurement. N Engl J Med. 2020;383:2477–8.
4. Zijlstra WG, Buursma A, Meeuwsen-van der Roest WP. Absorption spectra of human fetal and adult oxyhemoglobin, de-oxyhemoglobin, carboxyhemoglobin, and methemoglobin. Clin Chem. 1991;37:1633–8.
5. Kelman GR. Digital computer subroutine for the conversion of oxygen tension into saturation. J Appl Physiol. 1966;21:1375–6.
6. Sauthier M, Tuli G, Jouvet PA, Brownstein JS, Randolph AG. Estimated Pao2: a continuous and noninvasive method to estimate Pao2 and oxygenation index. Crit Care Explor. 2021;3:e0546.
7. Vincent JL. Monitoring tissue perfusion. Can J Anaesth. 1996;43:R55–60.
8. Bakker J, Postelnicu R, Mukherjee V. Lactate: where are we now? Crit Care Clin. 2020;36:115–24.
9. Kushimoto S, Akaishi S, Sato T, et al. Lactate, a useful marker for disease mortality and severity but an unreliable marker of tissue hypoxia/hypoperfusion in critically ill patients. Acute Med Surg. 2016;3:293–7.
10. Kallet RH, Matthay MA. Hyperoxic acute lung injury. Respir Care. 2013;58:123–41.
11. Turrens JF. Mitochondrial formation of reactive oxygen species. J Physiol. 2003;552:335–44.
12. Brueckl C, Kaestle S, Kerem A, et al. Hyperoxia-induced reactive oxygen species formation in pulmonary capillary endothelial cells in situ. Am J Respir Cell Mol Biol. 2006;34:453–63.
13. Littauer A, de Groot H. Release of reactive oxygen by hepatocytes on reoxygenation: three phases and role of mitochondria. Am J Phys. 1992;262:G1015–20.
14. Nakane M. Biological effects of the oxygen molecule in critically ill patients. J Intensive Care. 2020;8:95.
15. Kulkarni AC, Kuppusamy P, Parinandi N. Oxygen, the lead actor in the pathophysiologic drama: enactment of the trinity of normoxia, hypoxia, and hyperoxia in disease and therapy. Antioxid Redox Signal. 2007;9:1717–30.
16. Chandel NS, Budinger GR. The cellular basis for diverse responses to oxygen. Free Radic Biol Med. 2007;42:165–74.
17. de Jonge E, Peelen L, Keijzers PJ, et al. Association between administered oxygen, arterial partial oxygen pressure and mortality in mechanically ventilated intensive care unit patients. Crit Care. 2008;12:R156.
18. Boyle AJ, Holmes DN, Hackett J, et al. Hyperoxaemia and hypoxaemia are associated with harm in patients with ARDS. BMC Pulm Med. 2021;21:285.
19. Panwar R, Hardie M, Bellomo R, et al. Conservative versus liberal oxygenation targets for mechanically ventilated patients. A pilot multicenter randomized controlled trial. Am J Respir Crit Care Med. 2016;193:43–51.
20. Girardis M, Busani S, Damiani E, et al. Effect of conservative vs conventional oxygen therapy on mortality among patients in an intensive care unit: the oxygen-ICU randomized clinical trial. JAMA. 2016;316:1583–9.
21. Asfar P, Schortgen F, Boisrame-Helms J, et al. Hyperoxia and hypertonic saline in patients with septic shock (HYPERS2S): a two-by-two factorial, multicentre, randomised, clinical trial. Lancet Respir Med. 2017;5:180–90.
22. Mackle D, Bellomo R, Bailey M, et al. Conservative oxygen therapy during mechanical ventilation in the ICU. N Engl J Med. 2020;382:989–98.
23. Barrot L, Asfar P, Mauny F, et al. Liberal or conservative oxygen therapy for acute respiratory distress syndrome. N Engl J Med. 2020;382:999–1008.
24. Schjorring OL, Klitgaard TL, Perner A, et al. Lower or higher oxygenation targets for acute hypoxemic respiratory failure. N Engl J Med. 2021;384:1301–11.
25. Gelissen H, de Grooth HJ, Smulders Y, et al. Effect of low-normal vs high-normal oxygenation targets on organ dysfunction in critically ill patients: a randomized clinical trial. JAMA. 2021;326:940–8.
26. de Grooth HJ, Geenen IL, Girbes AR, Vincent JL, Parienti JJ, Oudemans-van Straaten HM. SOFA and mortality endpoints in randomized controlled trials: a systematic review and meta-regression analysis. Crit Care. 2017;21:38.

27. Young P, Mackle D, Bellomo R, et al. Conservative oxygen therapy for mechanically ventilated adults with sepsis: a post hoc analysis of data from the intensive care unit randomized trial comparing two approaches to oxygen therapy (ICU-ROX). Intensive Care Med. 2020;46:17–26.
28. Damiani E, Adrario E, Girardis M, et al. Arterial hyperoxia and mortality in critically ill patients: a systematic review and meta-analysis. Crit Care. 2014;18:711.
29. Chu DK, Kim LH, Young PJ, et al. Mortality and morbidity in acutely ill adults treated with liberal versus conservative oxygen therapy (IOTA): a systematic review and meta-analysis. Lancet. 2018;391:1693–705.
30. Chen XL, Zhang BL, Meng C, Huang HB, Du B. Conservative oxygen therapy for critically ill patients: a meta-analysis of randomized controlled trials. J Intensive Care. 2021;9:47.
31. Zhao X, Xiao H, Dai F, Brodie D, Meng L. Classification and effectiveness of different oxygenation goals in mechanically ventilated critically ill patients: network meta-analysis of randomised controlled trials. Eur Respir J. 2021;58:2002928.
32. The Mega Randomised Registry Trial Comparing Conservative vs. Liberal OXygenation Targets (Mega-ROX). Available at: https://www.anzctr.org.au/Trial/Registration/TrialReview.aspx?id=379432&isReview=true. Accessed 23 Oct 2021.
33. Intensive care unit randomised trial comparing two approaches to oxygen therapy (UK-ROX). Available at: https://www.isrctn.com/ISRCTN13384956. Accessed 23 Oct 2021.

Nebulized Therapeutics for COVID-19 Pneumonia in Critical Care

7

J. Dhanani and M. C. Reade

7.1 Introduction

Coronavirus disease 2019 (COVID-19) pneumonia is caused by infection with severe acute respiratory syndrome coronavirus-2 (SARS-CoV-2). The infection is transmissible by aerosol and causes various clinical phenotypes of pneumonia including the acute respiratory distress syndrome (ARDS). This infection has resulted in a worldwide pandemic affecting the majority of the human population. Severe disease is characterized by pneumonia and respiratory failure, resulting in death in about 0.5% of confirmed cases [1].

The various phenotypes of COVID-19 represent different phases of the infection from viral replication to the hyperimmune response (inflammatory cytokines interleukin [IL]-2, IL-6, IL-8, IL-10, and tumor necrosis factor [TNF]-α). Therapeutic options should therefore be selected based on the pathogenetic mechanism that is predominant at the time of need. Early stages of illness are the time of viral replication and shedding in the upper respiratory tract, making antiviral agents the logical

J. Dhanani (✉)
University of Queensland Centre of Clinical Research, Faculty of Medicine, The University of Queensland, St Lucia, QLD, Australia

Queensland University of Technology, School of Nursing, Brisbane City, QLD, Australia

Department of Intensive Care Medicine, Royal Brisbane and Women's Hospital, Herston, QLD, Australia
e-mail: j.dhanani@uq.edu.au

M. C. Reade
Department of Intensive Care Medicine, Royal Brisbane and Women's Hospital, Herston, QLD, Australia

School of Medicine, University of Queensland, St Lucia, QLD, Australia

Joint Health Command, Australian Defence Force, Canberra, ACT, Australia

J.-L. Vincent (ed.), *Annual Update in Intensive Care and Emergency Medicine 2022*, Annual Update in Intensive Care and Emergency Medicine,
https://doi.org/10.1007/978-3-030-93433-0_7

choice, whereas the cytokine mediated hyperinflammation in later stage disease suggests anti-inflammatory agents or immunomodulators would then be the most effective agents.

Many medications have demonstrated effective *in vitro* activity against the SARS-CoV-2 virus. Other potential COVID-19 pneumonia therapies, including anticoagulants, anti-inflammatory drugs, immunomodulators, and mucokinetics, have been assessed. Antibiotic use is also common due to the high prevalence of opportunistic lung infections. However, very few of these approaches have demonstrated sufficient effectiveness in large-scale trials. Consequently, COVID-19-associated mortality and morbidity remain high.

There are several possible causes for the failure of therapeutic agents that showed promise *in vitro* or by extrapolation of effectiveness in other lung conditions. Failure of systemic therapies could be due to their poor lung penetration, as seen with antibiotics such as aminoglycosides. Concerns regarding systemic toxicity could limit adequate drug dosing, as might be true of hydroxychloroquine. Systemic immunomodulation, especially if applied at a suboptimal time in the disease course, could lead to secondary infections.

Despite the recent development of effective vaccines, viral mutations and possible vaccine distribution and implementation issues may influence vaccine effectiveness. Hence, there is an urgent ongoing need to investigate effective therapy for COVID-19 pneumonia. Development of entirely novel therapeutics for COVID-19 takes a long time, hence the attraction of repurposing existing drugs, ideally specifically optimized for COVID-19.

7.2 Nebulized Therapeutics for COVID-19 Pneumonia

By delivering drugs directly to the lungs, it is possible to achieve high local concentrations whilst limiting systemic toxicity. Nebulized therapy offers the potential to repurpose existing drugs while avoiding many of their adverse effects. Nebulized drug therapy is commonly used for asthma, chronic obstructive lung disease, cystic fibrosis, and pneumonia. During the course of the COVID-19 pandemic, various research groups have investigated pulmonary drug administration. However, this remains a relatively under-explored field. Of 5641 trials related to COVID-19 registered on https://trialsearch.who.int/ (as of October 2021), only 126 (2.2%) were investigating nebulized therapy. Very few have yet reported their results. Nonetheless, this is a promising mode of drug administration that warrants greater attention.

7.3 Technical Aspects of Nebulized Drug Therapy

For effective drug therapy it is necessary to achieve optimal drug concentrations at sites of action. In COVID-19 pneumonia, the distal lung is the site of infection and associated disease. Several factors affect distal lung drug delivery. Of these, achieving a nebulized particle size of 1–5 μm (respirable fraction) is the major factor. This is primarily influenced by the physicochemical properties of the drug formulation, the type of nebulizer device, and humidification. Currently, there are no data specific to nebulized therapeutics in COVID-19 pneumonia, but extrapolation from other conditions such as asthma and distal lung infections is likely to be relevant.

Due to the inability of patients with severe disease to co-ordinate with device actuation and their limited inhalation capacity, metered dose inhalers (MDI) and dry powder inhalers (DPI) are unlikely to be appropriate. Hence, nebulizers are the most practical alternative. Nebulizers fall into three classes: those which use a gas jet to generate an aerosol, those which use ultrasonic vibration, and those which pass the liquid through a very fine vibrating mesh. Of these, the vibrating mesh nebulizer is deemed most efficient for generating particles of 1–5 μm and is recommended for nebulized therapy using antibiotics or bronchodilators [2].

Mechanical ventilatory support introduces additional complexity to nebulizer therapy. Published guidelines suggest placing the nebulizer in the inspiratory limb of the circuit, 15 cm from the Y-piece, turning off humidification, using a square flow waveform, prolonging the inspiratory time, and changing expiratory filters after nebulization [2]. Some ventilators incorporate specific devices and software algorithms to facilitate nebulization, as has been reviewed comprehensively elsewhere [3].

7.4 Current Clinical Trials on Nebulized COVID-19 Therapeutics in Critical Care

Nebulized pharmacological agents for the therapeutic use in COVID-19 pneumonia patients can be classified based on clinical effects, with some agents having more than one class of effect (Fig. 7.1). Many of these drugs are in clinical trials (Table 7.1). Those which have excited the greatest interest are discussed in detail below.

7.4.1 Antivirals

7.4.1.1 Chloroquine/Hydroxychloroquine

Rationale Chloroquine and hydroxychloroquine block proteolytic processing and endosomal acidification, inhibit autophagosome-lysosome fusion, inactivate enzymes required for viral replication, inhibit viral protein formation, and block viral entry into host cells through impairment of terminal glycosylation of the angiotensin-converting enzyme 2 (ACE2) enzyme receptor [4]. They may also reduce cytokine production.

Trials of chloroquine and hydroxychloroquine suggested higher mortality compared to placebo, possibly due to cardiac toxicity, and regulatory agencies have either revoked authorizations or recommended against its use [5]. Moreover, due to the complex pharmacokinetic (PK) mechanisms, including large volume of

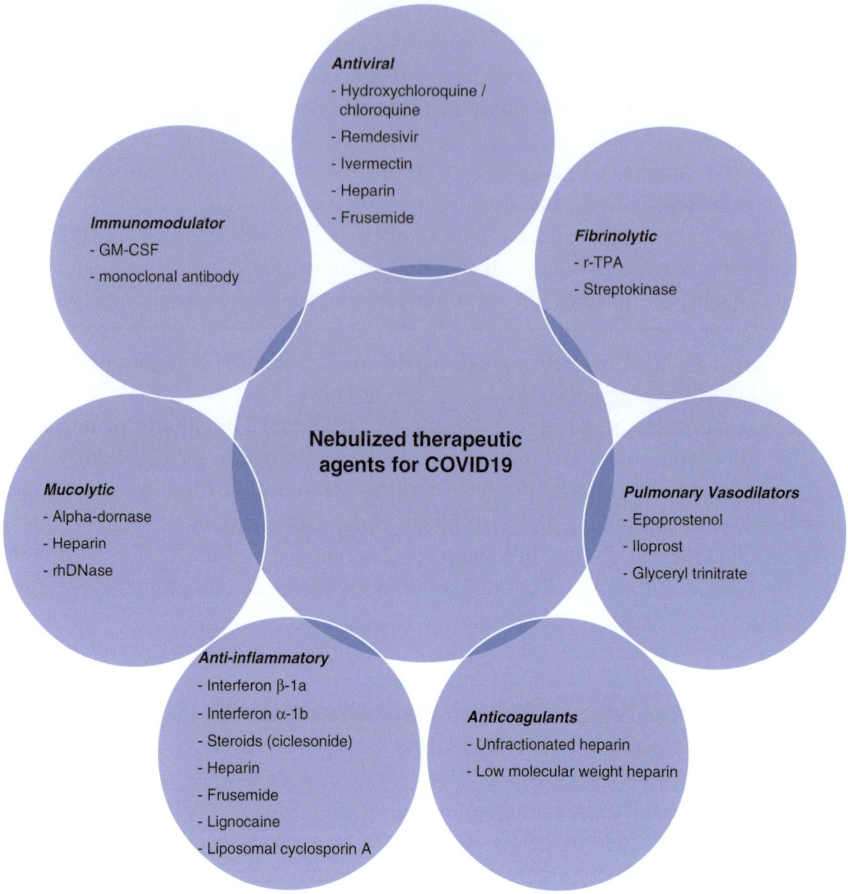

Fig. 7.1 Nebulized pharmacological agents as per their drug class used in the treatment of COVID-19 patients

distribution (~44,257 liters), orally administered hydroxychloroquine may not achieve adequate intracellular concentrations [6]. As its antiviral effect is achieved by blocking viral entry into the epithelial cells, direct delivery by inhalation is likely to be ideal. Given that the EC_{50} (half maximal effective concentration) for hydroxychloroquine against SARS CoV-2 is 6.14 μM, it is estimated that nebulized hydroxychloroquine doses as low as 10–20 mg/day would achieve the required drug concentrations in the lung [7]. In addition, ionization of hydroxychloroquine in the acidic pH of lysosomes in the lungs will reduce systemic exposure and hence toxicity of nebulized hydroxychloroquine. Thus, nebulized liposomal hydroxychloroquine can potentially achieve higher lung concentrations of hydroxychloroquine at small doses with limited adverse effects.

Table 7.1 Summary of currently registered clinical trials on nebulized therapeutics for COVID-19 (from https://trialsearch.who.int/ and www.clinicaltrials.gov as accessed on 05 October 2021)

Drug class	Total number of registered studies	Number of registered clinical trials with patient-centered endpoints	Number of registered studies completed
Antiviral			
Hydroxychloroquine	5	1	
Remdesivir	2	1	1
Niclosamide or levamisole or ivermectin (anti-helminthic)	3	1	
Neutralizing antibody	1	1	
Testosterone	1		
Modified ACE2	1		
4.2% sodium bicarbonate	2	2	
Monoclonal antibody	1		
Danoprevir + ritonavir	1	1	
Novaferon	1	1	
DAS 181	1	1	
Immunomodulator			
GM-CSF	2	1	
Dalargin (leu-enkephalin)	1	1	
Itraconazole	1	1	
Platelet lysate	1	1	
TLR agonist PUL-042	2	2	
JAK inhibitor TD-0903	1		
Anticoagulant			
Heparin	10	10	2
Enoxaparin	1		
Fibrinolytic			
Rt-PA	1	1	
Anti-inflammatory			
Interferon	6	5	
Steroid	9	9	
Retinoic acid	8	7	
Melphalan	1	1	
Furosemide	1		
Exosome	4	1	
Lidocaine	1	1	
Hyaluronan	1		
Magnesium	1	1	
Vasoactive intestinal polypeptide (VIP)	3	2	
Ibuprofen	1	1	
Acetylsalicylic acid	1	1	
Adenosine	1	1	
Alpha-1 antitrypsin	1	1	
AP-014 (Ampion; albumin)	2		
Azithromycin	1	1	
Ensifentrine	1	1	
Mucolytic			
N-acetylcysteine	2	2	
DNAase	6	6	1

(continued)

Table 7.1 (continued)

Drug class	Total number of registered studies	Number of registered clinical trials with patient-centered endpoints	Number of registered studies completed
Pulmonary vasodilator			
Iloprostenol/epoprostenol	2	2	
Glyceryl trinitrate	1	1	
Vaccine			
Vaccine or vaccine adjuvant	6	1	
Miscellaneous			
Surfactant	2	2	
Bacteriophage	1	1	

ACE angiotensin-converting enzyme, *GM-CSF* granulocyte-monocyte colony-stimulating factor, *JAK* janus kinase, *Rt-PA* recombinant tissue plasminogen activator, *TLR* toll-like receptor

Evidence Nebulized hydroxychloroquine has been used safely in asthmatic patients [8] and is well tolerated with limited cardiotoxicity and QTc prolongation, while increasing the therapeutic efficacy of the drug. A phase 1 trial of nebulized liposomal hydroxychloroquine for COVID-19 has been approved (ClinicalTrials.gov Identifier: NCT04697654). A pilot, randomized open label study of nebulized hydroxychloroquine for COVID-19 therapy (ClinicalTrials.gov Identifier: NCT04731051) is underway.

Recommendation Nebulized chloroquine and hydroxychloroquine should only be used as part of a clinical trial.

7.4.1.2 Remdesivir

Rationale Remdesivir is a prodrug metabolized to the active antiviral nucleoside triphosphate (Nuc-TP). It has broad spectrum antiviral activity through inhibition of viral RNA synthesis, with *in vitro* efficacy against other coronaviruses, such as Middle East Respiratory Syndrome coronavirus (MERS-CoV) in mice and monkeys. It has *in vitro* antiviral activity (IC_{50} 0.77 μM) against SARS-CoV-2. Oral administration is associated with high first pass metabolism and poor bioavailability, necessitating intravenous infusion. It is distributed into tissues and cells via passive diffusion where it is converted to nucleoside monophosphate (Nuc-MP) by intracellular hydrolases, ultimately forming the active Nuc-TP. Intravenous remdesivir is poorly distributed in tissues and in lungs as seen in monkey lungs [9]. Plasma PK studies of intravenous remdesivir 75 mg (over 30 min) in patients with Ebola demonstrated a short half-life ($t_{1/2}$), with an even lower area under the curve (AUC) of Nuc-TP in peripheral blood mononuclear cells. Therefore, remdesivir is unlikely to achieve a therapeutic concentration in the lungs [10]. Intravenous remdesivir is formulated with sulfobutylether-beta-cyclodextrin (SBECD) as a solubility enhancer, which is cleared by the kidneys and hence contraindicated in renal failure. Concern of hepatotoxicity also limits the dosing of remdesivir to 200 mg/day. Thus, currently, remdesivir is only administered to hospitalized patients. This is not ideal, as its antiviral effect is most likely to be effective very early in the disease course before patients otherwise require hospitalization. Nebulized remdesivir could be used early in patients with mild disease, or with contraindications for intravenous therapy. Early administration of nebulized remdesivir 50 mg for 30 min is likely optimal for antiviral activity [11].

Evidence A phase 1b/2A study (ClinicalTrials.gov Identifier: NCT04539262) in early stage COVID-19 to evaluate safety, efficacy, and PK of nebulized remdesivir is underway. Another placebo-controlled, randomized controlled trial (RCT) (ClinicalTrials.gov Identifier: NCT04480333) evaluating safety and PK of a nebulized nanoparticle formulation of remdesivir in healthy volunteers is ongoing.

Recommendation Nebulized remdesivir should only be used as part of a clinical trial.

7.4.1.3 Ivermectin

Rationale Ivermectin is an approved anthelminthic agent with antiviral properties. It is lipophilic and highly protein bound (~93%). It inhibits the formation of the importin-α (IMPα) and IMPβ1 subunit, which is used by the SARS-CoV-2 nucleoprotein to infiltrate the nucleus and establish optimal environment for viral replication and proliferation [12].

Evidence Ivermectin has demonstrated *in vitro* activity against SARS-CoV-2 with IC_{50} of 1750 ng/ml [13]. Oral ivermectin at prescribed safe doses did not achieve lung concentrations above this IC_{50} concentration [14]. Pulmonary bioavailability is likely to be low due to high protein binding, supporting the theoretical superiority of inhalation administration. A clinical trial (ClinicalTrials.gov Identifier: NCT04681053) is underway in COVID-19 patients.

Recommendation Should only be used as part of a clinical trial.

7.4.2 Immunomodulators

7.4.2.1 Granulocyte-Monocyte Colony-Stimulating Factor (GM-CSF)

Rationale: GM-CSF, a member of the colony stimulating superfamily, is a complex cytokine considered central to an integrated immune response. In healthy lungs, GM-CSF helps with maturation and function of alveolar macrophages and surfactant metabolism required to maintain lung function and cell mediated immunity in the lung. It also choreographs local and systemic inflammation.

Evidence A single-center cohort study of an anti GM-CSF receptor antibody in 13 COVID-19 patients suggested efficacy compared to standard care [15]. Conversely, nebulized sargramostim, a recombinant GM-CSF, is currently the subject of a RCT in comparison to standard care in patients (n = 80) with COVID-19 infection and severe respiratory failure (ClinicalTrials.gov Identifier: NCT04326920). Phase 2 studies to prevent ARDS in COVID-19 pneumonia (EUdraCT number:

2020-001654-21-DE, ClinicalTrials.gov Identifier: NCT04569877) are also underway. Timing of administration during the disease course is likely to be critical in understanding whether augmenting or inhibiting GM-CSF has any benefit.

Recommendation Should only be used as part of a clinical trial.

7.4.3 Anticoagulants

7.4.3.1 Heparin

Rationale SARS-Cov-2 binds to ACE2, which is widely expressed in the lungs on alveolar type 2 epithelial cells, bronchial epithelial cells, and arterial/venous endothelial cells, to gain cellular entry. ACE2 hijacking prevents angiotensin 2 degradation and the resulting high angiotensin 2 leads to vasoconstriction, endothelial injury, and coagulation cascade activation. COVID-19 infection is also associated with thromboembolic complications, often a cause of mortality in critically ill patients. Throughout the pandemic, systemic heparin for anticoagulation has been used effectively in the treatment of hospitalized COVID-19 patients. Although low molecular weight heparins (LMWHs) are seen to bind to SARS-CoV-2, *in vitro* studies suggest markedly lower potency compared to unfractionated heparin (UFH) [16] perhaps suggesting that higher molecular weight fractions (UFH 15650–19,100 Da vs LMWH 4200–6650 Da) are more effective due to the ability to bind to more receptor binding domain (RBD) and ACE2 sites of the virus.

- Antiviral effect

UFH binds to RBD sites of SARS-CoV-2 spike proteins leading to conformational change, inhibiting binding of the spike protein to cells [17]. With an IC_{50} of 0.6 μg/ml, *in vitro* studies with live SARS-CoV-2 and Vero E6 cells demonstrated up to 80% viral inhibition at 6.25–200 μg/ml [17]. However, the inhibitory concentration of heparin for wild type authentic live SARS-CoV-2 virus attenuation is unknown.

- Anti-inflammatory effect

Heparin exhibits a wide range of anti-inflammatory properties [18]. It neutralizes the cationic immune mediators IL-6, IL-8, and chemotaxins [19], which is thought to underly its mucolytic activity in cystic fibrosis. Nebulized heparin reduces pro-inflammatory cytokines in lung and nuclear factor-kappa B (NF-κB) and transforming growth factor (TGF)-β effectors in alveolar macrophages [20].

- Anti-coagulant effect

ARDS is marked by fibrin deposition in the alveolar space leading to hyaline membranes, along with pulmonary coagulopathy, which can be responsive to nebulized anticoagulants [21]. Heparin inhibits coagulation activation through several mechanisms: catalyzing antithrombin, promoting tissue factor pathway inhibitor (TFPI), and releasing plasminogen activator. Nebulized heparin has no systemic anticoagulation effect.

- Mucolytic effect

Neutrophil extracellular traps (NETs) in sputum contribute to sputum elasticity. Heparin de-aggregates DNA/actin bundles and activates endogenous DNAse to reduce sputum elasticity. Heparin also neutralizes the basic proteins (cytotoxic histones, neutrophil elastase, and IL-8) [22].

Evidence The United Kingdom ACCORD trial is investigating the effects of nebulized heparin 25,000 U q6h in hospitalized COVID-19 patients (EudraCT number: 2020-001736-95).

Recommendation Current evidence indicates that heparin is safe to use in mechanically ventilated patients with severe COVID-19. Where possible, participation in a clinical trial is desirable.

7.4.4 Fibrinolytics

7.4.4.1 Tissue Plasminogen Activator (t-PA)

Rationale Procoagulation is a feature of severe COVID-19 infection. Thromboembolism and pulmonary vascular thrombosis are common. Whilst systemic anticoagulation with heparin is commonly used in the prevention of these conditions, thrombolytic/fibrinolytic therapy has been recommended for treatment. t-PA is used for its fibrinolytic effect as well as anti-inflammatory action. However, the pathophysiology of COVID-19 also involves alveolar deposition of fibrin with hyaline membrane formation affecting gas exchange [23]. In addition, there is evidence that fibrinolysis may be hyperactivated in the advanced phase of COVID-19. Thus, systemic fibrinolytic therapy could cause significant bleeding [24]. Nebulized t-PA can be administered at any stage of COVID-19 without concerns about systemic bleeding [25]. Nebulized t-PA can dissolve fibrin thrombi in the microcirculation as well as alveolar exudates, thereby improving alveolar ventilation. Nebulized streptokinase demonstrated improved P/F ratios without increased bleeding in ARDS patients [26].

Evidence A pilot, open label, phase 2 clinical trial for nebulized recombinant t-PA (rt-PA) in COVID-19 ARDS patients (PACA trial) is underway (EudraCT number: 2020-001640-26-GB).

Recommendation Nebulized fibrinolytics should only be used as part of a clinical trial.

7.4.5 Anti-Inflammatory Agents

7.4.5.1 Interferon

Rationale Interferon (IFN) is an immune active protein with broad spectrum antiviral activity *in vivo*. IFNα is an antiviral agent effective against MERS-CoV *in vitro*. *In vitro* studies show that it inhibits severe cytopathology induced by MERS-coronavirus replication. MERS-CoV was 50–100 times more sensitive to recombinant IFNα (α2a, α2b, β1a and β1b) than SARS-CoV *in vitro*. IFNα binds receptors 1 and 2, followed by activation of Janus kinase/signal transducers and activators of the transcription (JAK/STAT) pathway and IFN-response genes. As SARS-CoV-2 causes inactivation of IFN regulatory factor 3 (IRF3), severe disease results in a significant decrease in IFN activity, especially in at-risk groups (elderly, immunosuppressive medications, comorbidities) [27]. IFN therapy could restore this dysregulated antiviral status. However, systemic IFN therapy can cause "interferonopathies": severe autoimmune disease exacerbations and other complications [28]. Nebulized IFN therapy could potentially achieve high lung concentrations without systemic adverse effects.

Evidence Zhou et al., in an observational study in patients with moderate COVID-19, used nebulized IFNα2b 5 mU twice a day for 10–14 days [29], finding that IFN was associated with reduced duration of detectable virus in the upper respiratory tract and reduced duration of elevated inflammatory biomarkers. SNG001 is a recombinant IFNβ for nebulized delivery that is well tolerated in patients with asthma and chronic obstructive pulmonary disease (COPD). A phase 2 RCT in hospitalized adult COVID-19 patients given SNG001 6 MIU for 14 days demonstrated that, compared to placebo, the drug was well tolerated and conferred greater odds of clinical improvement [30]. Multiple clinical trials using different forms of nebulized IFN in various stages of COVID-19 are underway (IFNα1b - ChiCTR number: 2000030480; recombinant supercompound IFN (rSIFN-co) - ChiCTR number: 2000029638; IFNβ1a - IRCT number: 2020-0511047396 N1, EudraCT number: 2020-001023-14-GB, EudraCT number: 2020-004743-83-GB; IFNβ1b - ClinicalTrials.gov Identifier: NCT04469491).

Recommendation Nebulized interferon should only be used as part of a clinical trial.

7.4.5.2 Steroids

Rationale Steroids could reduce coronavirus replication by affecting ACE2 expression on infected epithelial cells, in addition to their well-known anti-inflammatory effect. The results of the RECOVERY trial showed that oral or intravenous dexamethasone reduced 28-day mortality in mechanically ventilated COVID-19 patients [31]. However, systemic therapy is associated with significant adverse effects. Bloom et al. [32] showed that asthmatic patients on nebulized steroids had a reduced risk of death from COVID-19 compared to those not on nebulized steroids.

Evidence *In vitro* studies suggest that nebulized corticosteroids (ciclesonide, budesonide) downregulate the SARS-CoV-2 receptor ACE2 through suppression of type 1 IFN. Several RCTs are investigating the effect of nebulized steroids in COVID-19 patients (ClinicalTrials.gov Identifiers: NCT04355637, NCT04331470, NCT04377711, NCT04330586, and NCT04416399).

Recommendation Where possible consider enrolling in a clinical trial.

7.4.5.3 Retinoic Acid

Rationale Retinoids are biologically similar to all-trans retinol (vitamin A) and retinoic acid is the active retinoid metabolite that acts through retinoic acid receptors (RAR α, β, γ) to regulate gene expression involved in immune responses [33]. They also act as effectors of T-cell-mediated and innate immunity. Systemic therapy is associated with significant adverse effects [33].

Evidence Clinical data suggests that retinoids stimulate secretion and effects of IFN type 1. Currently there are clinical trials using 13-cis retinoic acid alone or in combination with testosterone (ClinicalTrials.gov Identifier: NCT04623385), captopril (ClinicalTrials.gov Identifier: NCT04578236), itraconazole (ClinicalTrials.gov Identifier: NCT04577378), all trans retinoic acid with tamoxifen (ClinicalTrials.gov Identifier: NCT04568096), isotretinoin (ClinicalTrials.gov Identifier: NCT04396067), and isotretinoin with recombinant ACE2 receptor-like enzyme (ClinicalTrials.gov Identifier: NCT04382950).

Recommendation Nebulized retinoic acid (13-cis retinoic acid, all-trans retinol) should only be used as part of a clinical trial.

7.4.6 Mucokinetics/Mucolytics

7.4.6.1 Dornase Alfa

Rationale Dornase alfa is a nebulized recombinant human DNase 1 and a safe mucolytic [34]. Approved for use in cystic fibrosis patients [34], it is also used in ARDS [35]. It improves ventilation by reducing DNA-mediated viscosity of neutrophil-rich secretions. NETs are a source of DNA in the sputum, which are increased in COVID-19 [36].

Evidence Targeting NETs is seen to reduce acute lung injury-related mortality in animal studies [37] and mucolytic treatment is also effective in COVID-19 patients [38]. It is seen to reduce the systemic inflammatory markers in patients with cystic fibrosis. In a five patient case series of mechanically ventilated COVID-19 patients, there was reduction in oxygen requirements, improvement in lung mechanics and 100% survival in patients treated with dornase alfa 2.5 mg BD [39]. Multiple studies are investigating the effect of dornase alfa in the management of COVID-19 pneumonia

(EudraCT number: 2020-001492-33-FR, EudraCT number: 2020-001849-39-SE, ClinicalTrials.gov Identifier: NCT04359654, EudraCT number: 2020-001937-11-GB, ClinicalTrials.gov Identifier: NCT04355364).

Recommendation Considering its safety profile and established role in clinical management of similar conditions, dornase alfa can be used in COVID-19. Where possible, consider as part of clinical trial.

7.4.7 Pulmonary Vasodilators

7.4.7.1 Epoprostenol, Iloprost

Rationale Nebulized pulmonary vasodilators (epoprostenol, iloprost) are used for refractory hypoxemia or ARDS with the rationale of improving the shunt fraction [40]. Although there is no evidence of mortality benefit, this improves oxygenation. Nebulized epoprostenol is equally effective but less expensive than nitric oxide (NO) [41]. A subset of COVID-19 patients has disproportionate hypoxemia relative to the abnormalities in imaging or lung mechanics, perhaps due to the vasculotropic component of the SARS-CoV-2. Nebulized pulmonary vasodilators might be particularly effective in such patients.

Evidence In COVID-19 patients, one study (n = 80) reported improved P/F ratio in 50% of mechanically ventilated patients treated with nebulized epoprostenol [42], while another study (n = 38) showed an effect of nebulized epoprostenol in only 41% patients but a trend toward benefit in hypoxemic patients with normal lung compliance compared to those with low compliance, reflecting a phenotypic subset that may respond to nebulized epoprostenol [43]. Iloprost is a safe and effective pulmonary vasodilator with a higher potency compared to epoprostenol (5:1).

Recommendation Considering established safety and efficacy in ARDS due to other causes, nebulized epoprostenol and iloprost could be used in the treatment of COVID-19 patients.

7.4.8 Miscellaneous

7.4.8.1 Surfactant

Rationale High viral tropism for type 2 alveolar cells that produce surfactant results in atelectasis and atelectotrauma in COVID-19, exacerbating ARDS. Exogenous surfactant therapy via intra-tracheal, bronchoscopic or nebulized routes improves oxygenation but not mortality in other forms of adult ARDS [44].

Evidence A retrospective study in seven patients showed the safety and efficacy of surfactant in patients with ARDS due to COVID-19 [45]. Phase 2 studies investigating the role of nebulized surfactant for the treatment of moderate to severe COVID-19 adult patients (EudraCT number: 2020-001886-35-GB, ClinicalTrials.gov Identifier: NCT04362059) and assessing the efficacy and tolerability of porcine surfactant (EudraCT number: 2020-002632-75-GB) and surfactant-BL (ClinicalTrials.gov Identifier: NCT04568018) in COVID-19 ARDS patients are underway.

Recommendation Considering the established safety of nebulized surfactant in ARDS due to other causes, this strategy could be used in COVID-19 patients. However, where possible consider enrolling as part of clinical trial.

7.5 Barriers to Safe and Effective Nebulized Therapy in COVID-19 Pneumonia in Critical Care

As the primary mode of transmission for SARS-CoV-2 is via the aerosol route, there is a concern that nebulization therapy in COVID-19 patients could result in transmission of infection. However, no definitive data guides practice. Consequently, regulatory authorities have taken varied approaches with some agencies in support [46] and others against [47] use of nebulizers in COVID-19 patients. Studies during the 2002-2003 SARS-CoV outbreaks showed no risk to healthcare workers from nebulizer therapy [48]. International experts have recommended mitigating strategies to reduce fugitive emissions and disease transmission risk [49]. The International Society of Aerosol Medicine (ISAM) provides guidance for safe nebulization therapy in COVID-19 patients [50] summarized in Table 7.2 and Figs. 7.2 (using nebulizers with mouthpiece and exhalation filter) and 7.3 (nebulization with high flow nasal prongs is safer and effective than using mask nebulization).

Table 7.2 Considerations for safe and effective nebulization in COVID-19 patients

Either nasal oxygen or no oxygen support	High flow nasal prongs	Non-invasive ventilator	Mechanical ventilator
1. Negative pressure room 2. Full PPE including N95 masks 3. Avoid using facemasks to prevent fugitive emissions 4. Use mouthpiece with expiratory HEPA filter to capture fugitive emissions	1. Negative pressure room 2. Full PPE including N95 masks 3. Surgical mask over the high flow nasal prongs 4. Placing nebulizer at the dry side of humidifier 5. Lowering gas flows to prevent fugitive emissions	1. Negative pressure room 2. Full PPE including N95 masks 3. Placing nebulizer either after the exhalation port or on the dry side of humidifier	1. Full PPE including N95 masks 2. Place nebulizer either 15 cm from Y-piece in inspiratory limb of the circuit or dry side of heated humidifier 3. Change expiratory filter post nebulization therapy

PPE personal protective equipment, *HEPA* high-efficiency particulate absorbing

While clinical trials are underway to investigate clinical effectiveness, it is also necessary to explore the PK and pharmacodynamic aspects of nebulized therapy to provide optimal dosing guidelines. Notwithstanding the attraction of the nebulized route, potential adverse effects, such as mucocutaneous irritation, cough and bronchoconstriction, must be sought in adequately powered trials before widespread adoption can be recommended.

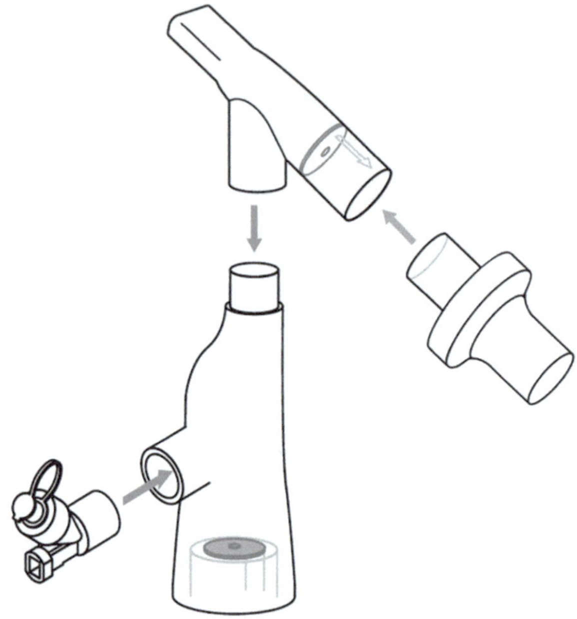

Fig. 7.2 A vibrating mesh nebulizer with mouthpiece and exhalation filter

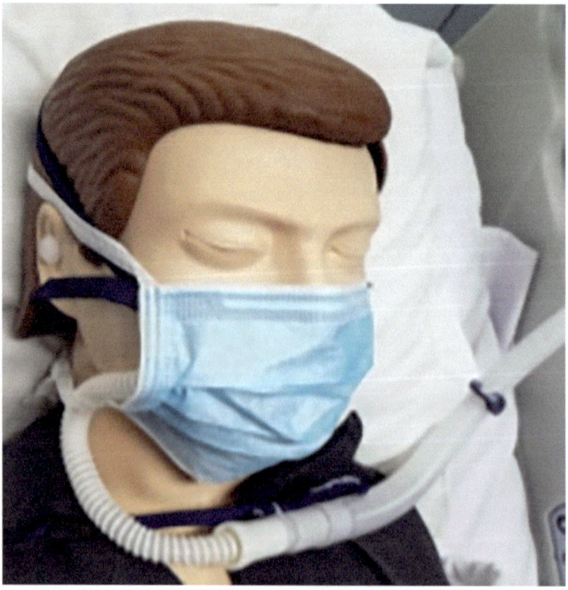

Fig. 7.3 High flow nasal prongs with surgical mask. The vibrating mesh nebulizer (not shown) is inserted at the dry end of the humidifier

7.6 Conclusion

Pending the results of ongoing RCTs, most nebulized therapies from drug classes such as antiviral, anti-inflammatory, immunomodulators, and thrombolytic agents should only be used in the context of participating in a clinical trial. Nebulized mucokinetics, anticoagulants, and pulmonary vasodilators can be safely used in the treatment of select COVID-19 patients, but effectiveness is still not clear. It is important to prioritize research in this promising field.

References

1. Salje H, Tran Kiem C, Lefrancq N, et al. Estimating the burden of Sars-Cov-2 in France. Science. 2020;369:208–11.
2. Dhanani J, Fraser JF, Chan HK, Rello J, Cohen J, Roberts JA. Fundamentals of aerosol therapy in critical care. Crit Care. 2016;20:269.
3. Dhand R. How should aerosols be delivered during invasive mechanical ventilation? Respir Care. 2017;62:1343–67.
4. Gbinigie K, Frie K. Should chloroquine and hydroxychloroquine be used to treat Covid-19? A rapid review. BJGP Open. 2020;4:bjgpopen20X101069.
5. FDA cautions against use of hydroxychloroquine or chloroquine for COVID-19 outside of the hospital setting or a clinical trial due to risk of heart rhythm problems. Available at: https://www.fda.gov/drugs/drug-safety-and-availability/fda-cautions-against-use-hydroxychloroquine-or-chloroquine-covid-19-outside-hospital-setting-or. Accessed December 28, 2021.
6. Garcia-Cremades M, Solans BP, Hughes E, et al. Optimizing hydroxychloroquine dosing for patients with Covid-19: an integrative modeling approach for effective drug repurposing. Clin Pharmacol Ther. 2020;108:253–63.
7. Yao X, Ye F, Zhang M, et al. In vitro antiviral activity and projection of optimized dosing design of hydroxychloroquine for the treatment of severe acute respiratory syndrome coronavirus 2 (Sars-Cov-2). Clin Infect Dis. 2020;71:732–9.
8. Charous BL, Halpern EF, Steven GC. Hydroxychloroquine improves airflow and lowers circulating ige levels in subjects with moderate symptomatic asthma. J Allergy Clin Immunol. 1998;102:198–203.
9. Warren TK, Jordan R, Lo MK, et al. Therapeutic efficacy of the small molecule gs-5734 against Ebola virus in rhesus monkeys. Nature. 2016;531:381–5.
10. Sun D. Remdesivir for treatment of Covid-19: combination of pulmonary and iv administration may offer additional benefit. AAPS J. 2020;22:77.
11. Knight V, McClung HW, Wilson SZ, et al. Ribavirin small-particle aerosol treatment of influ enza. Lancet. 1981;2:945–9.
12. Yang SNY, Atkinson SC, Wang C, et al. The broad spectrum antiviral ivermectin targets the host nuclear transport importin alpha/beta1 heterodimer. Antivir Res. 2020;177:104760.
13. Caly L, Druce JD, Catton MG, Jans DA, Wagstaff KM. The FDA-approved drug ivermectin inhibits the replication of Sars-Cov-2 in vitro. Antivir Res. 2020;178:104787.
14. Jermain B, Hanafin PO, Cao Y, Lifschitz A, Lanusse C, Rao GG. Development of a minimal physiologically-based pharmacokinetic model to simulate lung exposure in humans following oral administration of ivermectin for Covid-19 drug repurposing. J Pharm Sci. 2020;109:3574–8.
15. De Luca G, Cavalli G, Campochiaro C, et al. Gm-Csf blockade with mavrilimumab in severe Covid-19 pneumonia and systemic hyperinflammation: a single-Centre, prospective cohort study. Lancet Rheumatol. 2020;2:e465–73.

16. Partridge LJ, Urwin L, Nicklin MJH, et al. ACE2-independent interaction of SARS-CoV-2 spike protein with human epithelial cells is inhibited by unfractionated heparin. Cell. 2021;10:1419.
17. Mycroft-West CJ, Su D, Pagani I, et al. Heparin inhibits cellular invasion by Sars-Cov-2: structural dependence of the interaction of the spike s1 receptor-binding domain with heparin. Thromb Haemost. 2020;120:1700–15.
18. Mulloy B, Hogwood J, Gray E, Lever R, Page CP. Pharmacology of heparin and related drugs. Pharmacol Rev. 2016;68:76–141.
19. Lever R, Page CP. Non-anticoagulant effects of heparin: an overview. Handb Exp Pharmacol. 2012;207:281–305.
20. Chimenti L, Camprubi-Rimblas M, Guillamat-Prats R, et al. Nebulized heparin attenuates pulmonary coagulopathy and inflammation through alveolar macrophages in a rat model of acute lung injury. Thromb Haemost. 2017;117:2125–34.
21. Juschten J, Tuinman PR, Juffermans NP, Dixon B, Levi M, Schultz MJ. Nebulized anticoagulants in lung injury in critically ill patients-an updated systematic review of preclinical and clinical studies. Ann Transl Med. 2017;5:444.
22. Porto BN, Stein RT. Neutrophil extracellular traps in pulmonary diseases: too much of a good thing? Front Immunol. 2016;7:311.
23. Whyte CS, Morrow GB, Mitchell JL, Chowdary P, Mutch NJ. Fibrinolytic abnormalities in acute respiratory distress syndrome (ARDS) and versatility of thrombolytic drugs to treat Covid-19. J Thromb Haemost. 2020;18:1548–55.
24. Belen-Apak FB, Sarialioglu F. Pulmonary intravascular coagulation in Covid-19: possible pathogenesis and recommendations on anticoagulant/thrombolytic therapy. J Thromb Thrombolysis. 2020;50:278–80.
25. Piras AM, Zambito Y, Lugli M, et al. Repurposing of plasminogen: an orphan medicinal product suitable for Sars-Cov-2 inhalable therapeutics. Pharmaceuticals (Basel). 2020;13:425.
26. Abdelaal Ahmed Mahmoud A, Mahmoud HE, Mahran MA, Khaled M. Streptokinase versus unfractionated heparin nebulization in patients with severe acute respiratory distress syndrome (ARDS): a randomized controlled trial with observational controls. J Cardiothorac Vasc Anesth. 2020;34:436–43.
27. Hadjadj J, Yatim N, Barnabei L, et al. Impaired type I interferon activity and inflammatory responses in severe Covid-19 patients. Science. 2020;369:718–24.
28. Borg FA, Isenberg DA. Syndromes and complications of interferon therapy. Curr Opin Rheumatol. 2007;19:61–6.
29. Zhou Q, Chen V, Shannon CP, et al. Interferon-alpha2b treatment for Covid-19. Front Immunol. 2020;11:1061.
30. Monk PD, Marsden RJ, Tear VJ, et al. Safety and efficacy of inhaled nebulised interferon beta-1a (Sng001) for treatment of Sars-Cov-2 infection: a randomised, double-blind, placebo-controlled, phase 2 trial. Lancet Respir Med. 2021;9:196–206.
31. Group RC, Horby P, Lim WS, et al. Dexamethasone in hospitalized patients with Covid-19. N Engl J Med. 2021;384:693–704.
32. Bloom CI, Drake TM, Docherty AB, et al. Risk of adverse outcomes in patients with underlying respiratory conditions admitted to hospital with Covid-19: a national, multicentre prospective cohort study using the Isaric WHO clinical characterisation protocol UK. Lancet Respir Med. 2021;9:699–711.
33. Raverdeau M, Mills KH. Modulation of T cell and innate immune responses by retinoic acid. J Immunol. 2014;192:2953–8.
34. Yang C, Montgomery M. Dornase alfa for cystic fibrosis. Cochrane Database Syst Rev. 2018;9:CD001127.
35. Morris C, Mullan B. Use of dornase alfa in the management of ARDS. Anaesthesia. 2004;59:1249.
36. Middleton EA, He XY, Denorme F, et al. Neutrophil extracellular traps contribute to immunothrombosis in covid-19 acute respiratory distress syndrome. Blood. 2020;136:1169–79.

37. Thomas GM, Carbo C, Curtis BR, et al. Extracellular DNA traps are associated with the pathogenesis of TRALI in humans and mice. Blood. 2012;119:6335–43.
38. Earhart AP, Holliday ZM, Hofmann HV, Schrum AG. Consideration of dornase alfa for the treatment of severe Covid-19 acute respiratory distress syndrome. New Microbes New Infect. 2020;35:100689.
39. Weber AG, Chau AS, Egeblad M, Barnes BJ, Janowitz T. Nebulized in-line endotracheal dornase alfa and albuterol administered to mechanically ventilated Covid-19 patients: a case series. Mol Med. 2020;26:91.
40. Fuller BM, Mohr NM, Skrupky L, Fowler S, Kollef MH, Carpenter CR. The use of inhaled prostaglandins in patients with ARDS: a systematic review and meta-analysis. Chest. 2015;147:1510–22.
41. Ammar MA, Bauer SR, Bass SN, Sasidhar M, Mullin R, Lam SW. Noninferiority of inhaled epoprostenol to inhaled nitric oxide for the treatment of ARDS. Ann Pharmacother. 2015;49:1105–12.
42. Sonti R, Pike CW, Cobb N. Responsiveness of inhaled epoprostenol in respiratory failure due to Covid-19. J Intensive Care Med. 2021;36:327–33.
43. DeGrado JR, Szumita PM, Schuler BR, et al. Evaluation of the efficacy and safety of inhaled epoprostenol and inhaled nitric oxide for refractory hypoxemia in patients with coronavirus disease 2019. Crit Care Explor. 2020;2:e0259.
44. Meng SS, Chang W, Lu ZH, et al. Effect of surfactant administration on outcomes of adult patients in acute respiratory distress syndrome: a meta-analysis of randomized controlled trials. BMC Pulm Med. 2019;19:9.
45. Piva S, DiBlasi RM, Slee AE, et al. Surfactant therapy for covid-19 related ARDS: a retrospective case-control pilot study. Respir Res. 2021;22:20.
46. National Institute for Health and Care Excellence Covid-19 Rapid Guideline: Severe Asthma. Avaialble at: https://www.nice.org.uk/guidance/ng166. Accessed 8 October 2021.
47. Australian National Asthma Council Managing Asthma During the Covid-19 (Sars-Cov-2) Pandemic. Available at: https://www.asthmahandbook.org.au/clinical-issues/covid-19. Accessed 8 October 2021.
48. Tran K, Cimon K, Severn M, Pessoa-Silva CL, Conly J. Aerosol generating procedures and risk of transmission of acute respiratory infections to healthcare workers: a systematic review. PLoS One. 2012;7:e35797.
49. Ari A. Promoting safe and effective use of aerosol devices in Covid-19: risks and suggestions for viral transmission. Expert Opin Drug Deliv. 2020;17:1509–13.
50. Fink JB, Ehrmann S, Li J, et al. Reducing aerosol-related risk of transmission in the era of Covid-19: an interim guidance endorsed by the International Society of Aerosols in medicine. J Aerosol Med Pulm Drug Deliv. 2020;33:300–4.

Part III

Mechanical Ventilation

8 Positive End-Expiratory Pressure in Invasive and Non-invasive Ventilation of COVID-19 Acute Respiratory Distress Syndrome

L. Weaver, D. G. Bates, and L. Camporota

8.1 Introduction

Coronavirus disease 2019 (COVID-19) pneumonia has many clinical characteristics compatible with the definition of acute respiratory distress syndrome (ARDS), with bilateral lung infiltrates on chest radiology, an oxygenation defect with PaO_2/FiO_2 ratio <300 mmHg, and increased dead space ventilation. Positive end-expiratory pressure (PEEP) is routinely used as part of lung protective ventilation strategies in the management of ARDS [1, 2]. In the case of ARDS arising due to COVID-19 (CARDS), there is some debate as to whether atypical pathophysiological characteristics of the disease (i.e., moderate-severe hypoxemia despite preserved lung volumes at presentation, and minimal parenchymal consolidation) could warrant a different approach to ventilator management, particularly with regards to PEEP settings [3, 4]. Here we review the available evidence for the existence of a unique underlying lung pathophysiology in CARDS, and discuss the implications for standard approaches to setting PEEP, in both the invasive and non-invasive ventilation settings. We show how detailed computational models informed by this evidence can shed light on the available data, and help to explain recent results in the literature.

L. Weaver · D. G. Bates
School of Engineering, University of Warwick, Coventry, UK

L. Camporota (✉)
Department of Critical Care, Guy's and St Thomas' NHS Foundation Trust, London, UK

Centre for Human and Applied Physiological Sciences, School of Basic and Medical Biosciences, King's College London, London, UK
e-mail: luigi.camporota@gstt.nhs.uk

J.-L. Vincent (ed.), *Annual Update in Intensive Care and Emergency Medicine 2022*, Annual Update in Intensive Care and Emergency Medicine,
https://doi.org/10.1007/978-3-030-93433-0_8

8.2 Evidence for a Unique CARDS Pathophysiology

There is by now abundant evidence to suggest that several of the clinical features of CARDS, particularly in its early stages, are unique, or at the very least atypical, when compared to ARDS of standard etiologies. Early stage CARDS patients typically present with focal subpleural and peri-bronchovascular ground glass opacities, very limited amounts of alveolar collapse and atelectasis, low extravascular lung water (EVLW) accumulation, and relatively well preserved compliance, features which cannot fully explain the associated large shunt fraction and severe hypoxemia [5, 6]. Typically, in patients with ARDS, hypoxemia is proportional to the quantity of anatomical shunt (i.e., the fraction of non-aerated lung tissue mass in relation to the total tissue mass). The small proportion of consolidated lung tissue seems to distinguish patients with early CARDS from those with ARDS exhibiting similar PaO_2/FiO_2 ratios. A complete understanding of the pathophysiological mechanisms underlying CARDS is still to emerge; however, the etiology of the associated early respiratory failure and disproportionate hypoxemia is likely to be due to multiple factors affecting the distribution of pulmonary perfusion in relation to areas of the lung that are more or less aerated. These factors include:

- Pulmonary vasculopathy with loss of adaptive hypoxic pulmonary vasoconstriction and dysregulated pulmonary perfusion [7, 8]. Although the pivotal role angiotensin converting enzyme (ACE)2 receptors play in severe acute respiratory syndrome coronavirus 2 (SARS-CoV-2) transmission is well defined, their expression within the pulmonary endothelium and role in dysregulated pulmonary perfusion is now becoming apparent [7]. The carboxypeptidase ACE2 counteracts the renin-angiotensin-aldosterone system through conversion of angiotensin I and II to angiotensin-(1-9) and -(1-7), respectively; these then promote localized vasodilation and attenuation of the immune response [9]. The initial downregulation of ACE2 results in angiotensin II accumulation with resulting chemotactic effects and accelerated lymphocyte recruitment [7, 10]. The resulting pulmonary vascular inflammation results in an ACE1 'shedding' phenomenon where endothelial surface-bound ACE1 is released into the interstitium and ultimately results in sub-physiologic angiotensin II concentrations [10]. Low angiotensin II concentrations in this phase lead to vasodilation and worsened capillary leak. The alterations in pulmonary perfusion determine large ventilation/perfusion inequalities with greater presence of lung compartments with low ventilation/perfusion ratio. Some of the perfusion abnormalities are 'functional' consequent to a loss in hypoxic vasocontriction and inflammatory vasoplegia leading to hyper-perfusion of poorly ventilated lung tissue (increase in venous admixture); while others are more 'structural' anatomical changes caused by vascular enlargement or neovascularization within the poorly ventilated lung parenchyma. These regions with very low ventilation/perfusion ratio can become more numerous in the presence of high cardiac output (e.g., fever and hyperinflammation) leading to hyperperfusion of poorly ventilated alveolar units.
- The high incidence of pulmonary microvascular and macrovascular thrombosis offers insight into the high compliance, increased dead space, D-dimer elevation, and

right ventricular dysfunction frequently observed in COVID-19 and documented in post-mortem findings and histology [7, 11–14].

- The neurotropic potential of SARS-CoV-2 with altered central control of breathing mediated by pontine pneumotaxic center dysfunction and the relatively normal lung volume, which results in increased tidal volumes relative to ventilatory frequency. Although low pulmonary elastance partially explains the deceptively effortless work of breathing [15], infiltration of SARS-CoV-2 into the cerebrospinal fluid (CSF), carotid body sensing, and impaired brainstem autoregulation may also contribute [16, 17].
- Increased basal metabolic rate resulting in higher tissue oxygen extraction, lower mixed venous oxygen content, and increased venous admixture [18].
- Increased intrapulmonary shunt fraction with cardiac output elevation [19, 20]. Although high peripheral oxygen extraction partially explains the increased venous admixture observed in catabolic states, there may also be alterations in regional pulmonary blood flow distinct from this, related to increased cardiac output [18–20].

Despite the well documented pathophysiological features described above, many of which are unique to CARDS, there has been much controversy surrounding (a) the extent to which CARDS differs from standard ARDS, and (b) the resulting implications (if any) for clinical management. Case series and small observational studies early in the pandemic highlighted various atypical features of the disease [5, 21–24], focusing in particular on the higher than usual compliance (and lower than usual amount of gasless tissue) for the same PaO_2/FiO_2 in early-stage CARDS patients. However, subsequent studies that compared larger cohorts of CARDS patients with 'matched' cohorts of ARDS patients from previous studies failed to find significant differences [25, 26]. A possible explanation for these discrepancies is that CARDS exhibits a dynamic time-dependent disease profile, encompassing several stages (or phenotypes), which starts with the highly atypical presentation described above and culminates in a more standard ARDS presentation as the disease progresses [27]. Thus, data from CARDS patients that was collected over different (or later, i.e., post-intubation) stages in the disease course could mask the particular characteristics of the early-stage presentation [28]. This argument is supported by a recent study of 114 exclusively early-stage (pre-intubation) CARDS patients that clearly showed the posited unique pathophysiological features of this disease [29].

8.3 A Computational Simulator to Compare CARDS Versus ARDS Pathophysiology

Computer simulation offers a fresh approach to traditional medical research that is particularly well suited to investigating treatment of critical illness. Critically ill patients are routinely monitored in great detail, providing extensive high quality data-streams for model design and configuration and patient-matching. Models based on such data can incorporate very complex system dynamics that can be validated against patient responses for use as investigational surrogates. Crucially, simulation offers the potential to 'look inside' the patient, allowing unimpeded access to all variables of interest. In contrast to trials on both animal models and human patients, *in silico* models are completely configurable and reproducible; for example, different ventilator settings can be applied to an identical virtual patient, or the same settings applied to different patients, in order to understand their mode of action and quantitatively compare their effectiveness.

We have developed a multicompartmental computational model that simulates highly integrated pulmonary and cardiovascular physiologies together with a detailed representation of the effects of mechanical ventilation. The simulator offers several advantages, including the ability to define hundreds of alveolar compartments (each with its own individual mechanical characteristics), with configurable alveolar collapse, alveolar stiffening, disruption of alveolar gas exchange, pulmonary vasoconstriction and vasodilation, and airway obstruction. As a result, several defining clinical features of acute lung injury can be represented in the model, including varying degrees of ventilation-perfusion mismatch, physiological shunt and deadspace, alveolar gas trapping with intrinsic PEEP, collapse-reopening of alveoli, etc. The model has been successfully deployed in several previous studies investigating the pathophysiology and ventilatory management of conventional ARDS [30–35].

This model has recently been adapted to represent early-stage CARDS patients [36]. Based on data suggesting that early-stage COVID-19 patients have relatively well preserved lung gas volume and compliance [29], the model was set to have 8% of its alveolar compartments collapsed, i.e., non-aerated, by increasing the values of parameters representing alveolar extrinsic pressure and threshold opening pressure. To simulate the hyperperfusion of gasless tissue reported in [8, 37, 38], vasodilation was implemented in the collapsed units by decreasing their vascular resistance by 80%. Hypoxic pulmonary vasoconstriction (HPV) is normally incorporated in the simulator via a mathematical function—to simulate the hypothesized disruption of HPV in COVID-19, this function was disabled. Poor alveolar ventilation due to the effects of pneumonitis was modeled by disrupting alveolar–capillary gas equilibration in 20% of the alveolar compartments. As thrombotic complications have been reported to be a characteristic feature of COVID-19 [7, 11–14], the presence of microthrombi was simulated by increasing vascular resistance by a factor of 5 in 10% of the compartments.

The cardiopulmonary simulator can be configured to represent either mechanically ventilated [36] or spontaneously breathing [39] CARDS patients.

8.4 Setting PEEP in Invasive Mechanical Ventilation of CARDS Patients

Several studies have examined lung recruitability and the effects of PEEP in CARDS patients. In a study of 12 patients with severe CARDS who had received various days of non-invasive or invasive ventilatory support before the first day of observation [40], predominantly (83%) poor recruitability was observed, as measured at the bedside using the recruitment to inflation ratio (R/I ratio) [41], and poorly recruitable patients were ventilated with PEEP values between 5 and 10 cmH_2O. In a crossover physiologic study [42], multiple refined physiological measurements were performed to evaluate recruitability in 10 CARDS patients at different time points along their clinical course. Changing PEEP between 5 cmH_2O and 15 cmH_2O again revealed high inter-individual variability, with the increase in the lung volume due to a PEEP increase of 10 cmH_2O varying from 16% to 140%. Despite this variability, driving pressure increased, and respiratory system compliance decreased, on average across the cohort in response to higher PEEP, indicating the potential for significant PEEP-induced overdistension in those patients with poorly recruitable lungs.

Beloncle et al. [43] assessed gas exchange, compliance, and hemodynamics at two levels of PEEP (15 cmH_2O and 5 cmH_2O) within 36 h (day1) and from 4 to 6 days (day 5) after intubation in a cohort of 26 CARDS patients. These authors also found wide variation in recruitability, with PaO_2/FiO_2 ratio significantly increased at PEEP 15 cmH_2O compared to 5 cmH_2O only in the highly recruitable patients. Conversely, poorly recruitable patients exhibited a trend toward higher compliance at low PEEP compared to highly recruitable patients, again suggesting a risk of overinflation associated with high PEEP in these patients. The authors speculated that the small increase in PaO_2/FiO_2 ratio with PEEP observed in the poorly recruitable patients could be explained, at least in part, by a potential reduction in cardiac output induced by PEEP that may have contributed to decrease the shunt fraction.

Tsolaki et al., in a study of 17 patients with COVID-19 pneumonia fulfilling the Berlin criteria for severe ARDS on the second or third day of invasive mechanical ventilation [44], evaluated respiratory mechanics, arterial blood gases, and hemodynamics before and after PEEP was reduced from settings based on standard ARDSnet criteria by an average of 29%. Reducing PEEP resulted in significantly increased respiratory system compliance and reduced hypercapnia. PEEP reduction was not accompanied by lung derecruitment, and oxygenation did not deteriorate. The authors concluded that PEEP reduction decreased lung overdistension as interpreted by the increase in respiratory system compliance and decrease in dead space ventilation (reduced $PaCO_2$). The authors noted that, although a conservative or de-resuscitative fluid strategy is recommended in the management of patients with ARDS, in their CARDS patients application of PEEP levels based on the ARDSnet protocol was accompanied by substantial vasopressor dosage and 12-h fluid balance. PEEP de-escalation led to significant reduction in cumulative fluid balance during the subsequent 12 h and a three-fold decrease in vasopressor dosage. Decreased need for vasopressors and better fluid management translates into increased cardiac output and organ perfusion, accompanied by less fluid accumulation in the lungs.

Roesthuis et al. [3] assessed respiratory mechanics in 14 CARDS patients, all of whom had higher than expected lung compliance compared to standard ARDS. Reducing PEEP increased lung compliance in all but one of the patients, and reduced dead space ventilation in all patients. Finally, Ball et al. [45] analyzed the effects of varying PEEP in 44 mechanically ventilated patients with severe COVID-19 pneumonia using computed tomography (CT) scans. Minimal alveolar recruitment was induced by changes in PEEP from 8 cmH_2O to 16 cmH_2O. Higher PEEP improved oxygenation at FiO_2 of 0.5 but not 1.0, and decreased respiratory system compliance.

Although the above studies provide much compelling evidence, the interactions between hemodynamics (cardiac output and distribution of pulmonary blood flow) and alveolar recruitment with higher PEEP is difficult to establish at the bedside and can confound the discrepancy between changes seen in the oxygenation (improvement or deterioration) and the alteration in lung mechanics (either concordant or discordant). To shed further light on these issues, we configured our cardiopulmonary simulator to represent both the standard ARDS and hypothesized CARDS disease pathophysiology, as described in the previous section, and then compared its outputs, for the same ventilator settings, when PEEP was set at 5, 10 and 15 cmH_2O. As shown in Fig. 8.1, higher PEEP in the standard ARDS model leads to the typical benefits associated with recruitment of alveolar units in a lung suffering from significant levels of alveolar collapse: improved oxygenation, increased

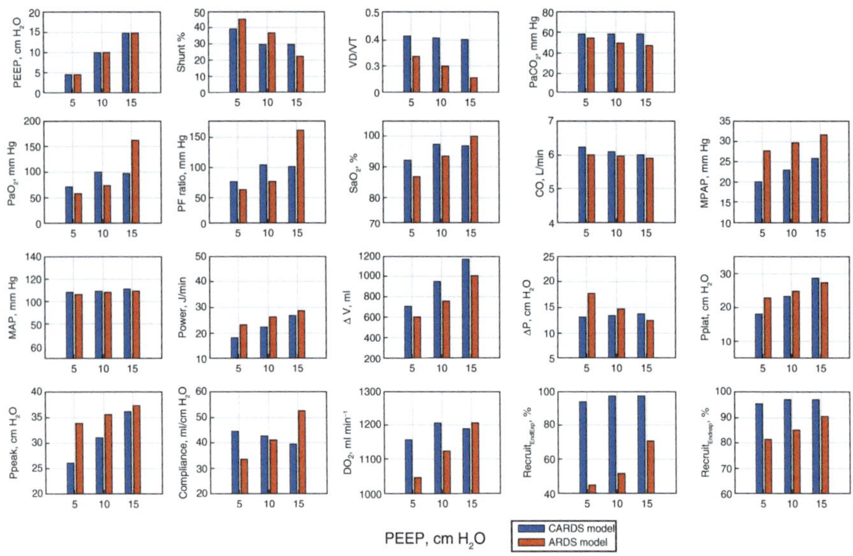

Fig. 8.1 Simulated responses of COVID-19 acute respiratory distress syndrome (CARDS) and standard ARDS models to different levels of positive end-expiratory pressure (PEEP). Other mechanical ventilator settings were fixed at tidal volume (V_T) = 470 ml (6.75 ml/kg), ventilation rate = 20 breaths/min, duty cycle = 0.33, FiO_2 = 100%. *MAP* mean arterial pressure, *CO* cardiac output, *DO_2* oxygen delivery, *MPAP* mean pulmonary artery pressure

compliance, and reduced driving pressure. In the CARDS model, however, no oxygenation benefits are observable above a PEEP of 10 cmH_2O, whereas compliance decreases and driving pressure increases as PEEP is increased. The change in lung volume ΔV (calculated as the end inspiratory lung volume - lung volume at FRC) is also significantly higher at each value of PEEP in the CARDS model compared to the standard ARDS model, indicating the potential for damaging levels of strain at higher PEEP.

8.5 Setting PEEP in Non-invasive Pressure Support Ventilation of CARDS Patients

The use of PEEP during non-invasive ventilation (NIV) of CARDS patients has been less well studied than in the case of invasive ventilation. Tonelli et al. compared inspiratory effort and respiratory mechanics in 30 spontaneously breathing patients receiving NIV for acute respiratory failure due to COVID-19 and a 'matched' cohort of standard ARDS patients [46]. In both cohorts, mean pressure support and PEEP values of 12 and 10 cmH_2O, respectively, were reported. Application of NIV allowed CARDS patients to reduce their respiratory effort – measured as esophageal pressure swings (ΔPes) from 12.4 to 7.6 cm H_2O, and respiratory rate reduced from 28 to 24 breaths/min, after 2 h of ventilatory support.

In a recent study of 114 early-stage CARDS patients treated with NIV, a recruitment maneuver involving increasing PEEP from 0 to 10 produced no improvement in oxygenation, but significantly increased an estimated value for total lung stress [29]. Tonelli et al. [27] reported waveform traces from an esophageal balloon catheter measuring Pes as a surrogate of pleural pressure (Ppl) in two spontaneously breathing patients with SARS-CoV-2 pneumonia undergoing NIV with helmet. CT scans of both patients confirmed the proposed CARDS phenotype, i.e., ground glass opacities with limited amounts of alveolar collapse and atelectasis. Patient 1 presented with modest respiratory effort (ΔPes of 11 cm H_2O, respiratory rate of 16 breaths/min) and subsequently exhibited progressive clinical and radiological improvement with ground glass resolutions, while Patient 2 had a significant respiratory effort (ΔPes of 32 cm H_2O, respiratory rate of 35 breaths/min) and subsequently required intubation and invasive mechanical ventilation.

To further investigate the effect of PEEP in NIV, we configured the simulator to match the ΔPes waveforms from the two CARDS patients reported in [27], under spontaneous breathing with a standard NIV pressure support value of 12 cmH_2O (Fig. 8.2 panels A and C). We then examined the effect of applying PEEP levels of 0, 2, 4, 6, 8, and 10 cmH_2O to both patients while maintaining their

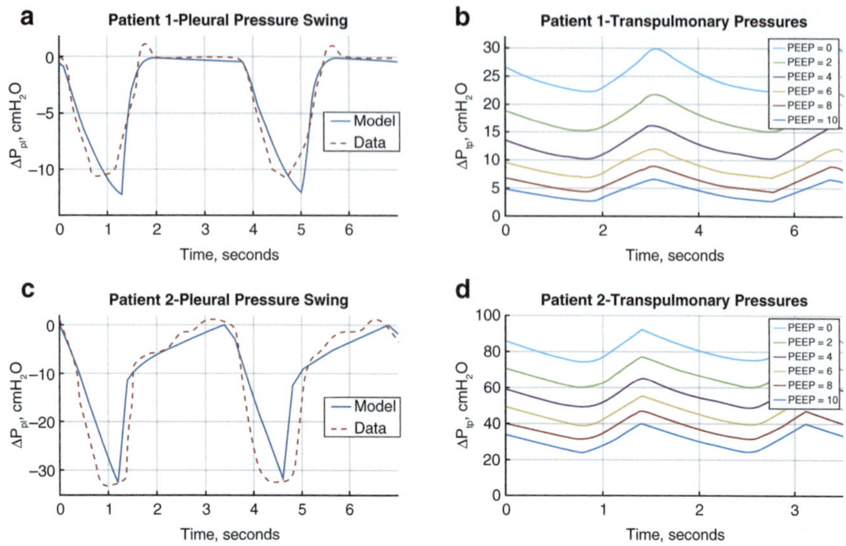

Fig. 8.2 (**a**) Simulated pleural pressure swings (ΔPpl) from the CARDS model compared with esophageal pressure waveforms (ΔPes) reported in [27], modest respiratory effort patient (Patient 1). (**b**) Simulated transpulmonary pressure (Ptp) swings for different levels of positive end-expiratory pressure (PEEP). (**c**) Simulated pleural pressure swings from the CARDS model compared with ΔPes waveforms reported in [27], high respiratory effort patient (Patient 2). (**d**) Simulated transpulmonary pressure swings for different levels of PEEP

spontaneous respiratory effort constant. As shown in Table 8.1, PEEP levels >2 cmH_2O produced no benefit in terms of oxygenation in either patient. The compliance of the lung and the respiratory system decreased markedly with increasing PEEP, while pleural and transpulmonary pressure swings (Fig. 8.2 panels B and D), total stress and total strain all increased (Table 8.1). Interestingly, in a study by Coppola et al. [29], increasing PEEP from 0 to 10 also produced no improvement in oxygenation; total lung stress was the only variable independently associated with negative outcome (intubation). In our simulations, an increase in PEEP from 0 to 10 produced large increases in total lung stress–from 6.5 to 29.8 cmH_2O in the patient experiencing modest respiratory effort, and from 40.0 to 92.6 cmH_2O in the patient experiencing significant respiratory effort (Table 8.1).

Table 8.1 Simulated outputs for patients with COVID-19 ARDS (CARDS) with moderate and high respiratory efforts undergoing non-invasive ventilation (NIV) (based on data in [27]) with varying levels of positive end-expiratory pressure (PEEP)

	Patient 1 (low inspiratory effort)						Patient 2 (high inspiratory effort)					
PEEP (cmH_2O)	0	2	4	6	8	10	0	2	4	6	8	10
Respiratory rate (bpm)	16	16	16	16	16	16	35	35	35	35	35	35
Muscle pressure (cmH_2O)	-13	-13	-13	-13	-13	-13	-21	-21	-21	-21	-21	-21
SaO_2 (%)	92.2	93.7	93.6	93.5	93.4	93.2	91.4	93.2	93.2	93.1	93.0	92.9
PaO_2 (mmHg)	60.6	65.9	65.9	65.7	65.7	66.7	58.2	63.7	63.6	63.7	63.7	63.9
Shunt (%)	33.4	30.7	30.7	30.7	30.7	30.7	34.5	31.5	31.5	31.6	31.6	31.6
$PaCO_2$ (mmHg)	18.2	20.0	22.8	26.2	31.0	37.7	16.1	17.3	19.1	21.3	24.3	28.1
SvO_2 (%)	63.9	65.4	65.2	65.0	64.7	64.4	62.8	64.7	64.6	64.4	64.3	64.1
Tidal volume (V_T) (ml)	965.1	870.0	769.3	672.3	579.1	490.2	600.3	556.8	508.9	462.6	416.7	371.8
V_T/kg (ml/kg)	13.8	12.4	11.0	9.6	8.3	7.0	8.6	8.0	7.3	6.6	6.0	5.3
Minute ventilation (ml/ min)	15.4	13.9	12.3	10.8	9.3	7.8	21.0	19.5	17.8	16.2	14.6	13.0
Driving pressure (cmH_2O)	10.6	10.6	10.6	10.7	10.9	11.1	19.9	19.9	20.0	20.1	20.2	20.3
Power (J/min)	3.0	3.1	3.2	3.2	3.1	3.0	16.2	15.4	14.4	13.4	12.4	11.3
Resp. system compliance (ml/ cmH_2O)	91.0	81.9	72.5	62.9	53.4	44.2	30.2	27.9	25.4	23.0	20.6	18.3
Lung compliance (ml/cmH_2O)	247.0	190.0	145.8	111.7	84.8	63.7	38.2	34.6	30.9	27.4	24.1	21.0
Dynamic strain	0.58	0.52	0.46	0.40	0.34	0.28	0.35	0.33	0.30	0.27	0.24	0.21
Static strain	0.09	0.19	0.29	0.38	0.47	0.55	0.26	0.35	0.43	0.51	0.58	0.65
Total strain	0.67	0.71	0.75	0.78	0.81	0.83	0.62	0.68	0.73	0.77	0.82	0.86
Pleural pressure swing (cmH_2O)	10.2	10.5	10.9	11.5	12.2	13.7	29.7	30.3	31.0	31.8	32.6	33.4
Transpulmonary pressure swing (cmH_2O)	3.9	4.6	5.3	6.0	6.8	7.7	15.7	16.1	16.5	16.9	17.3	17.7
Total stress (cmH_2O)	6.5	8.8	11.9	16.0	21.7	29.8	40.0	47.1	55.5	65.5	77.7	92.6

8.6 Conclusion

The clinical studies performed to date, further confirmed by our simulations, indicate that use of standard protocols employing high PEEP in early-stage CARDS patients (whether invasively or non-invasively ventilated) is unlikely to lead to alveolar recruitment, and may be injurious in some patients due to the risk of significantly increasing transpulmonary pressure swings and total lung stress and strain. The limited improvement in oxygenation that can be observed in these circumstances can be conceptualized as the consequence of changes in hemodynamic (cardiac output) rather than alveolar recruitment *per se*.

In the context of CARDS patients undergoing NIV, the argument that high PEEP is necessary to allow patients to reduce their respiratory effort is not supported by the available data.

The emphasis on the atypical features of COVID-19 has been questioned by some authors, who point out that ARDS is by definition heterogeneous. It has also been shown that some of the alterations seen in CARDS are features that have already been encountered in ARDS from mixed etiologies [47]. Although these general premises are certainly true and reasonable, the fact that the prevalence of these atypical features is much higher in COVID-19 than in ARDS should raise questions about the way that mechanical ventilation should be personalized, and what effects – beyond oxygenation– should be monitored. Specific pathophysiological considerations related to CARDS should also invite further clinical and physiological studies that evaluate the effects of PEEP on cardiopulmonary interactions, recruitability, and inspiratory effort, as well as on how PEEP (or NIV) can alter the disease's physiological trajectory over time. Ultimately, as we have learnt in the last 20 years of ARDS research, a strategy that leads to higher oxygenation may not be the most appropriate or safest strategy for every patient with ARDS, regardless of its etiology.

References

1. Fan E, Del Sorbo L, Goligher EC, et al. An official American Thoracic Society/European Society of Intensive Care Medicine/Society of Critical Care Medicine clinical practice guideline: mechanical ventilation in adult patients with acute respiratory distress syndrome. Am J Respir Crit Care Med. 2017;195:1253–63.
2. Papazian L, Aubron C, Brochard L, et al. Formal guidelines: management of acute respiratory distress syndrome. Ann Intensive Care. 2019;9:69.
3. Roesthuis L, van den Berg M, van der Hoeven H. Advanced respiratory monitoring in COVID-19 patients: use less PEEP! Crit Care. 2020;24:230.
4. Tsolaki V, Zakynthinos GE, Makris D. The ARDSnet protocol may be detrimental in COVID-19. Crit Care. 2020;24:351.
5. Gattinoni L, Coppola S, Cressoni M, Busana M, Rossi S, Chiumello D. COVID-19 does not lead to a "typical" acute respiratory distress syndrome. Am J Respir Crit Care Med. 2020;201:1299–300.
6. Sherren PB, Ostermann M, Agarwal S, Meadows CIS, Ioannou N, Camporota L. COVID-19-related organ dysfunction and management strategies on the intensive care unit: a narrative review. Br J Anaesth. 2020;125:912–25.

7. Ackermann M, Verleden SE, Kuehnel M. Pulmonary vascular endothelialitis, thrombosis, and angiogenesis in Covid-19. N Engl J Med. 2020;383:120–8.
8. Gattinoni L, Chiumello D, Caironi P. COVID-19 pneumonia: different respiratory treatments for different phenotypes? Intensive Care Med. 2020;46:1099–102.
9. Kuba K, Imai Y, Rao S. A crucial role of angiotensin converting enzyme 2 (ACE2) in SARS coronavirus-induced lung injury. Nat Med. 2005;11:875–9.
10. Leisman DE, Deutschman CS, Legrand M. COVID-19 in the ICU: vascular dysfunction, thrombosis, and dysregulated inflammation. Intensive Care Med. 2020;46:1105–8.
11. Copin MC, Parmentier E, Duburcq T, Poissy J, Mathieu D. The Lille COVID-19 ICU and Anatomopathology group. Time to consider histologic pattern of lung injury to treat critically ill patients with COVID-19 infection. Intensive Care Med. 2020;46:1124–6.
12. Cui S, Chen S, Li X, Liu S, Wang F. Prevalence of venous thromboembolism in patients with severe novel coronavirus pneumonia. J Thromb Haemost. 2020;18:1421–4.
13. Klok FA, Kruip MJHA, van der Meer NJM. Incidence of thrombotic complications in critically ill ICU patients with COVID-19. Thromb Res. 2020;191:145–7.
14. Zhang T, Sun LX, Feng RE. Comparison of clinical and pathological features between severe acute respiratory syndrome and coronavirus disease 2019. Zhonghua Jie He He Hu Xi Za Zhi. 2020;43:496–502.
15. Vaporidi K, Akoumianaki E, Telias I, Goligher EC, Brochard L, Georgopoulos D. Respiratory drive in critically ill patients: pathophysiology and clinical implications. Am J Respir Crit Care Med. 2020;201:20–32.
16. Li YC, Bai WZ, Hashikawa T. The neuroinvasive potential of SARS-CoV2 may play a role in the respiratory failure of COVID-19 patients. J Med Virol. 2020;92:552–5.
17. Montalvan V, Lee J, Bueso T, De Toledo J, Rivas K. Neurological manifestations of COVID-19 and other coronavirus infections: a systematic review. Clin Neurol Neurosurg. 2020;194:105921.
18. Takala J. Hypoxemia due to increased venous admixture: influence of cardiac output on oxygenation. Intensive Care Med. 2007;33:908–11.
19. Lynch JP, Mhyre JG, Dantzker DR. Influence of cardiac output on intrapulmonary shunt. J Appl Physiol Respir Environ Exerc Physiol. 1979;46:315–21.
20. Dantzker DR, Lynch JP, Weg JG. Depression of cardiac output is a mechanism of shunt reduction in the therapy of acute respiratory failure. Chest. 1980;77:636–42.
21. Gattinoni L, Chiumello D, Rossi S. COVID-19 pneumonia: ARDS or not? Crit Care. 2020;24:154.
22. Gattinoni L, Meissner K, Marini JJ. The baby lung and the COVID-19 era. Intensive Care Med. 2020;46:1438–40.
23. Marini JJ, Gattinoni L. Management of COVID-19 respiratory distress. JAMA. 2020;323:2329–30.
24. Marini JJ. Dealing with the CARDS of COVID-19. Crit Care Med. 2020;48:1239–41.
25. Ziehr DR, Alladina J, Petri CR, et al. Respiratory pathophysiology of mechanically ventilated patients with covid-19: a cohort study. Am J Respir Crit Care Med. 2020;201:1560–4.
26. Grasselli G, Tonetti T, Protti A, et al. Pathophysiology of COVID-19-associated acute respiratory distress syndrome: a multicentre prospective observational study. Lancet Respir Med. 2021;9:e5–6.
27. Tonelli R, Marchioni A, Tabbì L, et al. Spontaneous breathing and evolving phenotypes of lung damage in patients with COVID-19: review of current evidence and forecast of a new scenario. J Clin Med. 2021;10:975.
28. Chiumello D, Busana M, Coppola S, et al. Physiological and quantitative CT-scan characterization of COVID-19 and typical ARDS: a matched cohort study. Intensive Care Med. 2020;46:2187–96.
29. Coppola S, Chiumello D, Busana M, et al. Role of total lung stress on the progression of early COVID-19 pneumonia. Intensive Care Med. 2021;47:1130–9.
30. Das A, Cole O, Chikhani M, et al. Evaluation of lung recruitment maneuvers in acute respiratory distress syndrome using computer simulation. Crit Care. 2015;19:8.

31. Chikhani M, Das A, Haque M, et al. High PEEP in acute respiratory distress syndrome: quantitative evaluation between improved arterial oxygenation and decreased oxygen delivery. Br J Anaesth. 2016;117:650–8.
32. Das A, Haque M, Chikhani M, et al. Hemodynamic effects of lung recruitment maneuvers in acute respiratory distress syndrome. BMC Pulm Med. 2017;17:34.
33. Das A, Camporota L, Hardman JG, et al. What links ventilator driving pressure with survival in the acute respiratory distress syndrome? A computational study. Respir Res. 2019;20:29.
34. Saffaran S, Das A, Hardman JG, et al. High-fidelity computational simulation to refine strategies for lung-protective ventilation in paediatric acute respiratory distress syndrome. Intensive Care Med. 2019;45:1055–7.
35. Saffaran S, Das A, Laffey JG, et al. Utility of driving pressure and mechanical power to guide protective ventilator settings in two cohorts of adult and pediatric patients with acute respiratory distress syndrome: a computational investigation. Crit Care Med. 2020;48:1001–8.
36. Das A, Saffaran S, Chikhani M, et al. In silico modeling of coronavirus disease 2019 acute respiratory distress syndrome: pathophysiologic insights and potential management implications. Crit Care Expl. 2020;2:pe0202.
37. Lang M, Som A, Mendoza DP, et al. Hypoxaemia related to COVID-19: vascular and perfusion abnormalities on dual-energy CT. Lancet Infect Dis. 2020;20:1365–6.
38. Albarello F, Pianura E, Di Stefano F, et al. 2019-novel coronavirus severe adult respiratory distress syndrome in two cases in Italy: an uncommon radiological presentation. Int J Infect Dis. 2020;93:192–7.
39. Weaver L, Das A, Saffaran S, et al. High risk of patient self-inflicted lung injury in COVID-19 with frequently encountered spontaneous breathing patterns: a computational modelling study. Ann Intensive Care. 2021;11:109.
40. Pan C, Chen L, Lu C, et al. Lung recruitability in SARS-CoV-2 associated acute respiratory distress syndrome: a single-center, observational study. Am J Respir Crit Care Med. 2020;201:1294–7.
41. Chen L, Del Sorbo L, Grieco DL, et al. Potential for lung recruitment estimated by the recruitment-to-inflation ratio in acute respiratory distress syndrome. A clinical trial. Am J Respir Crit Care Med. 2020;201:178–87.
42. Mauri T, Spinelli E, Scotti E, et al. Potential for lung recruitment and ventilation-perfusion mismatch in patients with the acute respiratory distress syndrome from coronavirus disease 2019. Crit Care Med. 2020;48:1129–34.
43. Beloncle FM, Pavlovsky B, Desprez C, et al. Recruitability and effect of PEEP in SARS-Cov-2-associated acute respiratory distress syndrome. Ann Intensive Care. 2020;10:55.
44. Tsolaki V, Siempos I, Magira E, Kokkoris S, Zakynthinos GE, Zakynthinos S. PEEP levels in COVID-19 pneumonia. Crit Care. 2020;24:303.
45. Ball L, Robba C, Maiello L, et al. Computed tomography assessment of PEEP-induced alveolar recruitment in patients with severe COVID-19 pneumonia. Crit Care. 2021;25:81.
46. Tonelli R, Busani S, Tabbì L, et al. Inspiratory effort and lung mechanics in spontaneously breathing patients with acute respiratory failure due to COVID-19: a matched control study. Am J Respir Crit Care Med. 2021;204:725–8.
47. Panwar R, Madotto F, Laffey JG, van Haren FMP. Compliance phenotypes in early acute respiratory distress syndrome before the COVID-19 pandemic. Am J Respir Crit Care Med. 2020;202:1244–52.

Personalized Mechanical Ventilation Settings: Slower Is Better!

9

P. L. Silva, P. R. M. Rocco, and P. Pelosi

9.1 Introduction

Under controlled mechanical ventilation, the ventilator must overcome elastic and resistive forces, which are represented by the classic equation of motion [P(t) = V/C(t) + RV'(t) + P0] (where at any time, t, P is applied pressure, V is volume, C is compliance, *R* is resistance, V′ is flow, and P_0 is the pressure corresponding to transpulmonary pressure at end expiration), to provide respiratory movement. The model is characterized by a dashpot and a spring, representing resistive and elastic properties, respectively [1]. The resistive-elastic model does not explain the slow airway pressure decay after sudden interruption in airflow due to lung deformation (stress relaxation) or the slow increase in lung deformation after continuous stress application (creep). To explain such phenomena, the viscoelastic model should be used because it better represents the behavior of the lung structure. The viscoelastic model adds a third component to the resistive-elastic model, the Maxwell body, in which a dashpot (viscous element) lies in series with a spring (elastic element) [2]. Superior models have been considered, such as the constant-phase model by Hantos et al. [3], describing the viscoelastic properties of lung tissue. Nevertheless, whichever model is used, time should be taken into account in a way that can explain why the alveoli do not immediately close or instantaneously

P. L. Silva · P. R. M. Rocco
Laboratory of Pulmonary Investigation, Institute of Biophysics Carlos Chagas Filho, Federal University of Rio de Janeiro, Rio de Janeiro, Brazil

P. Pelosi (✉)
Department of Surgical Sciences and Integrated Diagnostics, University of Genoa, Genoa, Italy

Anesthesia and Critical Care, San Martino Policlinico Hospital, IRCCS for Oncology and Neurosciences, Genoa, Italy
e-mail: paolo.pelosi@unige.it

J.-L. Vincent (ed.), *Annual Update in Intensive Care and Emergency Medicine 2022*, Annual Update in Intensive Care and Emergency Medicine,
https://doi.org/10.1007/978-3-030-93433-0_9

become full of air after deformation. Changes in time, that is, how fast the clinician changes the ventilator variables on the mechanical ventilator, can have profound biological effects. In this chapter, we discuss the experimental and clinical evidence showing that slowing the changes in tidal volume, respiratory rate (RR), airway pressure when increasing or decreasing positive end-expiratory pressure (PEEP), and flow-controlled ventilation may minimize ventilator-induced lung injury (VILI) and improve respiratory function.

9.2 Strain, Stress, and Strain Rate: Insights from Polymeric Material

In physics, stress is the force acting on the unit area of a material, and strain is defined as the difference between the initial and the final distance for two points divided by the initial distance. In other words, the relationship between stress and strain can be described according to the following equation: stress = $K[\ln(\text{strain})]^n$ where K is the strength coefficient and n is the index of material behavior, that is, the power dissipation. In terms of respiratory physiology, stress is the transpulmonary pressure, and strain is the variation in tidal volume according to the resting position, end-expiratory lung volume (EELV). The strain rate is the rate at which the material is expanding or shrinking (expansion rate). Translating to the respiratory system, the strain rate is the rate at which strain occurs. Strain and strain rate are mathematically expressed according to tidal volume (V_T):

$$\text{Strain} = \Delta V_T - \text{EELV} / \text{EELV} \tag{9.1}$$

$$\begin{aligned} \text{Strain rate} &= \text{strain} / dt \\ &= \left[\Delta V_T - \text{EELV} / \text{EELV}\right] / dt \\ &= \Delta V_T - \text{EELV} / dt / \text{EELV} \\ &= d\upsilon(t) / \text{EELV} \end{aligned} \tag{9.2}$$

where υ is the speed at which the tidal volume is moving away from the resting position (EELV) and dt is the change in time. If different ventilatory parameters, either static or dynamic, can change the strain, the strain rate can expand to changes over time of tidal volume, PEEP, and inspiratory and expiratory flows. The strain rate is inversely correlated with time. For the same stress, longer times (slow changes in mechanical ventilator variables) are related to lower strain rates, and shorter times (fast changes in mechanical ventilator variables) are related to higher strain rates (Fig. 9.1). Assuming the strain rate reacts to temperature like for polymeric material, lower strain rates mimic the behavior observed at higher temperatures, and higher strain rates reflect the behavior at lower temperatures. As the speed increases, the yield strength and modulus also increase. The material appears to be stronger and stiffer simply due to the increase in the strain rate (Fig. 9.2).

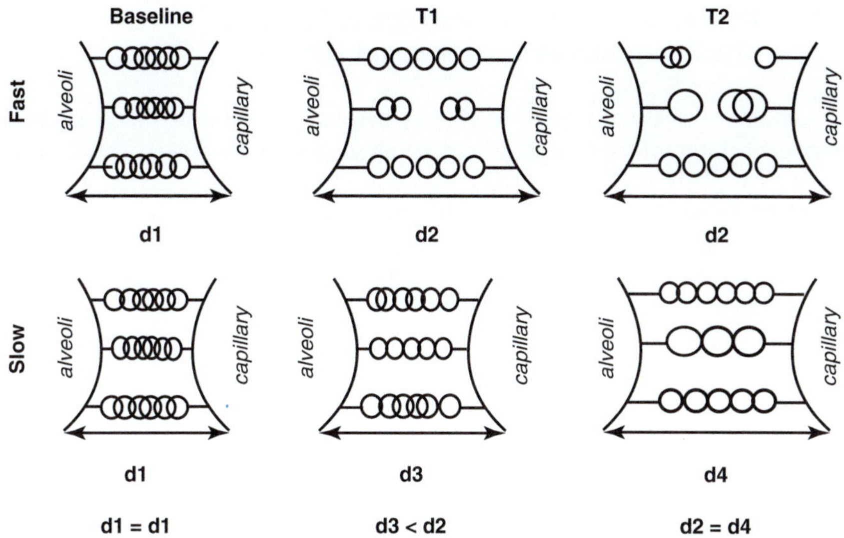

Fig. 9.1 Representative schema showing the alveolar capillary membrane subjected to fast and slow changes during mechanical ventilation. At fast changes, the baseline displacement is given as d1. At T1, d2 > d1, the fracture of interstitial alveolar structures can be seen due to fast displacement, mainly in the central area with little accommodation of strain, static or dynamic. At T2, further fractures of alveolar structures occur. At slow changes, the baseline displacement is also given as d1. At T1, d3 < d2, the interstitial alveolar structures are preserved due to better accommodation of strain, with a low strain rate, static or dynamic. At T2, although the alveoli are heterogeneous, fractures of alveolar structures are less likely

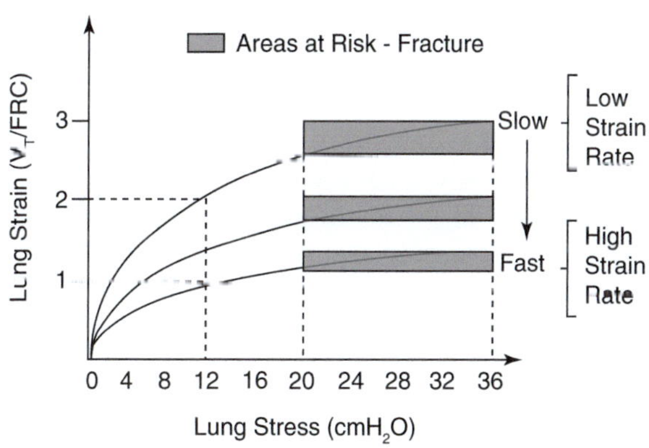

Fig. 9.2 Relationship between lung strain (tidal volume/ functional residual capacity [V_T/FRC] and stress. If slow changes in ventilatory parameters are made, meaning a low strain rate, the dangerous range of stress is achieved only at higher overall strain. On the other hand, if fast changes in ventilatory parameters are made, meaning a high strain rate, a dangerous range of stress is achieved even at lower overall strain. The resulting manageable area for changes is reduced and there is a high risk of fracture. Thus, the strain rate determines the threshold for stress injury

9.3 Origins of the Mechanical Power Formula: The Components Must Respect Time

In addition to measurements of respiratory mechanics, ventilatory variables have been pooled toward the concept of generation of mechanical power. This concept relies on the delivery of mechanical energy within each respiratory cycle, by multiplying by the number of respiratory cycles per minute (RR), in a way that mechanical power can be reached. The most simplified version of the mechanical power formula [4], which has been generated based on the classic equation of motion [5], is as follows:

Volume-controlled ventilation:

$$\text{Mechanical power} = 0.098 \times V_T \times RR \times \left(P\text{peak},_{RS} - \Delta P,_{RS} /2 \right) \tag{9.3}$$

Pressure-controlled ventilation:

$$\text{Mechanical power} = 0.098 \times V_T \times RR \times \left(\Delta P,_{RS} + \text{PEEP} \right) \tag{9.4}$$

In the ARDS Network trial [6], the low tidal volume group (6 ml/kg predicted body weight [PBW]) showed a mean RR of 29 bpm on day 1 and 30 bpm on day 7 compared with 16 bpm on day 1 and 20 bpm on day 7 in the high tidal volume group (12 ml/kg PBW). On day 1, the mechanical power was 30.6 J/min in the low tidal volume group and 33.1 J/min in the high tidal volume group. No difference in $PaCO_2$ was observed between the groups over time. With a reduction in tidal volume toward the protective range, an increase in RR is expected to maintain minute ventilation at safe levels to avoid acidosis. In terms of mechanical power, no major differences were observed between the low and high tidal volume groups: both are in the injurious range [7]. When patients were recruited (1996-1999) for the ARDS Network trial, there was no discussion about mechanical power, and the contribution of such an increased RR to cause harm to the respiratory system of critically ill patients was unknown. Recently, it has been acknowledged that RR is an independent predictor of mortality in patients with acute respiratory distress syndrome (ARDS) [8]. Nevertheless, one additional point of interest is how fast the changes occur in ventilator settings. For example, as previously mentioned, the mechanical power formula is based on the classic equation of motion, which may not account for different time constants at both inspiration and expiration, as well as inhomogeneity and heterogeneous ventilation of several different alveolar units. Even in healthy lungs, alveolar units do not inflate or deflate at equivalent periods in a way that 'fast alveoli' (low inspiratory time constant) easily become full, and 'slow alveoli' (high inspiratory time constant) demand more time to fill. For example, as RR increases, slow alveoli with relatively high time constants will have less time to undergo volume changes. Like RR changes, stepwise increases in tidal volume according to EELV may induce lung injury when the strain exceeds a critical level, and this is intensified when transpulmonary pressure, or stress, is repeated excessively [9, 10]. In relation to PEEP and recruitment maneuvers, it has been shown that stepwise increases in airway pressure, allowing slow alveolar units with different opening pressures to become fully expanded, may protect lungs from additional injury inherent to mechanical ventilation. More recently, flow-controlled ventilation, which represents a new form of ventilation, avoids zero-flow conditions, which means that airflows at inspiration and expiration phases are both constant. The resulting constant flow coupled with direct intratracheal pressure measurements allows a much more precise analysis of individual lung mechanics than is possible in conventional ventilation modes. Here, we enumerate how changes in ventilatory settings could be smoothed to protect the lungs from further damage. Table 9.1 summarizes the preclinical studies on different ventilatory variables.

9.4 Slow the Changes in Tidal Volume during Mechanical Ventilation

Different from the resistive and elastic unicompartmental model, lungs are more likely to behave as a viscoelastic system: for example, when they are deformed and held constant, the lungs relieve tension, so-called "stress relaxation" [1]. Due to their mechanical nature, it is conceivable that different parenchymal distortions may occur depending on how fast tidal volume or strain is modified for a period of time. By comparing low (1.8/s) and high (4.6/s) strain rates at similar overall strain (2.1), Protti et al. [10] showed that high strain rates may increase the risk of pulmonary edema possibly because they augment lung viscoelastic behavior (parenchymal energy dissipation) [10]. In the high strain rate group, inspiratory flow was also higher because of the ventilatory settings used in the two study groups. Inspiratory flow has been independently associated with lung injury [11, 12]. In heterogeneous alveolar units with varying regional aeration, tidal energy can concentrate on a small mass of pulmonary tissue, spreading lung damage with successive cycles. In the clinical setting, changes in tidal volume are usually applied abruptly. The extracellular matrix requires an adaptive "stress relaxation" time to mitigate the damaging strain associated with large tidal excursions. These internal adjustments occur over both short (over a respiratory cycle) and extended time scales [1], depending on the degree of lung injury. Felix et al. [13] showed that increasing strain gradually (shorter adaptation time) rather than abruptly (no adaptation time) attenuated lung injury, likely by preemptive adaptation of the epithelial cells and extracellular matrix. However, a more gradual increase in tidal strain (longer adaptation time) compared with the shorter adaptation time led to more cumulative transfer of mechanical power and did not prevent lung damage, suggesting that the longer adaptation time strategy initiated injurious strain at an earlier timepoint. This preclinical study shed light on mechanical power calculation. At the end of 2 h of mechanical ventilation, total mechanical power was similar among the groups that had their tidal strains changed. On the other hand, early exposure to tidal volume increments, which in turn increased the cumulative mechanical power, was the main factor associated with lung damage. Therefore, should mechanical power be calculated as a snapshot at a specific moment, or should mechanical power be calculated

Table 9.1 Effects of changes in different ventilatory variables at slow and high rates on lung injury: preclinical studies

Study	Animals	Interventions	Outcomes
Tidal volume			
Protti et al., 2016 [10]	Piglets	(1) Low (1.8/s) and (2) high (4.6/s) strain rate. At high strain rate, inspiratory flow was threefold higher than low strain rate	High strain rates increased the risk of pulmonary edema
Felix et al., 2019 [13]	Rats	(1) $V_T = 6$ ml/kg for 2 h (control); (2) $V_T = 6$ ml/kg during hour 1 followed by an abrupt increase to $V_T = 22$ ml/kg during hour 2; (3) $V_T = 6$ ml/kg during the first 30 min followed by a gradual increase in V_T up to 22 ml/kg for 30 min, then constant $V_T = 22$ ml/kg during hour 2; (4) more gradual increase in V_T, from 6 to 22 ml/kg during hour 1 followed by $V_T = 22$ ml/kg during hour 2	Lung damage was lower in the shorter adaptation time compared with the no adaptation time group. Extending the adaptation period increased cumulative mechanical power and did not prevent lung damage
Inspiratory flow			
Rich et al., 2000 [11]	Sheep	(1) PCV, RR = 15 breaths/min, PIP = 25 cmH_2O; (2) PCV, RR = 15 breaths/min, PIP = 50 cmH_2O; (3) PCV, RR = 5 breaths/min, PIP = 50 cmH_2O, IT = 6 s; (4) PCV, RR = 5 breaths/min, PIP = 50 cmH_2O, IT = 2 s; and (5) limited inspiratory flow VCV, RR = 5 breaths/min, pressure-limit = 50 cmH_2O, flow = 15 l/min	Reduction of inspiratory flow at similar PIP provides pulmonary protection
Maeda et al., 2004 [12]	Rabbit	(1) PRVC with IT set at 20% of total cycle time; (2) VCV with 20% IT of total cycle time; and (3) VCV with 50% IT of total cycle time. V_T was 30 ml/kg, RR was 20 breaths/min, and PEEP was 0 cmH_2O	At an injurious V_T, the lung damage appeared to be marked at a high peak inspiratory flow
Expiratory flow			
Schmidt et al., 2018 [45]	Pigs	(1) Expiratory ventilation assistance mode; and (2) VCV for 5 h with PEEP = 5 cmH_2O and $V_T = 8$ ml/kg. RR adjusted for a target end-tidal CO_2 of 4.7 to 6 kPa	Expiratory ventilation assistance mode improved lung aeration and arterial oxygenation at similar PEEP and PIP
Borgmann et al., 2018 [46]	Pigs	(1) 2 min of conventional VCV; (2) 2 min of VCV with FLEX; (3) 1 min again of conventional VCV	FLEX shifts regional ventilation toward dependent lung areas in healthy and injured pig lungs
Spraider et al., 2020 [44]	Pigs	(1) FCV settings were individualized by compliance-guided PEEP and PIP titration; (2) PCV was performed with a PEEP of 5 cmH_2O and PIP was set to achieve a $V_T = 7$ ml/kg	Individualized FCV improved gas exchange and lung tissue aeration without signs of overinflation compared with PCV

Table 9.1 (continued)

Study	Animals	Interventions	Outcomes
Schmidt et al., 2020 [47]	Pigs	(1) FCV; and (2) VCV (control group) with identical $V_T = 7$ ml/kg and PEEP = 9 cmH_2O	FCV enhanced lung aeration in the dependent lung region and consequently improved gas exchange and attenuated lung injury
Wittenstein et al., 2020 [48]	Pigs	(1) Intravascular normovolemia; and (2) intravascular hypovolemia, combined with VCV-FCV or FCV-VCV (60 min per mode)	Mechanical power was lower during FCV compared with VCV. The efficacy of ventilation was higher during FCV compared with VCV during normovolemia
PEEP increment			
Lim et al., 2004 [35]	Pigs	(1) Sustained inflation; (2) extended sigh; (3) incremental PEEP and PCV	Recruitment by PCV is equivalent or superior to sustained inflation, with the same PIP, despite its lower mean airway pressure and reduced risk for hemodynamic compromise
Silva et al., 2011 [34]	Rats	(1) Non-recruited; (2) RMs with CPAP for 15 s; (3) RMs with CPAP for 30 s; (4) RMs with STEP to targeted maximum within 15 s; and (5) RMs with STEP within 30 s	Longer-duration RMs with slower airway pressure increase efficiently improved lung function, while minimizing the biological impact on lungs
Silva et al., 2013 [36]	Rats	(1) CPAP for 30 s; (2) STEP (5 cm H_2O/step, 8.5 s at each step) over 51 s (STEP-51) to achieve a pressure–time product similar to that of CPAP-30; and (3) STEP (5 cm H_2O/step, 5 s at each step) over 30 s with maximum pressure sustained for a further 30 s (STEP-30/30)	RMs improved respiratory mechanics, but stepwise RM without sustained airway pressure appeared to have less biological impact on lungs
Santos et al., 2016 [37]	Rats	(1) Non-recruited; (2) RM with CPAP (30 cm H_2O for 30 s; $CPAP_{RM}$ or fast RM); and (3) RM with STEP (5 cm H_2O/step, 8.5 s/step, 6 steps, 51 s; $STEP_{RM}$ or slow RM), with a maximum pressure hold for 10 s	Compared with $CPAP_{RM}$, $STEP_{RM}$ reduced biological markers associated with endothelial cell damage and ultrastructural endothelial cell injury in both moderate and severe sepsis-induced acute lung inflammation

(continued)

Table 9.1 (continued)

Study	Animals	Interventions	Outcomes
Wittenstein et al., 2021 [38]	Pigs	(1) PROVHILO strategy, V_T was increased stepwise by 4 ml/kg at a fixed PEEP of 12 cmH_2O until a plateau pressure of 30–35 cmH_2O was reached; (2) iPROVE strategy, at fixed driving pressure of 20 cmH_2O, PEEP was increased up to 20 cmH_2O followed by PEEP titration according to the lowest E_{RS}	iPROVE strategy compared with the PROVHILO strategy increased dorsal Ptrans at the cost of lower MAP during RMs, and decreased E_{RS}
PEEP decrement			
Katira, 2018 [41]	Rats	Low V_T = 6 ml/kg and randomized to (1) control, PEEP = 3 cmH_2O; (2) PEEP = 3 toward 11 cmH_2O over 70 min, followed by abrupt deflation to zero PEEP	Abrupt deflation after sustained inflation can cause acute lung injury. Injury did not occur with gradual deflation
Rocha et al., 2021 [42]	Rats	(1) Standard (10 ml/kg/h) or (2) high (30 ml/kg/h) fluid infusion regimen followed by abrupt or gradual (0.2 cmH_2O/min for 30 min) PEEP decrease from 9 to 3 cmH_2O	Decreasing PEEP abruptly increased pulmonary arterial hypertension. The combination of abrupt PEEP decrease and high fluid administration led to greater lung and kidney damage

CPAP continuous positive airway pressure, *FCV* flow-controlled ventilation, *FLEX* flow-controlled expiration, *IT* inspiration time, *MAP* mean arterial pressure, *PCV* pressure-controlled ventilation, *PEEP* positive end-expiratory pressure, *PIP* peak inspiratory pressure, *PRVC* pressure-regulated volume control, *RM* recruitment maneuver, *RR* respiratory rate, *STEP* stepwise increase in airway pressure, *VCV* volume-controlled ventilation

over the period of early connection to the mechanical ventilator, with mechanical power exposure the cornerstone factor? Similar approaches associated with exposure have been taken with other ventilator variables, such as inspired fraction of oxygen (FiO_2) [14].

9.5 Slow the Changes in Respiratory Rate during Mechanical Ventilation

Little attention has been paid to RR, but experimental evidence [11, 15–18] suggests it has a significant role in the generation of VILI. Theoretically, if a certain safe level of strain is passed, it is expected that lung damage will be greater as the number of injurious respiratory cycles is higher. Recently, it was shown in 4549 patients with ARDS that RR was an independent predictor of mortality [8]. The average RR was 25.7 ± 7.4 breaths/min, which is a common value observed in the intensive care unit (ICU). The authors showed that the impact of ΔP on mortality was four times greater than that of the RR, but the RR was still independently associated with mortality. They suggested, according to theoretical and practical issues at the bedside, the concept of using 4 × ΔP + 1 × RR (4ΔPRR) to quantify the impact of changes in ventilatory strategy on VILI [8]. On the other hand, it has been argued that the simplicity of 4ΔPRR is not superior to the simplicity of the bedside calculation of mechanical power through simplified formulas [19]. In addition to the best way to estimate lung damage, one important point is the recognition that RR has finally been considered to be an essential determinant of VILI. In clinical practice, if RR needs to be adjusted to higher levels for adequate minute ventilation due to low tidal volume, the adjustments are usually done abruptly. By doing so, several other ventilator parameters are abruptly dragged to new levels, such as inspiratory time and airflow.

9.5.1 Prolonged Versus Short Inspiratory Time?

In a model of mild acute lung inflammation, it was shown that prolonging the inspiratory time to the detriment of reducing expiratory time increased the gene expression of biological markers associated with inflammation and alveolar epithelial cell injury, and reducing the inspiratory time to the detriment of prolonging expiratory time increased markers of endothelial cell damage [20]. Similar results have been observed in other preclinical studies using high tidal volume and prolonged inspiratory time [21].

9.5.2 High Versus Low Inspiratory Flow?

Inspiratory airflow is closely associated with shear stress at the top of the cells within the respiratory bronchi. *In situ* experiments have shown that healthy lungs support magnitudes of shear stress (15 dyn/cm^2) at all alveolar opening velocities in the physiologic range. However, for a lung with increased viscosity of intra-alveoli fluid, shear stress may increase by several orders of magnitude, enough to induce epithelial cell injury [22]. In addition to the shear stress, the pressure gradient is an important factor acting toward development of hydraulic airway epithelial cell fracture or denudation. Some reports have associated high inspiratory flow profiles with gas exchange, the work of breathing, cardiovascular function, and lung damage [23–25]. For example, when inspiratory airflow was increased by 20%, mechanical power increased by 37% in experimental settings [4]. Due to its importance in the development of VILI, inspiratory flow has been incorporated in a new proposed formula to estimate mechanical power under volume-controlled ventilation:

$$\text{Mechanical power} = V'E \times \left(P\text{peak},_{RS} + \text{PEEP} + F/6\right)/20 \qquad (9.5)$$

where V'E is minute ventilation. In a preclinical study, the relationship between the unadjusted proposed mechanical power (Eq. 9.5) and the reference formula (Eq. 9.3) showed linear regression ($R^2 = 0.98$), with a bias of -2.45 J/min [26]. Besides the adjustments in inspiratory time and airflow that happen after an abrupt increase in

RR, the biological impact of abrupt increases in RR is unknown. An increment from 15 to 26 breaths/min is not unusual in the ICU and represents an increment of 73% in RR. However, should this increase be slow to better accommodate tidal strain and not increase cyclic stress for different time constants of alveolar units? Some clinical trials comparing high and low tidal volume have used higher RRs in the low tidal volume group. For example, in the ARDS Network trial [6], the RR in the low tidal volume group was 81% higher than in the high tidal volume group. Villar et al. [27] showed that when the PEEP level was set above Pflex at low tidal volume, RR was increased 37% compared with a high tidal volume strategy. These changes are required to keep similar levels of $PaCO_2$. If permissive hypercapnia is established in the protocol, the difference in RR will be smoothed, as shown by other trials comparing low and high tidal volumes [28]. We believe that how RR is adjusted over time in heterogeneous lungs deserves attention because alveolar units have different time constants.

9.6 Stepwise Increase in Airway Pressure during Recruitment Maneuvers

Recruitment maneuvers (RMs) have been associated with improvement in oxygenation and lung mechanics during mechanical ventilation [29]. However, RMs are effective only if the airway pressure exceeds the critical opening pressure of the small airways [30]. Alveoli recruit with differing time constants in injured lungs, therefore some time is required for the critical opening pressure to open each alveolar unit [30]. This was observed when application of 30 cmH_2O to a lung inflated at 5 cmH_2O for 2 s opened approximately 75% of alveoli and continuation of 30 cmH_2O for 40 s gradually increased the proportion of open alveoli to 85% [31]. Time is an important variable in both alveolar recruitment and stabilization; therefore, the pattern of increase in airway pressure (rapid versus slow increase) must also be considered [32]. Theoretically, sudden changes in airway pressure and inspiratory flow cause transient higher stress, worsening lung damage [33]. It was shown in a sepsis-induced model of acute lung injury that RMs with gradual (rather than abrupt) increases in airway pressure to the same target airway pressure improved lung function and minimized the biological impact on lungs [33]. This finding has been corroborated by other preclinical studies [35–37]. One recent translational preclinical study compared the RMs performed with the PROVHILO strategy with those of the iPROVE strategy in a random sequence [38]. In the PROVHILO strategy, tidal volume was increased stepwise by 4 ml/kg at a fixed PEEP of 12 cmH_2O until a plateau pressure of 30-35 cmH_2O was reached, whereas with the iPROVE strategy, at a fixed driving pressure of 20 cmH_2O, PEEP was increased up to 20 cmH_2O followed by PEEP titration according to the lowest elastance of the respiratory system. The authors showed that, compared with the PROVHILO strategy, the iPROVE strategy increased dorsal transpulmonary pressure at the cost of lower mean arterial pressure during RMs, and decreased the elastance of the respiratory system thereafter, without consistent improvement in oxygenation. In clinical settings in patients without ARDS, Ferrando et al. [39] investigated the preventive role of intraoperative ventilation with stepwise RMs plus an open lung approach on postoperative pulmonary complications. The authors showed that 55% patients subjected to an open lung approach were more likely to achieve an open lung condition than those receiving standard ventilation using low PEEP (33%). In addition, Ball et al. [40] performed a meta-analysis of unselected patients with ARDS who were mechanically ventilated with protective low tidal volume. The use of stepwise increments in PEEP and/or RMs did not result in a reduction in mortality or in the incidence of barotrauma compared with a strategy using a PEEP level aimed at achieving minimal acceptable oxygenation goals. Although stepwise RMs have been used in many preclinical and clinical studies, to date, their efficacy in terms of robust clinical outcomes has not been confirmed.

9.7 Slow Decreases in PEEP Levels and Lung Damage

Beyond the inspiratory phase of the pressure-volume curve, less attention has been given to the expiratory phase either in one respiratory cycle or during the overall expiratory phase of the pressure-volume curve. This aspect was highlighted by Katira et al. [41] in an elegant experimental study, which showed that lung damage can occur after sustained inflation followed by abrupt deflation. The mechanism may rely on increased left ventricular preload and afterload, which increases pulmonary microvascular pressure; this directly injures the endothelium and causes edema, which is potentiated by the surge in pulmonary perfusion. Furthermore, the authors showed that a gradual decrease, notwithstanding the same exposure to increased airway pressure during sustained inflation, was not associated with lung injury, in contrast to rapid deflation. The mechanism may be explained by no surge in cardiac output (and any increase in cardiac output would have been gradual). Rocha et al. [42] evaluated the effects of abrupt versus gradual PEEP release combined with standard or high fluid volumes. The authors showed that animals treated with high levels of fluid and abrupt decrease in PEEP exhibited greater diffuse alveolar damage and higher expression of genes associated with lung inflammation and endothelial cell damage compared with other groups. Abrupt reduction in PEEP, regardless of fluid status, led to greater epithelial cell damage and pulmonary arterial pressure (as indicated by the ratio of pulmonary acceleration time to pulmonary ejection time). Kidney injury molecule-1 (KIM-1) also increased in those animals with high versus standard fluid administration, during both abrupt and gradual decrease in PEEP. There are different clinical situations in which abrupt deflation from high airway pressure can occur, such as ventilator disconnection, patient transport, sustained high pressure RMs, and even airway pressure release ventilation [43]. These situations can be extreme when respiratory muscle tonus is absent, such as during paralysis. Elegant editorials have highlighted the additional mechanisms by which sudden airway pressure decay may contribute to lung damage [9]. One potential contribution of previous preclinical studies has been to shed light on expiratory events that may elicit lung damage through mechanisms related to hemodynamic changes.

9.8 Smooth the Expiration Phase: Does It Matter?

Less attention is given to the expiration phase than to inspiration during controlled mechanical ventilation. Nevertheless, de-pressurization of the respiratory system predisposes closure of the distal airway and generation of atelectasis areas. Flow-controlled ventilation avoids zero-flow conditions. During this form of ventilation, airflows at the inspiration and expiration phases are both constant. The resulting constant flow coupled with direct intratracheal pressure measurements allows much more precise analysis of individual lung mechanics than is possible in conventional ventilation modes, where flow varies over a wide range and intratracheal pressure is not directly accessible [44]. Preclinical studies have been conducted on healthy pigs on short-term ventilation [45] and on long-term ventilation [44], lung-injured pigs [46, 47], as well as during one lung ventilation under normovolemia and hypovolemia [48]. In addition, Wittenstein et al. [48] showed that regardless of fluid status, flow-controlled ventilation, compared with volume-controlled ventilation, reduced the mechanical power mainly due to the resistive component. By actively controlling the expiratory phase, the appearance of intrinsic PEEP may be avoided, which in turn promotes better air exhalation among alveoli with different time constants. Passive expiratory flow combined with reduced mean airway pressure may predispose to airway narrowing and limitation of expiratory flow. This phenomenon may have a negative impact on subsequent ventilator cycles. It is difficult to precisely measure airway closure in a large cross-sectional area, but, intuitively, flow-controlled ventilation may stay longer above the airway closure level compared with passive expiration as observed in volume-controlled ventilation. One of the fundamentals of flow-controlled ventilation is to physically reduce dissipated energy applied to lung tissue as much as possible [49]. By keeping the gas flow constant and active during the entire respiratory cycle, whether at inspiration or expiration, the dissipated energy is minimized to the lowest possible level [49]. Therefore, tidal volume may increase within lung mechanical limits to reduce dead space ventilation but simultaneously decrease the risk of atelectasis and/or overdistension. The increase in tidal volume is explained by the viscoelastic properties of lung tissue, because keeping a constant flow, lung tissue has more time to deform and increase the tidal volume ("creep") while relieving stress during flow-controlled ventilation. In a study by Spraider et al. [44], a further refinement was done, so-called "individualized flow-controlled ventilation". This approach combines the measurement of direct intratracheal pressure and a constant flow, which allows dynamic compliance to be measured during ventilation and pressure settings to be adjusted accordingly. The novelty in individualized flow-controlled ventilation is that tidal volume is naturally strongly related to individual lung compliance as a result of the individualization process, thereby representing the ventilation of the available aerated lung tissue. This can lead to a higher tidal volume in lung healthy individuals (as shown in this study) but would also result in decreased tidal volume if the compliance of an injured lung is reduced. However, a recent case report from the same group has shown that individualized flow-controlled ventilation may not work properly in patients with severely impaired lung function, such as the most severe coronavirus disease 2019 (COVID-19) phenotypes [50].

9.9 Conclusion

Slowing changes in ventilator parameters may prevent further lung damage in ARDS lungs, mainly because of the viscoelastic nature of pulmonary tissue in which elements of the extracellular matrix as well as epithelial/endothelial cells require an adaptive "stress relaxation" time to mitigate the damaging strain/stress.

References

1. Faffe DS, Zin WA. Lung parenchymal mechanics in health and disease. Physiol Rev. 2009;89:759–75.
2. Hildebrandt J. Pressure-volume data of cat lung interpreted by a plastoelastic, linear viscoelastic model. J Appl Physiol (1985). 1970;28:365–72.
3. Hantos Z, Daroczy B, Suki B, Nagy S, Fredberg JJ. Input impedance and peripheral inhomogeneity of dog lungs. J Appl Physiol (1985). 1992;72:168–78.
4. Gattinoni L, Tonetti T, Cressoni M, et al. Ventilator-related causes of lung injury: the mechanical power. Intensive Care Med. 2016;42:1567–75.
5. Otis AB, Fenn WO, Rahn H. Mechanics of breathing in man. J Appl Physiol (1985). 1950:2:592–607.
6. Brower RG, Matthay MA, Morris A, Schoenfeld D, Thompson BT, Wheeler A. Ventilation with lower tidal volumes as compared with traditional tidal volumes for acute lung injury and the acute respiratory distress syndrome. N Engl J Med. 2000;342:1301–8.
7. Parhar KKS, Zjadewicz K, Soo A, et al. Epidemiology, mechanical power, and 3-year outcomes in acute respiratory distress syndrome patients using standardized screening. An observational cohort study. Ann Am Thorac Soc. 2019;16:1263–72.
8. Costa ELV, Slutsky AS, Brochard LJ, et al. Ventilatory variables and mechanical power in patients with acute respiratory distress syndrome. Am J Respir Crit Care Med. 2021;204:303–11.
9. Marini JJ, Gattinoni L. Energetics and the root mechanical cause for ventilator-induced lung injury. Anesthesiology. 2018;128:1062–4.
10. Protti A, Maraffi T, Milesi M, et al. Role of strain rate in the pathogenesis of ventilator-induced lung edema. Crit Care Med. 2016;44:e838–45.
11. Rich PB, Reickert CA, Sawada S, et al. Effect of rate and inspiratory flow on ventilator-induced lung injury. J Trauma. 2000;49:903–11.
12. Maeda Y, Fujino Y, Uchiyama A, Matsuura N, Mashimo T, Nishimura M. Effects of peak inspiratory flow on development of ventilator-induced lung injury in rabbits. Anesthesiology. 2004;101:722–8.
13. Felix NS, Samary CS, Cruz FF, et al. Gradually increasing tidal volume may mitigate experimental lung injury in rats. Anesthesiology. 2019;130:767–77.
14. Aggarwal NR, Brower RG. Targeting normoxemia in acute respiratory distress syndrome may cause worse short-term outcomes because of oxygen toxicity. Ann Am Thorac Soc. 2014;11:1449–53.
15. Hotchkiss JR Jr, Blanch L, Murias G, et al. Effects of decreased respiratory frequency on ventilator-induced lung injury. Am J Respir Crit Care Med. 2000;161:463–8.
16. Conrad SA, Zhang S, Arnold TC, Scott LK, Carden DL. Protective effects of low respiratory frequency in experimental ventilator-associated lung injury. Crit Care Med. 2005;33:835–40.

17. Vaporidi K, Voloudakis G, Priniannakis G, et al. Effects of respiratory rate on ventilator-induced lung injury at a constant PaCO2 in a mouse model of normal lung. Crit Care Med. 2008;36:1277–83.
18. Retamal J, Borges JB, Bruhn A, et al. High respiratory rate is associated with early reduction of lung edema clearance in an experimental model of ARDS. Acta Anaesthesiol Scand. 2016;60:79–92.
19. Camporota L, Busana M, Marini JJ, Gattinoni L. The 4DPRR index and mechanical power: a step ahead or four steps backward? Am J Respir Crit Care Med. 2021;204:491–2.
20. Spieth PM, Silva PL, Garcia CS, et al. Modulation of stress versus time product during mechanical ventilation influences inflammation as well as alveolar epithelial and endothelial response in rats. Anesthesiology. 2015;122:106–16.
21. Muller-Redetzky HC, Felten M, Hellwig K, et al. Increasing the inspiratory time and I:E ratio during mechanical ventilation aggravates ventilator-induced lung injury in mice. Crit Care. 2015;19:23.
22. Chen ZL, Song YL, Hu ZY, Zhang S, Chen YZ. An estimation of mechanical stress on alveolar walls during repetitive alveolar reopening and closure. J Appl Physiol (1985). 2015;119:190–201.
23. Smith RA, Venus B. Cardiopulmonary effect of various inspiratory flow profiles during controlled mechanical ventilation in a porcine lung model. Crit Care Med. 1988;16:769–72.
24. Al-Saady N, Bennett ED. Decelerating inspiratory flow waveform improves lung mechanics and gas exchange in patients on intermittent positive-pressure ventilation. Intensive Care Med. 1985;11:68–75.
25. Garcia CS, Abreu SC, Soares RM, et al. Pulmonary morphofunctional effects of mechanical ventilation with high inspiratory air flow. Crit Care Med. 2008;36:232–9.
26. Giosa L, Busana M, Pasticci I, et al. Mechanical power at a glance: a simple surrogate for volume-controlled ventilation. Intensive Care Med Exp. 2019;7:61.
27. Villar J, Kacmarek RM, Perez-Mendez L, Aguirre-Jaime A. A high positive end-expiratory pressure, low tidal volume ventilatory strategy improves outcome in persistent acute respiratory distress syndrome: a randomized, controlled trial. Crit Care Med. 2006;34:1311–8.
28. Amato MB, Barbas CS, Medeiros DM, et al. Effect of a protective-ventilation strategy on mortality in the acute respiratory distress syndrome. N Engl J Med. 1998;338:347–54.
29. Fan E, Wilcox ME, Brower RG, et al. Recruitment maneuvers for acute lung injury: a systematic review. Am J Respir Crit Care Med. 2008;178:1156–63.
30. Suki B, Barabasi AL, Hantos Z, Petak F, Stanley HE. Avalanches and power-law behaviour in lung inflation. Nature. 1994;368:615–8.
31. Albert SP, DiRocco J, Allen GB, et al. The role of time and pressure on alveolar recruitment. J Appl Physiol (1985). 2009;106:757–65.
32. Odenstedt H, Lindgren S, Olegard C, et al. Slow moderate pressure recruitment maneuver minimizes negative circulatory and lung mechanic side effects: evaluation of recruitment maneuvers using electric impedance tomography. Intensive Care Med. 2005;31:1706–14.
33. Nucci G, Suki B, Lutchen K. Modeling airflow-related shear stress during heterogeneous constriction and mechanical ventilation. J Appl Physiol (1985). 2003;95:348–56.
34. Silva PL, Moraes L, Santos RS, et al. Impact of pressure profile and duration of recruitment maneuvers on morphofunctional and biochemical variables in experimental lung injury. Crit Care Med. 2011;39:1074–81.
35. Lim SC, Adams AB, Simonson DA, Dries DJ, Broccard AF, Hotchkiss JR, et al. Intercomparison of recruitment maneuver efficacy in three models of acute lung injury. Crit Care Med. 2004;32:2371–7.
36. Silva PL, Moraes L, Santos RS, et al. Recruitment maneuvers modulate epithelial and endothelial cell response according to acute lung injury etiology. Crit Care Med. 2013;41:e256–65.
37. Santos RS, Moraes L, Samary CS, et al. Fast versus slow recruitment maneuver at different degrees of acute lung inflammation induced by experimental sepsis. Anesth Analg. 2016;122:1089–100.

38. Wittenstein J, Huhle R, Scharffenberg M, et al. Effects of two stepwise lung recruitment strategies on respiratory function and haemodynamics in anaesthetised pigs: a randomised crossover study. Eur J Anaesthesiol. 2021;38:634–43.
39. Ferrando C, Librero J, Tusman G, et al. Intraoperative open lung condition and postoperative pulmonary complications. A secondary analysis of iPROVE and iPROVE-O2 trials. Acta Anaesthesiol Scand. 2021:66:30–9.
40. Ball L, Serpa Neto A, Trifiletti V, et al. Effects of higher PEEP and recruitment manoeuvres on mortality in patients with ARDS: a systematic review, meta-analysis, meta-regression and trial sequential analysis of randomized controlled trials. Intensive Care Med Exp. 2020;8(Suppl 1):39.
41. Katira BH, Engelberts D, Otulakowski G, et al. Abrupt deflation after sustained inflation causes lung injury. Am J Respir Crit Care Med. 2018;198:1165–76.
42. Rocha NN, Samary CS, Antunes MA, et al. The impact of fluid status and decremental PEEP strategy on cardiac function and lung and kidney damage in mild-moderate experimental acute respiratory distress syndrome. Respir Res. 2021;22:214.
43. Nieman GF, Al-Khalisy H, Kollisch-Singule M, et al. A physiologically informed strategy to effectively open, stabilize, and protect the acutely injured lung. Front Physiol. 2020;11:227.
44. Spraider P, Martini J, Abram J, et al. Individualized flow-controlled ventilation compared to best clinical practice pressure-controlled ventilation: a prospective randomized porcine study. Crit Care. 2020;24:662.
45. Schmidt J, Wenzel C, Mahn M, et al. Improved lung recruitment and oxygenation during mandatory ventilation with a new expiratory ventilation assistance device: a controlled interventional trial in healthy pigs. Eur J Anaesthesiol. 2018;35:736–44.
46. Borgmann S, Schmidt J, Goebel U, Haberstroh J, Guttmann J, Schumann S. Dorsal recruitment with flow-controlled expiration (FLEX): an experimental study in mechanically ventilated lung-healthy and lung-injured pigs. Crit Care. 2018;22:245.
47. Schmidt J, Wenzel C, Spassov S, et al. Flow-controlled ventilation attenuates lung injury in a porcine model of acute respiratory distress syndrome: a preclinical randomized controlled study. Crit Care Med. 2020;48:e241–e8.
48. Wittenstein J, Scharffenberg M, Ran X, et al. Comparative effects of flow vs. volume-controlled one-lung ventilation on gas exchange and respiratory system mechanics in pigs. Intensive Care Med Exp. 2020;8(Suppl 1):24.
49. Barnes T, van Asseldonk D, Enk D. Minimisation of dissipated energy in the airways during mechanical ventilation by using constant inspiratory and expiratory flows - flow-controlled ventilation (FCV). Med Hypotheses. 2018;121:167–76.
50. Spraider P, Putzer G, Breitkopf R, et al. A case report of individualized ventilation in a COVID-19 patient - new possibilities and caveats to consider with flow-controlled ventilation. BMC Anesthesiol. 2021;21:145.

Spontaneous Breathing in Acute Respiratory Failure

10

E. Chiodaroli and D. Chiumello

10.1 Introduction

Physiology must provide understanding of emergent phenomena and explore deeper levels of natural organization. In terms of respiratory physiology and mechanical ventilation of heterogeneously injured lungs, only a deeper knowledge of the complex regional behaviors regulating unstable airways and lung units –not merely an investigation of length of stay and mortality [1]– can lead to significant improvements in therapeutic strategies and individualized respiratory care [2]. The last decades have brought important insights into the mechanisms of lung injury. Substantial progress has been made in the ventilator management of severely lung-injured patients [3]. However, the recognition that further injury can result from incongruous ventilatory settings leading to ventilator-induced lung injury (VILI) has opened a vast area of research, which still encompasses many unexplored and controversial issues [4]. Randomized controlled trials (RCTs) have confirmed that large tidal volumes and high driving pressures are among the main determinants of VILI [5, 6]. Moreover, assisted ventilation is one of the more complex and unpredictable ventilator conditions. In this case, VILI is called patient self-inflicted lung injury (P-SILI) [7]. Studying the interaction between lung mechanics and diaphragm function during assisted ventilation is extremely important for understanding mechanical ventilation in patients who preserve their own respiratory drive.

E. Chiodaroli
Department of Anesthesia and Intensive Care, ASST Santi Paolo e Carlo, San Paolo University Hospital, Milan, Italy

D. Chiumello (✉)
Department of Anesthesia and Intensive Care, ASST Santi Paolo e Carlo, San Paolo University Hospital, Milan, Italy

Department of Health Sciences, University of Milan, Milan, Italy
e-mail: davide.chiumello@unimi.it

J.-L. Vincent (ed.), *Annual Update in Intensive Care and Emergency Medicine 2022*, Annual Update in Intensive Care and Emergency Medicine,
https://doi.org/10.1007/978-3-030-93433-0_10

Unfortunately, complex patient-ventilator interactions during assisted ventilation are still largely unexplored.

Despite a clear improvement in ventilatory strategies brought about through large randomized trials, we still lack knowledge that could make mechanical ventilation fully protective. Insufficient information regarding regional lung mechanics and deformation at the acinar level is likely the main determinant of these unresolved issues [8].

10.2 Acute Respiratory Distress Syndrome

The acute respiratory distress syndrome (ARDS) is an acute, diffuse, edematous inflammation of lung tissue induced by increased permeability of the alveolar-capillary membrane. Clinically, ARDS is characterized by impaired oxygenation due to increased venous admixture, decreased lung compliance, increased physiological dead space, and bilateral radiographic opacities [9, 10]. The underlying cause of the syndrome is a reaction by the pulmonary parenchyma to a variety of serious conditions, the most frequent of which are sepsis, severe pneumonia, peritonitis, and multiple trauma [11]. According to the Berlin definition, ARDS can be divided into mild, moderate, and severe, depending on the PaO_2/FiO_2 values [10].

Before the Berlin definition, population-based estimates of the yearly incidence of moderate and severe ARDS ranged from 3 to 88 per 100,000 people. In critically ill patients hospitalized in intensive care units (ICUs), the prevalence of ARDS has been estimated to be about 5-15% [12]. The overall mortality is 15-50% in all major series, although several RCTs, some including mild cases, have reported a better survival in selected ARDS patients [13, 14]. On gross pathological examination, the lungs of patients who have not survived ARDS are heavy because of atelectasis, interstitial and alveolar edema, and hyaline membranes [14]. On examination with laser confocal imaging, ARDS lungs have both collapsed and over-distended alveoli with a range of air pockets of various sizes surrounded by fluid and foam [15].

Tissue damage during ARDS involves disruption of endothelial and epithelial surfaces, flooding of alveolar spaces, inactivated surfactant, and an inflammatory reaction. The lung inflammation in ARDS is initiated, amplified, and modulated by a complex network of cytokines and other pro-inflammatory mediators produced by a variety of cell types in the lungs, including fibroblasts, epithelial cells, and inflammatory cells [16].

With regard to lung function in ARDS, hypoxemia is the most prominent feature and is the result of extensive collapsed and poorly ventilated lung areas with shunt and ventilation-perfusion (V/Q) mismatch [17]. In addition, dead space is markedly increased, which increases ventilatory demand [18]. Alterations in lung mechanics include decreased compliance due to the significantly large proportion of the lungs that is functionally lost because of collapse, consolidation, and flooding [19]. Thus, ventilation takes place in functionally small lungs (a condition termed “baby lung”) [20]. In addition, there is marked heterogeneity in regional aeration. However, bronchoalveolar lavage (BAL) studies indicate that even normally aerated areas are substantially inflamed [21].

10.3 Mechanical Ventilation and VILI

Mechanical ventilation is intended as supportive treatment of respiratory function, ensuring gas exchange while allowing the respiratory muscles to rest. Ventilatory support was first introduced during the polio epidemic in Copenhagen in 1952, decreasing mortality from over 80% to 40% [22]. Despite the clear benefits and a normalized gas exchange, many patients still died. Among all the possible causal factors, direct complications of mechanical ventilation, such as barotrauma due to structural damage of the lung, could be observed [23]. Lung damage as a consequence of mechanical ventilation is now referred to as VILI [20]. Recognition of the importance of VILI has led to considerable changes in ventilatory strategy. The main target was initially related to gas exchange optimization, but now a new target has been introduced: minimizing VILI, even if this means accepting a higher partial pressure of arterial carbon dioxide ($PaCO_2$). RCTs have clearly shown that large tidal volumes and/or high driving pressures are among the main determinants of VILI [5, 6, 24, 25]. Thus, a ventilation strategy characterized by low tidal volume, high positive end-expiratory pressure (PEEP) and low driving pressure is now considered state of the art in terms of protective ventilation. However, fully protective mechanical ventilation is still far from being reality.

10.4 Stress, Strain, and Stress Raisers

The structure responsible for bearing the mechanical stress of respiration and giving support to the endothelial and epithelial cells is a skeleton made up of elastin and fibrillary collagen [26]. Secondary to non-physiological deformation, cells can react by secreting cytokines and pro-inflammatory molecules that can initiate an inflammatory reaction. These cells can be activated through direct damage or by mechanotransduction signaling [27]. In addition, the fibroelastic skeleton can be disrupted and these fragments can work as damage-associated molecular patterns (DAMPs) and activate an inflammatory response via Toll-like receptors [26–28]. Lung distention is commonly inferred from tidal volume (ml/kg of ideal body weight) and end-inspiratory (plateau) airway pressure [25]. However, neither of these two variables reliably reflects tissue deformation, especially during acute lung injury when relationships between body weight and functional residual capacity (FRC) and between airway and transpulmonary pressure become unpredictable [29, 30]. A practical way of approaching the real tissue deformation is by assessing the volumetric strain, understood as the ratio of change of volume and the resting lung volume ($\Delta V/V0$). In this ratio, ΔV corresponds to tidal volume, and V0 corresponds to the resting volume, usually estimated as the FRC volume [26, 30, 31].

Protti and coworkers showed that high strain levels were associated with VILI when they exceeded a threshold of 1.5-2.5. In addition, the same group showed that dynamic strain was the main determinant of VILI [30, 31]. This approach to the volumetric strain is global, summarizing the mechanical behavior of whole lungs. However, at the regional level, the situation is probably different, with multiple regional strains of different magnitudes. When an alveolus collapses, the traction forces exerted on its walls by adjacent expanded units increase and become concentrated. These forces may promote re-expansion of the alveolus at the expense of potentially harmful stresses at the interface between the collapsed and the expanded units. These inhomogeneities are also known as pressure multipliers or stress raisers [26, 29]. This conceptual framework was described by Mead and coworkers in 1970 and is essentially related to alveolar interdependence phenomena [29]. In their theoretical analysis, Mead et al. estimated that the alveolar pressure at the junction of the fully collapsed and expanded alveoli could be as high as 4-5 times the applied pressure. This landmark estimation of approximately four times local amplification was recently confirmed using synchrotron-based X-ray tomographic microscopy in a rat lung preparation. There is also clinical information that supports this theoretical model. Cressoni and coworkers showed that inhomogeneities assessed by computed tomography (CT) image analysis were associated with overall disease severity and mortality. In addition, ventilatory techniques like higher PEEP or the prone position, decrease lung inhomogeneity and, consequently, reduce the extent of stress rise by keeping open previously collapsed regions. This in turn reduces the risk of VILI and may potentially improve survival of ARDS patients [32].

10.5 P-SILI and Assisted Ventilation

Assisted ventilatory modalities have been developed with the purpose of optimizing the interface between mechanical ventilation and a patient's pattern of spontaneous breathing, thus enhancing the comfort of the patient during the weaning phase. Spontaneous breathing during mechanical ventilation has been shown to be beneficial in those subjects who have a partially preserved respiratory capacity [33–35]. Theoretically, optimally ventilated healthy lungs would expand isotropically, having nearly homogenous time constants and being exposed only to equally distributed distending pressures [36, 37]. However, unpredictable phenomena of local overstretch have been demonstrated to characterize some spontaneous breathing settings under mechanical ventilation [38–40], mainly in injured lungs [7, 41–43], but also in healthy ones [44]. To this day, very little is known about regional mechanics in spontaneously breathing patients.

In recent years, experts in the field of lung injury and mechanical ventilation have expressed their concerns regarding spontaneous breathing, discouraging it in patients with ARDS because of the risk of P-SILI [7, 43]. Controlled mechanical ventilation under deep sedation and muscle paralysis is encouraged instead. The main reason behind concerns regarding spontaneous breathing is the unpredictability of injurious events due to a lack of monitoring to ensure safe spontaneous

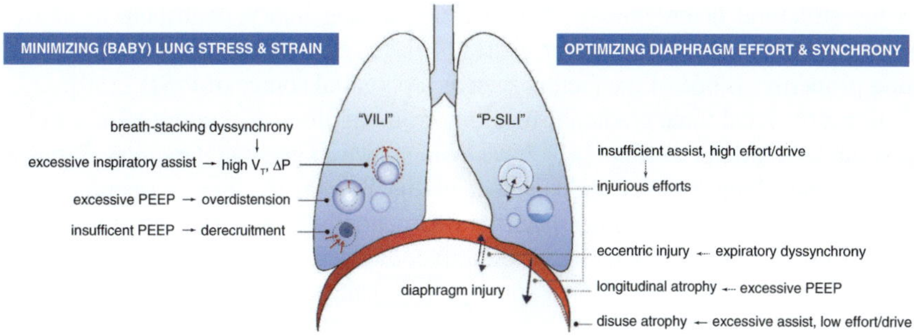

Fig. 10.1 Principles of lung and diaphragm-protective ventilation. *ΔP* change in airway pressure during inspiration, *PEEP* positive end-expiratory pressure, *P-SILI* patient self-inflicted lung injury, *VILI* ventilator-induced lung injury, V_T tidal volume (reproduced from [44] with permission)

breathing ventilation. By introducing monitoring tools based on a deeper physiopathological understanding of patient-ventilator interaction, safe control of spontaneous breathing may be reached. Spontaneous breathing could, if optimized, be a viable and safe alternative to passive mechanical ventilation.

While the importance of lung-protective ventilation is now well-established, the concept of diaphragm-protective ventilation has recently been introduced (Fig. 10.1) and scientific evidence related thereto is currently being gathered. The diaphragm plays a crucial role during the weaning phase, enabling patients to gradually take full control of ventilation. Controlled ventilation, as well as over-assistance during spontaneous breathing, combined with critical illness such as poly-neuromyopathy and/or systemic inflammatory cascades, can lead to diaphragmatic weakness and, consequently, to substantial morbidity and mortality in ventilated patients [44]. Several pathophysiological mechanisms have been indicated as possible causes leading to four different forms of ventilator-induced diaphragm dysfunction (VIDD): (1) cross-sectional atrophy from excessive support and over-assistance; (2) longitudinal atrophy from excessive PEEP; (3) concentric loading, which occurs when the muscle contracts against an excessive load during the contraction phase, e.g., in case of insufficient support; and (4) eccentric loading, which occurs when the muscle contracts against an excessive load during the relaxation phase.

10.6 Lung Mechanics and Pulmonary Heterogeneity

Respiratory mechanics measured at the airway opening constitutes a simplified parameter that does not necessarily reflect regional lung properties. A simplistic visualization of acute lung injury, at least its early phases, could be based on an elastic sponge: following injury, an excessive tissue mass, equally distributed in all lung regions, is exposed to the combined action of a gravitational field and to increased superimposed hydrostatic pressure due to lung edema [45, 46]. Intrinsic proprieties of the pulmonary structures, such as gravitational forces [47, 48], as well as the structural heterogeneity characterizing a lung injury, contribute to uneven regional distribution of gas and pressures [49]. Excessive heterogeneity of regional lung properties is one of the factors seen as a potential source of P-SILI [50].

Recently, local force gradients, resulting from vigorous inspiratory efforts and/or unsuitable ventilator settings [42], have been shown to generate large gas displacement among lung regions, independent of the flow at the airway opening. This dynamic gas redistribution has been named pendelluft, even if it does not occur under static conditions. Dynamic pendelluft could be a cause of unpredictable overstretch in mechanically ventilated heterogeneous lungs, activating an inflammatory cascade [43].

The prevalence and impact of dynamic pendelluft in clinical settings remain uncertain. Furthermore, the regional lung mechanics behind regional gas redistribution have neither been investigated nor quantified before.

10.7 Conclusion

A better understanding of pathophysiological mechanisms is fundamental to improving therapeutic strategies and patient outcomes in ARDS. The key to fully protective assisted ventilation of lung-injured critically ill patients is a deeper investigation of respiratory physiology. At the moment, we still lack full monitoring and understanding of potentially injurious regional events. Further research studies are necessary for deeper investigation of the complex regional behaviors regulating unstable airways and lung units in order to make spontaneous breathing fully protective in patients with ARDS.

References

1. Hedenstierna G, Edmark L, Perchiazzi G. Postoperative lung complications: have multicentre studies been of any help? Br J Anaesth. 2015;114:541–3.
2. Winkler T, Venegas JG, Harris RS. Mathematical modeling of ventilation defects in asthma. Drug Discov Today Dis Model. 2015;15:3–8.
3. Slutsky AS. History of mechanical ventilation. From Vesalius to ventilator induced lung injury. Am J Respir Crit Care Med. 2015;191:1106–15.
4. Slutsky AS, Ranieri VM. Ventilator-induced lung injury. N Engl J Med. 2013;369:2126–36.
5. Amato MBP, Meade MO, Slutsky AS, et al. Driving pressure and survival in the acute respiratory distress syndrome. N Engl J Med. 2015;372:747–55.
6. Amato MBP, Barbas CSV, Medeiros DM, et al. Effect of a protective-ventilation strategy on mortality in the acute respiratory distress syndrome. N Engl J Med. 1998;338:347–54.
7. Brochard L, Slutsky A, Pesenti A. Mechanical ventilation to minimize progression of lung injury in acute respiratory failure. Am J Respir Crit Care Med. 2017;195:1–16.
8. Hubmayr RD. Perspective on lung injury and recruitment: a skeptical look at the opening and collapse story. Am J Respir Crit Care Med. 2002;165:1647–53.
9. Costa EL, Amato MB. The new definition for acute lung injury and acute respiratory distress syndrome: is there room for improvement? Curr Opin Crit Care. 2013;19:16–23.
10. Ranieri VM, Rubenfeld GD, Thompson BT, et al. Acute respiratory distress syndrome: the Berlin definition. JAMA. 2012;307:2526–33.

11. Gattinoni L, Pelosi P, Suter PM, Pedoto A, Vercesi P, Lissoni A. Acute respiratory distress syndrome caused by pulmonary and extrapulmonary disease. Different syndromes? Am J Respir Crit Care Med. 1998;158:3–11.
12. Brun-Buisson C, Minelli C, Bertolini G, et al. Epidemiology and outcome of acute lung injury in European intensive care units. Results from the ALIVE study. Intensive Care Med. 2004;30:51–61.
13. Kushimoto S, Endo T, Yamanouchi S, et al. Relationship between extravascular lung water and severity categories of acute respiratory distress syndrome by the Berlin definition. Crit Care. 2013;17:R132.
14. Villar J, Sulemanji D, Kacmarek RM. The acute respiratory distress syndrome: incidence and mortality, has it changed? Curr Opin Crit Care. 2014;20:3–9.
15. Biehl M, Kashiouris MG, Gajic O. Ventilator-induced lung injury: minimizing its impact in patients with or at risk for ARDS. Respir Care. 2013;58:927–37.
16. Matthay MA, Ware LB, Zimmerman GA. The acute respiratory distress syndrome. J Clin Invest. 2012;122:2731–40.
17. Cressoni M, Caironi P, Polli F, et al. Anatomical and functional intrapulmonary shunt in acute respiratory distress syndrome. Crit Care Med. 2008;36:669–75.
18. Coffey RL, Albert RK, Robertson HT. Mechanisms of physiological dead space response to PEEP after acute oleic acid lung injury. J Appl Physiol Respir Environ Exerc Physiol. 1983;55:1550–7.
19. Kallet RH, Katz JA. Respiratory system mechanics in acute respiratory distress syndrome. Respir Care Clin N Am. 2003;9:297–319.
20. Gattinoni L, Pesenti A. The concept of "baby lung". Intensive Care Med. 2005;31:776–84.
21. Pittet JF, Mackersie RC, Martin TR, Matthay MA. Biological markers of acute lung injury: prognostic and pathogenetic significance. Am J Respir Crit Care Med. 1997;155:1187–205.
22. Lassen HCA. A preliminary report on the 1952 epidemic of poliomyelitis in Copenhagen with special reference to the treatment of acute respiratory insufficiency. Lancet. 1953;1:37–41.
23. Avignon PD, Hedenstrom G, Edman C. Pulmonary complications in respirator patients. Acta Med Scand Suppl. 1956;316:86–90.
24. Mead J, Takishima TL, D. Stress distribution in lungs: a model of pulmonary elasticity. J Appl Physiol. 1970;28:596–608.
25. ARDSnetwork. Ventilation with lower tidal volumes as compared with traditional tidal volumes for acute lung injury and the acute respiratory distress syndrome. N Engl J Med. 2000;342:1301–8.
26. Gattinoni L, Carlesso E, Caironi P. Stress and strain within the lung. Curr Opin Crit Care. 2012;18:42–7.
27. Plataki M, Hubmayr RD. The physical basis of ventilator-induced lung injury. Expert Rev Respir Med. 2010;4:373–85.
28. O'Neill LA. TLRs play good cop, bad cop in the lung. Nat Med. 2005;11:1161–2.
29. Chiumello D, Carlesso E, Cadringher P, et al. Lung stress and strain during mechanical ventilation for acute respiratory distress syndrome. Am J Respir Crit Care Med. 2008;178:346–55.
30. Protti A, Votta E, Gattinoni L. Which is the most important strain in the pathogenesis of ventilator-induced lung injury: dynamic or static? Curr Opin Crit Care. 2014;20:33–8.
31. Protti A, Andreis DT, Monti M, et al. Lung stress and strain during mechanical ventilation: any difference between statics and dynamics? Crit Care Med. 2013;41:1046–55.
32. Gattinoni L, Carlesso E, Langer T. Towards ultraprotective mechanical ventilation. Curr Opin Anaesthesiol. 2012;25:141–7.
33. Putensen C, Zech S, Wrigge H, et al. Long-term effects of spontaneous breathing during ventilatory support in patients with acute lung injury. Am J Respir Crit Care Med. 2001;164:43–9.
34. Wrigge H, Zinserling J, Neumann P, et al. Spontaneous breathing improves lung aeration in oleic acidinduced lung injury. Anesthesiology. 2003;99:376–84.
35. Levine S, Nguyen T, Taylor N, et al. Rapid disuse atrophy of diaphragm fibers in mechanically ventilated humans. N Engl J Med. 2008;358:1327–13.

36. Milic-Emili J. Ventilation distribution. In: Hamid Q, Shannon J, Martin J, editors. Physiologic basis of respiratory disease. Ontario: BC Decker; 2005. p. 133–40.
37. Krueger JJ, Bain T, Patterson JL. Elevation gradient of intrathoracic pressure. J Appl Physiol. 1961;16:465–8.
38. Gama de Abreu M, Cuevas M, Spieth PM, et al. Regional lung aeration and ventilation during pressure support and biphasic positive airway pressure ventilation in experimental lung injury. Crit Care. 2010;14:R34.
39. Neumann P, Wrigge H, Zinserling J, et al. Spontaneous breathing affects the spatial ventilation and perfusion distribution during mechanical ventilatory support. Crit Care Med. 2005;33:1090–5.
40. Perlman CE, Lederer DJ, Bhattacharya J. Micromechanics of alveolar edema. Am J Respir Cell Mol Biol. 2010;44:34–9.
41. Yoshida T, Uchiyama A, Matsuura N, Mashimo T, Fujino Y. Spontaneous breathing during lung-protective ventilation in an experimental acute lung injury model: high transpulmonary pressure associated with strong spontaneous breathing effort may worsen lung injury. Crit Care Med. 2012;40:1578–85.
42. Yoshida T, Roldan R, Beraldo MA, et al. Spontaneous effort during mechanical ventilation: maximal injury with less positive end- expiratory pressure. Crit Care Med. 2016;44:1–11.
43. Yoshida T, Fujino Y, Amato M, Kavanagh B. Fifty years of research in ARDS. Spontaneous breathing during mechanical ventilation - risks, mechanisms & management. Am J Respir Crit Care Med. 2017;195:985–92.
44. Goligher EC, Annemijn H, Jonkman AH, Dianti J, et al. Clinical strategies for implementing lung and diaphragm-protective ventilation: avoiding insufficient and excessive effort. Intensive Care Med. 2020;46:2314–26.
45. Gattinoni L, Pesenti A, Carlesso E. Body position changes redistribute lung computed-tomographic density in patients with acute respiratory failure: impact and clinical fallout through the following 20 years. Intensive Care Med. 2013;39:1909–15.
46. Gattinoni L, Pelosi P, Vitale G, Pesenti A, D'Andrea L, Mascheroni D. Body position changes redistribute lung computed-tomographic density in patients with acute respiratory failure. Anesthesiology. 1991;74:15–23.
47. Ma B, Sanderson M, Bates JHT. Airway-parenchymal interdependence in the lung slice. Respir Physiol Neurobiol. 2013;185:211–6.
48. Milic-Emili J, Henderson JA, Dolovich MB, Trop D, Kaneko K. Regional distribution of inspired gas in the lung. J Appl Physiol. 1966;21:749–59.
49. Winkler T, Suki B. Emergent structure–function relations in emphysema and asthma. Crit Rev Biomed Eng. 2011;39:263–80.
50. Gattinoni L, Tonetti T, Quintel M. Regional physiology of ARDS. Crit Care. 2017;21:9–14.

Laryngeal Injury: Impact on Patients in the Acute and Chronic Phases

11

E. Kelly, S. Wallace, and Z. Puthucheary

11.1 Introduction

The endotracheal tube (ETT) passes through a vulnerable anatomical region for laryngeal function. Iatrogenic effects of intubation may result in injury to these structures, resulting in an altered upper airway or compromised communication and swallow function. These injuries have a negative impact on the patient both in the acute and chronic phase. This narrative review addresses the key concerns for clinicians working in this setting, delineating current practices in assessment and management, and future directions.

11.2 Laryngeal Injury

11.2.1 Endotracheal Intubation

Intubation is an essential intervention in the critical care unit, though its impact on the larynx is known to be associated with laryngeal injury [1]. Laryngeal injury in the acute phase may result in significant consequences for the patient, such as the

E. Kelly (✉)
Adult Critical Care Unit, Royal London Hospital, Barts Health, London, UK
e-mail: eileen.kelly3@nhs.net

S. Wallace
Critical Care, Wythenshawe Hospital Manchester, Manchester University NHS Foundation Trust, Manchester, UK

Z. Puthucheary
William Harvey Research Institute, Barts and The London School of Medicine and Dentistry, Queen Mary University of London, London, UK

Department of Intensive Care, Royal London Hospital, Barts Health NHS Trust, London, UK

J.-L. Vincent (ed.), *Annual Update in Intensive Care and Emergency Medicine 2022*, Annual Update in Intensive Care and Emergency Medicine,
https://doi.org/10.1007/978-3-030-93433-0_11

need for re-intubation, nosocomial pneumonia and prolonged length of intensive care unit (ICU) stay [1, 2]. More than twice as many patients who undergo endotracheal intubation will sustain moderate or severe injury, manifesting as airway, voice or swallowing impairment, than will have no injury [1]. Delayed assessment of these injuries and their severity may result in a protracted ICU and hospital stay [1].

Laryngeal trauma may occur at the time the ETT is placed or later during the period of intubation. Passing orally through the larynx and eventually to the trachea, the ETT contacts the base of the tongue, epiglottis, cricoarytenoid joints, posterior glottis, arytenoid cartilages, vocal folds, and subglottis [3, 4]. Additionally, it is recognized that urgent or emergency intubation increases the risk of laryngeal injury. Many who are admitted to the ICU present with known airway obstruction or difficult airway, reported in up to 6% of ICU patients, which may pose further risk of laryngeal trauma during the intubation phase [4, 5].

Depending on the reason for intubation, mechanical ventilation via the ETT may be transient or prolonged. Although duration of intubation has been shown to be associated with laryngeal injury, with increased severity of injury noted in those intubated for >5 days, even transient intubation can result in laryngeal injury [1, 4, 6]. Complications increase with the size of the tracheal tube used and vary with the design of the tube and cuff [4]. For those who require prolonged mechanical ventilation, complications increase with the duration of intubation [1]. The risk of vocal fold paralysis increases two-fold in patients intubated for longer than 6 h, and the risk of laryngeal stenosis increases to 5% for those intubated for up to 10 days [4]. Prolonged intubation via an ETT may damage the laryngeal structures through the impact of the pressure of the tube itself or the cuff on the submucosa, perichondrium and cartilage [4]. Due to the configuration of the glottis and the path of the ETT, main injuries tend to occur in the posterior portion of the larynx and vocal processes [4]. If the ETT cuff sits too high or the cuff pressure exceeds capillary perfusion pressure, the recurrent laryngeal nerve responsible for innervating laryngeal musculature may be compressed [4]. Patient movement, coughing, or patient-attempted extubation may further compound the risk of laryngeal injury.

11.2.2 Identification and Management of Laryngeal Injury in the Acute Phase

Identification of laryngeal injury and its associated symptoms typically occurs after extubation. In the majority of settings, laryngeal function is not directly evaluated prior to extubation. The presence of the ETT precludes direct visualization of the upper airway; however, the cuff leak test has been used to predict the presence of laryngeal edema or airway obstruction with excellent specificity [7]. The role of laryngeal ultrasound in predicting extubation success has been explored, however its sensitivity for detecting upper airway obstruction falls below that of the cuff leak test and caution is advised in applying this diagnostic tool without further research [8].

Laryngeal injury therefore may only be detected following extubation. Laryngeal edema, airway obstruction, post-extubation stridor, arytenoid dislocation, vocal fold injury (palsy or paresis) or laryngeal stenosis have all been reported as consequences of injury in the acute phase [1, 4, 7]. These injuries may result in the need for re-intubation, which is associated with an increase in morbidity, duration of mechanical ventilation, and ICU stay [9]. Laryngeal injury may also manifest as post-extubation dysphagia, a significant complication which is associated with poorer patient outcomes, such as pneumonia, in-hospital mortality, and requirement for feeding tubes [10].

Despite the high incidence rates of laryngeal injury reported post-extubation and its negative consequences, there is no international consensus on the most appropriate timing or method of assessment of laryngeal function [1]. Identifying the nature and severity of laryngeal injury is imperative to establishing appropriate management. Timely assessment can be coordinated by the ICU multidisciplinary team and involve a variety of other disciplines [1]. Direct visualization of the larynx enables definitive appreciation of its structures and their function. Fiberoptic endoscopic evaluation of swallowing (FEES) can evaluate secretion management, vocal fold mobility, detect aspiration, and provide detailed assessment of the function of the pharynx and larynx [4]. FEES is a portable, sensitive diagnostic tool that can be carried out at the bedside by speech and language therapists. The ICU medical team, affiliated medical or surgical teams, nursing staff, physiotherapists, dietitians, and the patient can view FEES images at the bedside, promoting multidisciplinary team discussion and decision making. Findings can be discussed immediately, resulting in timely interventions and onward referrals to specialist teams, such as ear nose and throat (ENT) surgeons. Individualized management can be initiated at this point, and may include prescription of glucocorticoids, anti-reflux medications, surgical intervention by ENT surgeons and therapy by speech and language therapists for dysphagia and voice, improving management of laryngeal injury within the acute ICU phase [1]. Figure 11.1 illustrates some common laryngeal injuries visualized on FEES.

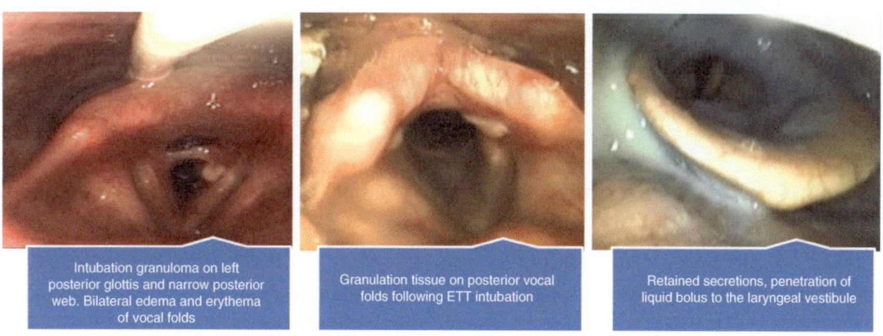

Fig. 11.1 Laryngeal injury as seen on fiberoptic endoscopic evaluation of swallowing. *ETT* endotracheal tube

11.3 Impact of Laryngeal Injury on the Patient in the Acute Phase

11.3.1 Swallowing and Return to Oral Intake

Laryngeal injury may manifest as post-extubation dysphagia. The reported incidence rates of dysphagia following mechanical ventilation are highly variable, with a range of 3-62% [1, 11, 12]. For those requiring ICU admission for acute respiratory failure, conservative estimates put the incidence of post-extubation dysphagia in the range of 20% [13]. The etiology of the dysphagia is the strongest determinant of the duration of dysfunction [13, 14]. Factors associated with dysphagia immediately post-extubation have been reported as prolonged intubation via ETT, repeated intubations, age, female sex, obesity, diabetes mellitus, hypertension, laryngopharyngeal reflux and malnutrition [4, 13, 15].

Post-extubation dysphagia is characterized by impaired secretion management, airway penetration/aspiration, delayed swallow onset, and post-swallow residue [16]. Post-extubation dysphagia may be compounded by ICU-acquired weakness, which can affect peripheral and respiratory muscles [17]. The incidence of ICU-acquired weakness may be as high as 46% in the septic or prolonged mechanical ventilation cohort, with up to 30% muscle mass loss reported to occur within the first 10 days [18]. Additionally, a combination of these factors may contribute to sarcopenia-related dysphagia, which has been demonstrated in elderly patients, highlighting the association between polyneuropathy and dysphagia in the ICU [19, 20].

Up to 36% of critically ill patients with post-extubation dysphagia present with silent aspiration [13]. Silent aspiration, alongside dependence for oral hygiene, poor mobility and respiratory compromise, may result in aspiration pneumonia. Aspiration pneumonia leads to negative health outcomes, such as mortality and increased length of hospital stay [2]. Early referral for comprehensive evaluation allows for identification of post-extubation dysphagia and selection of the most accurate assessment method. Diagnosis of dysphagia may be reached by clinical bedside evaluation or through the use of instrumental evaluation of swallow, such as FEES. Identification of silent aspiration using instrumental assessment early in the patient's journey can minimize setbacks and conversely reduce patients being placed 'nil by mouth' unnecessarily, reducing the need for tube feeding [4].

11.3.2 Communication in the ICU

Inability to vocalize during critical illness can be a significant contributing factor to delirium, anxiety and psychological distress. Research evaluating patient experience during ICU admission reports this as one of the most frustrating and anxious experiences for mechanically ventilated patients [21]. Patients who have experienced loss of communication have reported feeling trapped, caged, and with a loss of personhood and control [21]. Facilitating communication is a responsibility for all the multidisciplinary team and is vital for the patient's engagement in rehabilitation on the ward.

Change in vocal function following endotracheal intubation may result in difficulty communicating. Symptoms of post-extubation dysphonia may include hoarseness, reduced volume, or a complete absence of voice in those with severe injuries. Dysphonia incidence rates in the post-extubation population are reported to be as high as 76% [1]. Compromised respiratory function may also contribute to vocal quality, with the impact of breathlessness or vocal fatigue a potential exacerbating factor for vocal fold pathology [22]. While alternative communication devices such as picture boards, whiteboards or technology may assist with basic commands, they cannot replace restoration of voice and should only be used if natural communication is not possible [23].

Loss of voice may contribute to delirium in the ICU. Delirium is characterized by impaired cognitive function, resulting in reduced ability to receive, process, and store information. Delirium impacts negatively on the acute phase of illness, and is associated with poor outcomes including increased length of hospital stay and higher mortality rates [24]. Delirium can occur in up to 83% in those who are mechanically ventilated [24]. Reduced ability to communicate in this setting results in poorer pain management, lack of engagement in treatment and rehabilitation strategies, and the inability to communicate basic needs [25]. Early identification of communication impairment, especially prior to extubation, aims to identify and support those with language or voice impairments in this early stage of care [26].

11.4 Impact of Laryngeal Injury on the Patient in the Chronic Phase

The long-term consequences of critical illness have gained traction in recent years, as the short-term mortality after critical illness decreases [27]. The majority of ICU patients have expectations beyond survival [28]. Patients have reported reduced ability to undertake activities of daily living, which may include social interactions or gainful employment [29]. Airway, swallow, and voice impairment are known to impact on quality of life; however, laryngeal injury is not routinely screened for in ICU follow-up clinics. Previous research identifying the incidence of laryngeal injury following extubation has focused on the acute phase, and data pertaining to persistent features is lacking [1, 2, 12, 30].

Dysphagia has been shown to persist beyond hospital discharge in those with severe sepsis, with almost 21% requiring restricted oral intake and partial tube-assisted nutrition [31]. Laryngotracheal stenosis can occur in up to 5% of patients following prolonged intubation, and may result in compromised airway, dyspnea, stridor, or even respiratory failure [4]. This serious complication often requires multiple surgical procedures. The breathlessness experienced by patients also impacts on swallowing and can result in dysphagia [32]. Post-ICU follow up clinics and those working in primary care should screen for airway and laryngeal problems when breathlessness, dysphonia, or dysphagia are reported in those who have undergone ETT intubation and/or tracheostomy [4].

Despite widely acknowledged recognition of the need for post-ICU follow up services, there remains a lack of standardization of service delivery, clinical measurement of patient outcomes, and identification of tools for rehabilitation needs in this cohort [33]. In the United Kingdom, the post-ICU presentation screen (PICUPS) has been developed to address this need [33]. The PICUPS tool aims to identify the needs of patients stepping down from the ICU to acute wards, and to signpost referrals to areas of ongoing need. Laryngeal injury is a key component of the PICUPS tool, with clinicians asked to consider its function across a range of domains including tracheostomy, communication, breathing, voice, and swallowing. Beyond the acute phase, vocal changes, which may manifest as hoarseness, vocal fatigue, breathlessness, or resonance changes, may impact on an individual's return to work and daily interactions. Specialist follow-up clinics may be required to manage dysphonia and its impact on return to work and quality of life [34]. However, the role of laryngeal function assessments in follow-up clinics is ill-defined. There are opportunities to re-design care pathways for this cohort, as the most effective method of delivering follow up ICU services has not been established [17]. There is a paucity of research pertaining to the longer-term consequences of laryngeal injury beyond ICU, with an absence of patient-reported outcomes and quality of life measures discussed in the available research. Determining the impact of laryngeal injury on the ability to return to work, participate in social engagements and daily activities will greater support the rationale for screening in ICU clinics. It is unlikely that persistent features of laryngeal injury exist in isolation from other post-intensive care symptoms, given that more than half of all ICU patients present with a new disability at 6 months post-hospital discharge [35]. Understanding the trajectory of recovery and the follow-up services required may further guide discussions regarding post-intensive care follow-up and aid prognostication for this complex patient cohort.

11.5 Laryngeal Injury in the ICU and beyond

11.5.1 Clinical Assessment: Future Directions

Given the large numbers of critically ill patients requiring ETT intubation, it is not feasible to complete an instrumental assessment such as FEES for all patients [2]. Specialist diagnostic swallow assessments such as FEES are typically delivered by speech and language therapists, who may not be present in all ICUs or, if present, have restricted availability. In the United Kingdom, the Guidelines for Provision of Intensive Care Services (GPICS) provide minimum staffing recommendations for speech and language therapist input in critical care and advocate for timely assessment [36].

In the absence of assessment by speech and language therapists, bedside screening tools exist to detect dysphagia. However, all bedside screening tools have issues with sensitivity and specificity and there is no universally accepted screening tool for dysphagia in the ICU population [12, 37]. A systematic review in this area supported the use of the Water Swallow Test (WST), which may be a starting point for identifying patients at risk of dysphagia in the ICU cohort [38]. Implementation of an appropriate screening tool in the ICU may reduce time to return to oral intake for patients when speech and language therapist services are not available in a timely manner. However, patients silently aspirating remain difficult to detect at the bedside and pose a greater medical risk for aspiration pneumonia, and these patients require specialist assessment. The clinician should also remain cognizant that around one-third of tracheostomized patients who 'pass' a bedside swallow assessment are at risk of aspiration or failed decannulation [4].

Laryngeal ultrasound has been discussed as an exploratory non-invasive clinical tool for identifying laryngeal and supra-stomal abnormalities and could be explored in the process of tracheostomy decannulation or swallow evaluations. There is increasing interest in ultrasound development for diagnostic and monitoring purposes, due to its safety, lack of radiation, rapid application, and real-time dynamic feedback [39]. The severe acute respiratory syndrome coronavirus 2 (SARS-CoV-2) global pandemic has challenged clinicians' abilities to complete instrumental assessments such as endoscopy, secondary to the risk of completing aerosol generating procedures affecting transmissibility of the disease. This challenge has encouraged clinicians to explore alternative approaches to clinical care, including developments in laryngeal ultrasound. However, a recent rapid review by an international expert panel recommended caution for its use as a comprehensive swallow assessment [40]. An emerging role in assessment of laryngeal structures associated with swallow function has been identified; however in the absence of a standardized, evidence-based protocol the current literature does not support its use as a tool in isolation [40].

Screening for other features of laryngeal injury, such as dysphonia or laryngotracheal stenosis remains less defined. Typically, dysphonia will present as loss of voice, hoarseness, reduced volume, or impaired cough [4]. Use of a post-ICU screening tool, such as the PICUPS tool, can support identification of complications associated with the upper airway. In the follow up setting, patient-reported outcome questionnaires, such as the Voice Handicap Index-10 [41], may guide clinicians to the most appropriate specialist onward referral.

11.5.2 Laryngeal Rehabilitation

Promotion and restoration of laryngeal function to enable swallowing and communication is a key principle of management [4]. Rehabilitation may take the form of tailored voice and swallowing exercises, targeting vocal fold closure, increased breath support for speech, secretion clearance and management and biomechanical swallow exercises. These may include established rehabilitation exercises or newer equipment-based therapies such as pharyngeal electrical stimulation and expiratory muscle strength training. Pharyngeal electrical stimulation is indicated for patients with sensory dysphagia, which is frequently the main component in laryngeal dysfunction in critical illness. Research in this population is in its early stages but indications are that it may be beneficial for return to oral intake [42]. A prospective study examining the implementation of pharyngeal electrical stimulation in stroke patients with tracheostomy demonstrated expedited decannulation times in those who received the treatment within 1 month of their stroke [43]. The use of compensatory strategies as directed by speech and language therapists can also support return to safe oral intake, including altering bolus size and delivery, and diet and fluid modification.

Dysphagia and dysphonia in critical care may be the result of direct laryngeal trauma, ICU-acquired weakness, and altered sensation in the upper airway [44]. Identification of the most appropriate interventions to target the impaired swallow mechanism remains an area of ongoing development. According to a recent systematic review evaluating interventions for oropharyngeal dysphagia in the ICU, there is a wide variability in the methods of intervention, reported outcomes, and duration of rehabilitation provided [44].

11.5.3 Community Follow Up of Critical Illness Survivors

The optimal provision of laryngeal assessment in ICU follow-up clinics remains unclear. For those already working with ICU patients in follow-up clinics, assessment should be guided by a biopsychosocial model of care that evaluates structure and function, limitations in activities, and restrictions as a result of airway, voice, and swallow impairment. While it is unlikely given the abundance of screening tools available that a newly designed tool is needed, consideration for the validity and reliability of the tool selected is pertinent [38]. For the cognitively intact patient, use of validated patient-reported outcomes, such as the Voice Handicap IndexVHI-10 [41] and the Eating Assessment Tool (EAT-10) [45], may be useful tools to identify those needing onward referrals to specialist services.

In the context of coronavirus disease 2019 (COVID-19), there have been increased calls for symptoms of laryngeal injury to be considered in follow-up clinics. A global collaboration of experts concluded the need for well-resourced rehabilitation within and beyond the ICU [46]. Prior to the pandemic, an international stakeholders task force focusing on respiratory cohorts identified problems relating to the larynx, voice, and swallowing after extubation and their connection to long term impairments as another research gap [27]. Clarity is needed as to the best method of implementing services in this population, and remains an area for future research. Comprehensive multidisciplinary team follow up, using frameworks to identify areas of ongoing patient need, may allow for referral to specialist services.

11.6 Conclusion

Laryngeal injury following endotracheal intubation is associated with negative health consequences for patients in the ICU, such as mortality, aspiration pneumonia, delayed resumption of oral intake, and malnutrition. As well as the associated healthcare costs, these complications have a negative impact on patient quality of life and result in prolonged ICU and hospital lengths of stay. Early consideration, identification, and management of laryngeal injury in the acute and chronic phases is the first step towards improving patient outcomes in this cohort.

References

1. Brodsky MB, Levy MJ, Jedlanek E, et al. Laryngeal injury and upper airway symptoms after oral endotracheal intubation with mechanical ventilation during critical care: a systematic review. Crit Care Med. 2018;46:2010–7.
2. McIntyre M, Doeltgen S, Dalton N, Koppa M, Chimunda T. Post-extubation dysphagia incidence in critically ill patients: a systematic review and meta-analysis. Aust Crit Care. 2021;34:67–75.
3. Mota LA, de Cavalho GB, Brito VA. Laryngeal complications by orotracheal intubation: literature review. Int Arch Otorhinolaryngol. 2012;16:236–45.
4. Wallace S, McGrath BA. Laryngeal complications after tracheal intubation and tracheostomy. BJA Educ. 2021;21:250–7.
5. Higgs A, McGrath BA, Goddard C, et al. Guidelines for the management of tracheal intubation in critically ill adults. Br J Anaesth. 2018;120:323–52.
6. Shinn JR, Kimura KS, Campbell BR, et al. Incidence and outcomes of acute laryngeal injury after prolonged mechanical ventilation. Crit Care Med. 2019;47:1699–706.
7. Kuriyama A, Jackson JL, Kamei J. Performance of the cuff leak test in adults in predicting post-extubation airway complications: a systematic review and meta-analysis. Crit Care. 2020;24:640.
8. Sahbal M, Kamel M, Zaghla H, Kenawy M. Laryngeal ultrasound versus cuff leak test in prediction of post-extubation stridor. Egypt J Crit Care Med. 2017;5:83–6.
9. Frutos-Vivar F, Esteban A, Apezteguia C, et al. Outcome of reintubated patients after scheduled extubation. J Crit Care. 2011;26:502–9.
10. Macht M, Wimbish T, Clark BJ, Benson AB, Burnham EL, Williams A, Moss M. Postextubation dysphagia is persistent and associated with poor outcomes in survivors of critical illness. Crit Care. 2011;15:R231.
11. Schefold JC, Berger D, Zürcher P, et al. Dysphagia in mechanically ventilated icu patients (DYnAMICS): a prospective observational trial. Crit Care Med. 2017;45:2061–9.
12. Skoretz SA, Flowers HL, Martino R. The incidence of dysphagia following endotracheal intubation: a systematic review. Chest. 2010;137:665–73.
13. Macht M, White SD, Moss M. Swallowing dysfunction after critical illness. Chest. 2014;146:1681–9.
14. Martino R, Foley N, Bhogal S, Diamant N, Speechley M, Teasell R. Dysphagia after stroke: incidence, diagnosis, and pulmonary complications. Stroke. 2005;36:2756–63.
15. Tadié JM, Behm E, Lecuyer L, et al. Post-intubation laryngeal injuries and extubation failure: a fiberoptic endoscopic study. Intensive Care Med. 2010;36:991–8.
16. Scheel R, Pisegna JM, McNally E, Noordzij JP, Langmore SE. Endoscopic assessment of swallowing after prolonged intubation in the ICU setting. Ann Otol Rhinol Laryngol. 2016;125:43–52.

17. Hermans G, Van den Berghe G. Clinical review: intensive care unit acquired weakness. Crit Care. 2015;19:274.
18. Appleton RT, Kinsella J, Quasim T. The incidence of intensive care unit-acquired weakness syndromes: a systematic review. J Intensive Care Soc. 2015;16:126–36.
19. Zhao WT, Yang M, Wu HM, Yang L, Zhang XM, Huang Y. Systematic review and meta-analysis of the association between sarcopenia and dysphagia. J Nutr Health Aging. 2018;22:1003–9.
20. Ponfick M, Linden R, Nowak DA. Dysphagia--a common, transient symptom in critical illness polyneuropathy: a fiberoptic endoscopic evaluation of swallowing study. Crit Care Med. 2015;43:365–72.
21. Ford DW, Martin-Harris B. I miss the sound of your voice: earlier speech in tracheostomy patients. Crit Care Med. 2016;44:1234–5.
22. Royal College of Speech and Language Therapists. Position Statement: Speech and language therapists working in adult and paediatric critical care units. Available from https://www.rcslt.org/wp-content/uploads/media/docs/clinical-guidance/rcslt-position-statement-critical-care.pdf?la=en&hash=42823C17957D4848818438CBCD5DC3998EF0CDF7. Accessed 21 Oct 2021.
23. Sutt AL, Fraser JF. Patients want to be heard-loud and clear! Crit Care. 2017;21:6.
24. Ely EW, Inouye SK, Bernard GR, et al. Delirium in mechanically ventilated patients: validity and reliability of the confusion assessment method for the intensive care unit (CAM-ICU). JAMA. 2001;286:2703–10.
25. Barr J, Fraser GL, Puntillo K, et al. Clinical practice guidelines for the management of pain, agitation, and delirium in adult patients in the intensive care unit. Crit Care Med. 2013;41:263–306.
26. Royal College of Speech and Language Therapists. COVID-19 Speech and language therapy rehabilitation pathway: Part of the Intensive Care Society Rehabilitation Framework. Available at: https://www.rcslt.org/wp-content/uploads/media/docs/Covid/RCSLT-COVID-19-SLT-rehab-pathway_15-July-2020_FINAL.pdf?la=en&hash=29A7914A98103BDDF61ECAA072A70C80FBF50551 Accessed 21Oct 2021.
27. Needham DM, Davidson J, Cohen H, et al. Improving long-term outcomes after discharge from intensive care unit: report from a stakeholders' conference. Crit Care Med. 2012;40:502–9.
28. Bose S, Hoenig B, Karamourtopoulos M, et al. Beyond survival: identifying what matters to survivors of critical illness. Crit Care. 2021;25:129.
29. Moloney J, Walshe M. Managing and supporting quality-of-life issues in dysphagia: a survey of clinical practice patterns and perspectives in the UK, Ireland and South Africa. Int J Lang Commun Disord. 2019;54:41–9.
30. Brodsky MB, Akst LM, Jedlanek E, et al. Laryngeal injury and upper airway symptoms after endotracheal intubation during surgery: a systematic review and meta-analysis. Anesth Analg. 2021;132:1023–32.
31. Zielske J, Bohne S, Brunkhorst FM, Axer H, Guntinas-Lichius O. Acute and long-term dysphagia in critically ill patients with severe sepsis: results of a prospective controlled observational study. Eur Arch Otorhinolaryngol. 2014;271:3085–93.
32. Clunie GM, Roe JWG, Alexander C, Sandhu G, McGregor A. Voice and swallowing outcomes following airway reconstruction in adults: a systematic review. Laryngoscope. 2021;131:146–57.
33. Turner-Stokes L, Corner EJ, Siegert RJ, et al. The post-ICU presentation screen (PICUPS) and rehabilitation prescription (RP) for intensive care survivors part I: development and preliminary clinimetric evaluation. J Intensive Care Soc. 2021; Feb 18, https://doi.org/10.1177/1751143720988715, Epub ahead of print.
34. Royal College of Speech and Language Therapists. Position statement: speech and language therapists working with individuals with voice disorders. Available at: https://www.rcslt.org/wp-content/uploads/media/docs/clinical-guidance/voice-position-statement.pdf Accessed 21 Oct 2021.
35. Higgins AM, Neto AS, Bailey M, et al. Predictors of death and new disability after critical illness: a multicentre prospective cohort study. Intensive Care Med. 2021;47:772–81.

36. The Faculty of Intensive Care Medicine. Guidelines for the Provision of Intensive Care Services. Available at https://www.ficm.ac.uk/sites/default/files/gpics-v2.pdf. Accessed 21 Oct 2021.
37. Zuercher P, Moret CS, Dziewas R, et al. Dysphagia in the intensive care unit: epidemiology, mechanisms, and clinical management. Crit Care. 2019;23:103.
38. Brodsky MB, Suiter DM, González-Fernández M, Michtalik HJ, Frymark TB, Venediktov R, Schooling T. Screening accuracy for aspiration using bedside water swallow tests: a systematic review and meta-analysis. Chest. 2016;150:148–63.
39. Ding LW, Wang HC, Wu HD, Chang CJ, Yang PC. Laryngeal ultrasound: a useful method in predicting post-extubation stridor. A pilot study. Eur Respir J. 2006;27:384–9.
40. Allen JE, Clunie GM, Slinger C, et al. Utility of ultrasound in the assessment of swallowing and laryngeal function: a rapid review and critical appraisal of the literature. Int J Lang Commun Disord. 2021;56:174–204.
41. Rosen CA, Lee AS, Osborne J, Zullo T, Murry T. Development and validation of the voice handicap index-10. Laryngoscope. 2004;114:1549–56.
42. Wallace S, Knight S, McGrath B, Templeton R. Efficacy of pharyngeal electrical stimulation treatment (PES) for dysphagia in critical care patients. Dysphagia. 2020;35:173.
43. Dziewas R, Stellato R, van der Tweel I, et al. Pharyngeal electrical stimulation for early decannulation in tracheotomised patients with neurogenic dysphagia after stroke (PHAST-TRAC): a prospective, single-blinded, randomised trial. Lancet Neurol. 2018;17:849–59.
44. Duncan S, McAuley DF, Walshe M, McGaughey J, Anand R, Fallis R, Blackwood B. Interventions for oropharyngeal dysphagia in acute and critical care: a systematic review and meta-analysis. Intensive Care Med. 2020;46:1326–38.
45. Belafsky PC, Mouadeb DA, Rees CJ, Pryor JC, Postma GN, Allen J, Leonard RJ. Validity and reliability of the eating assessment tool (EAT-10). Ann Otol Rhinol Laryngol. 2008;117:919–24.
46. Freeman-Sanderson A, Ward EC, Miles A, et al. A consensus statement for the management and rehabilitation of communication and swallowing function in the ICU: a global response to COVID-19. Arch Phys Med Rehabil. 2021;102:835–42.

Part IV

Fluids and Electrolytes

Fluid Responsiveness as a Physiologic Endpoint to Improve Successful Weaning

12

R. Castro, P. Born, and J. Bakker

12.1 Introduction

The recommended therapeutic strategy for hypotensive patients with poor tissue perfusion is rapid fluid resuscitation, usually performed with goal-directed endpoints [1, 2]. However, current fluid administration practice in critically ill patients is highly variable, not just aiming at restoring oxygen delivery or correcting hypovolemia, but also pursuing a variety of other objectives that are not always physiologically supported [3]. After resuscitation, it is frequent to find that patients received more fluid than required. In patients with septic shock, Rivers et al. showed that 4.9 l of crystalloids were given in the first 6 h and 13.4 l in the first 72 h [1]. In our study on organ dysfunction and septic shock, the fluid balance reached up to 1.6 ± 3.0 l at 72 h [4]. Fluid overload, which has been defined as a fluid accumulation greater than 10% of the patient's baseline body weight [5, 6], is usually associated with some degree of pulmonary and peripheral edema, together with preload

R. Castro · P. Born
Departamento de Medicina Intensiva, Facultad de Medicina, Pontificia Universidad Católica de Chile, Santiago, Chile

J. Bakker (✉)
Departamento de Medicina Intensiva, Facultad de Medicina, Pontificia Universidad Católica de Chile, Santiago, Chile

Department of Intensive Care Adults, Erasmus MC University Medical Center, Rotterdam, The Netherlands

Department of Pulmonary and Critical Care, New York University School of Medicine, New York, NY, USA

Division of Pulmonary, Allergy, and Critical Care Medicine, Columbia University College of Physicians and Surgeons, New York, NY, USA
e-mail: jb3387@cumc.columbia.edu

J.-L. Vincent (ed.), *Annual Update in Intensive Care and Emergency Medicine 2022*, Annual Update in Intensive Care and Emergency Medicine,
https://doi.org/10.1007/978-3-030-93433-0_12

unresponsiveness [7]. Fluid balance, which is the arithmetic difference between input (resuscitation and non-resuscitation fluids) and output (diuresis, bleeding, surgical drains, etc.), is routinely computed in the intensive care unit (ICU). A positive fluid balance is associated with increased morbidity and mortality in critically ill patients [6, 8] and in patients with acute kidney injury [9], among other deleterious effects [10, 11]. Conversely, achieving a negative fluid balance may increase survival in patients with septic shock [12] and decrease the duration of the weaning process [13].

Critically ill patients, by definition, exhibit an evolving life-threatening multisystemic process usually characterized by severe respiratory, cardiovascular, or neurological derangement, often in combination leading to significant morbidity and mortality. In this scenario, mechanical ventilation may be a life-saving intervention but its application is also associated with serious complications and costs, often linked to its duration [14, 15].

Weaning from mechanical ventilation is the process of gradually withdrawing ventilatory support that is normally started once the original cause of cardio/respiratory failure has improved. Extubation failure is an important contributor to adverse outcomes in critically ill patients, such as longer time on mechanical ventilation, longer ICU and hospital stays, and higher mortality [16, 17]. Therefore, shortening the mechanical ventilation period and successful extubation are crucial steps for every ICU patient [18–23]. Patients benefit from a reduction in ventilator- and ICU-related complications, as well as contributing to a reduction in healthcare costs accruing from a reduction in duration of ICU stay [24].

12.2 Weaning from Mechanical Ventilation

As mentioned, as soon as the underlying cause that led to mechanical ventilation has improved sufficiently, the clinician should start evaluating the potential for weaning and assess the probability of weaning success (Fig. 12.1). This is a process of iterative evaluations in order to build assurance around a safe and timely extubation [18]. In this sequence, the spontaneous breathing trial (SBT) is a simple, efficient, safe, and effective strategy [18] and there are standardized guidelines to perform it [25]. The aim of the SBT is to challenge the cardiovascular and respiratory systems, determining whether the patient is ready to be separated from the ventilator. Importantly, the patient's response to the SBT determines subsequent steps. If the patient is able to sustain spontaneous breathing and proper gas exchange, then extubation follows [26]. Careful clinical monitoring during the SBT is mandatory to desist from the trial when the patient does not tolerate it. Furthermore, monitoring may assist in the identification of the mechanisms leading to the SBT failure (e.g., increased systolic blood pressure, tachyarrhythmias, clinical signs of diaphragmatic dysfunction).

Despite its importance, the weaning process has not been rigorously defined, especially for those patients who exhibit fluid overload after several days in the

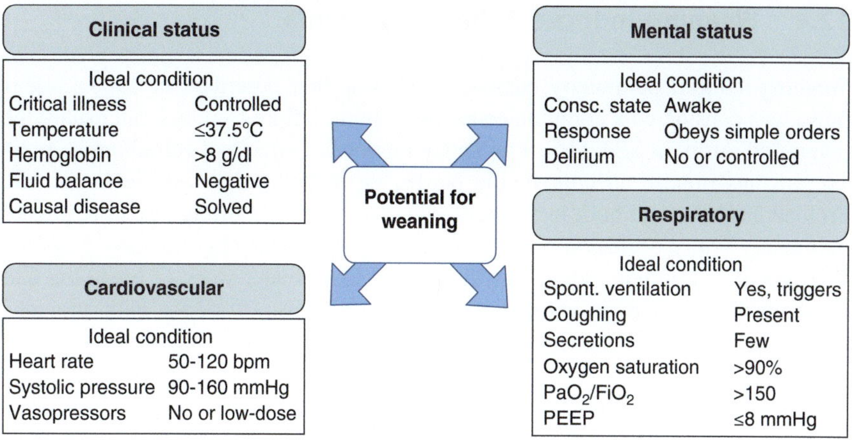

Fig. 12.1 To assess the potential for weaning or readiness to wean on a daily basis, at least four systems must be evaluated: clinical, respiratory, mental, and cardiovascular. Each of them can potentially determine weaning failure and must be properly addressed [27, 28]. *PEEP* positive end-expiratory pressure

ICU. In general, weaning definitions and practices are variable with only limited consensus on the topic [26]. From a hemodynamic perspective, weaning from mechanical ventilation could be seen as a cardiovascular stress test, equivalent to significant exercise [29]. The cardiac stress induced by the abrupt transition from mechanical ventilation to spontaneous breathing can induce both left and right ventricular dysfunction due to change in loading conditions, myocardial ischemia and, ultimately, cardiogenic pulmonary edema [30]. In fact, switching from mechanical ventilation to spontaneous breathing, causes intrathoracic pressure to go from uniformly positive across the ventilatory cycle to markedly negative, promoting both an increase in venous return and possibly impeding left ventricular (LV) ejection secondary to increased transmural pressure [31]. All these events are significantly aggravated when fluid overload is present, as a preload-independent heart will not be able to handle the increased venous return [32].

12.3 Weaning Failure

About 20% to 30% of mechanically ventilated patients are difficult to wean [26]. Weaning failure has been classically defined as the failure to pass an SBT or the need for reintubation within 48 h [53]. Failure of an SBT is often related to cardiovascular dysfunction or inability of the respiratory pump to support the load of breathing [18]. Extubation failure may be related to the same causes [18] with the addition of upper airway obstruction and excessive secretions [33].

12.4 Weaning-Induced Pulmonary Edema

Weaning-induced pulmonary edema, which was first described in 1988 [34], is nowadays considered a common cause of weaning failure [35] and can usually be diagnosed during a SBT [36]. Previously mentioned effects of intrathoracic pressure swings impose an unfavorable burden on both the right and left ventricle. Preload and afterload both increase, leading to greater LV filling pressure, greater pulmonary artery occlusion pressure (PAOP), and greater transcapillary pressure. The progressively more edematous lungs lead to a greater work of breathing and subsequently greater myocardial oxygen consumption. Patients with previous chronic heart or lung conditions represent a group particularly sensitive to this phenomenon [35].

A pragmatic and sequential approach has been proposed by Vignon [37], based on ultrasound as a diagnostic tool and a means to titrate therapy. Absence of increased filling pressure and volume overload surrogates as determined by echocardiography are potential endpoints of depletive therapy, but no threshold values have yet been properly validated.

The above discussed mechanisms are summarized in Fig. 12.2.

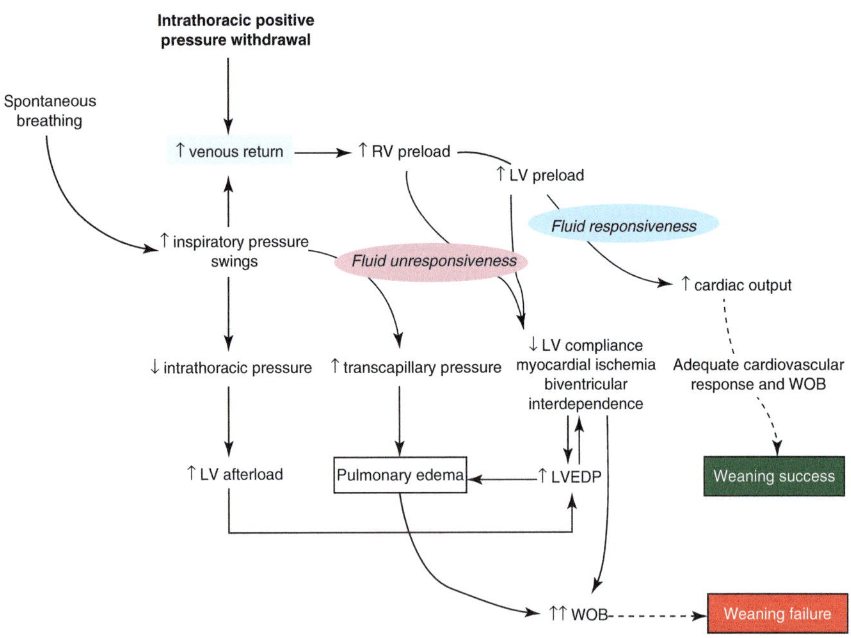

Fig. 12.2 Pathophysiology of weaning induced pulmonary edema and a probable role of fluid unresponsiveness as a determinant. *RV* right ventricular, *LV* left ventricular, *LVEDP* LV end-diastolic pressure, *WOB* work of breathing

12.5 De-Resuscitation

Although there is wide consensus on the need to deplete critically ill patients once the resuscitation phase has been completed [6, 38], there are no guidelines on how to de-resuscitate fluid overloaded patients [39]. Because fluid overload has been usually defined based on body weight increase [5], de-resuscitation is frequently intuitively driven by weight loss endpoints. An arbitrary negative fluid balance within a predefined time is pursued, usually by means of diuretics. However, overly enthusiastic fluid removal and resulting hypovolemia may give rise to convective problems causing regional hypoperfusion, tissue hypoxia, metabolic and acid-base alterations [6]. This may induce a new hit on a previously injured and dysfunctional organ, namely the "D" hit of the fluid stewardship model [40].

A restrictive fluid regimen with negative fluid balance combining high levels of positive end-expiratory pressure (PEEP), albumin administration, and furosemide or ultrafiltration was tested in patients receiving mechanical ventilation because of respiratory insufficiency. These patients had high extravascular lung water index (EVLWI) and intraabdominal pressure (IAP) values [41]. After 1 week of treatment, this approach showed beneficial effects on EVLWI, IAP, and organ function, resulting in a shorter duration of mechanical ventilation and lower 28-day mortality. No assessment of hypoperfusion, fluid responsiveness, cardiac function, or other dynamic parameters was performed. In addition, the authors recognized the presence of many selection biases. Notably, renal function deteriorated using this approach. Another study tested different depletive approaches in patients with acute decompensated heart failure [42]. Again, the endpoint was focused on fluid balance and treatment efficacy on weight loss achieved at 48 h. Authors reported that diuretic infusion resulted in comparable depletion to ultrafiltration in net fluid balance and weight loss. However, important cardiovascular and neurological adverse events were reported. Another study [43] evaluated the use of furosemide for fluid depletion in patients with early acute kidney injury. In this study, electrolyte abnormalities were frequent and important (hypokalemia, hypomagnesemia, hypernatremia), as well as pH alterations (metabolic alkalosis) that were relevant enough to discontinue the intervention.

These studies were intended to evaluate the efficacy and safety of different strategies on fluid depletion, and not to assess potential physiologic determinants of weaning failure. There is a lack of prospective studies looking for optimal clinical, physiological, biochemical, or organ-specific endpoints to guide the initiation and discontinuation of fluid removal strategies where an operational endpoint such as fluid balance seems unsuited given the complexity of heart-lung interactions.

In another approach, Dessap et al., in a randomized clinical trial, showed a significantly shorter time to successful extubation using a brain natriuretic peptide (BNP)-driven fluid depletion strategy when compared to a physician-driven usual care approach [13]. Patients with LV systolic dysfunction showed the greater benefit.

Regarding resuscitation, dynamic assessment of fluid responsiveness has been shown to improve patient-related outcomes. In the recent FRESH randomized clinical trial [44], patients whose fluid therapy was guided by passive leg raise (PLR, a diagnostic tool for prediction of fluid responsiveness) showed less fluid accumulation, less renal replacement therapy requirement, and shorter duration on mechanical ventilation. This study estimated fluid responsiveness by a non-invasive bioreactance monitor, which can estimate fluid responsiveness by means of a PLR or a fluid challenge, both of which can be used during spontaneous breathing.

These two studies show the potential benefits of what would be a physiology-based strategy, addressing the importance of fluid responsiveness using both ultrasound and bioreactance.

12.6 Physiology-Based Fluid Depletion

Having recognized the importance and impact of weaning-induced pulmonary edema on weaning failure, we hypothesize that, in mechanically ventilated patients, reaching a state of fluid responsiveness before starting a SBT will result in better outcomes when compared to the standard fluid balance approach. This hypothesis is supported by a study assessing preload dependence and risk of weaning-induced cardiovascular dysfunction. In this report, preload unresponsiveness prior to SBT predicted weaning failure due to cardiovascular dysfunction (97% sensitivity, 81% specificity) [28]. Hence, clinicians have been encouraged to test preload responsiveness to guide fluid removal before starting an SBT, to avoid weaning failure [45]. Furthermore, this physiologically-driven strategy may be less aggressive than the purely arithmetic negative fluid balance strategy. In practical terms, this strategy could be accomplished by two means: first, by optimizing the capacity of the fluid overloaded patient to handle the rise in venous return after cessation of positive pressure. We think that this optimal condition is a state of preload-responsiveness regardless of the fluid balance or weight change. Second, by assuring that the other organ systems are in the best possible condition after the primary injury and resuscitative therapies. This implies lowering the risk of hypoperfusion, regional ischemia, and new-onset organ dysfunction.

Studies designed to demonstrate that this approach is not just physiologically plausible but clinically relevant are needed. Less weaning-induced heart failure should result in earlier weaning, and less aggressive fluid depletion might preserve organs from iatrogenic secondary injury. Moreover, shorter weaning time will benefit many patients by a shorter duration of mechanical ventilation and, consequently, less exposure to the risks of a longer ventilation time (infections, delirium), metabolic alterations, needless sedation, etc. From a broader standpoint, the prevention of serious complications and rationalization in general healthcare costs is a mandate for the future provision of care in the ICU [46]. Hopefully, the ongoing FLOW trial (ClinicalTrials.gov Identifier: NCT04496583) will be able to answer some of these questions. Putting this all together we propose a general flowchart for optimal fluid unloading to facilitate weaning from mechanical ventilation (Fig. 12.3).

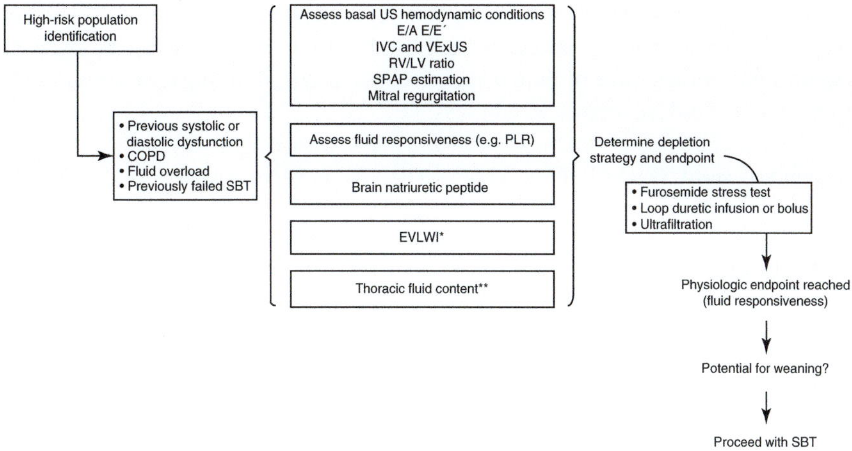

Fig. 12.3 A physiologic approach proposed to assess fluid depletion prior to a spontaneous breathing test (SBT) based on physiologic endpoints. Current evidence does not support one approach over another. Choosing more than one will likely reduce the risk of developing weaning-induced pulmonary edema, although aiming to reach more endpoints might unnecessarily delay SBT. *US* ultrasound, *EVLWI* extravascular water index, *PLR* passive leg raise, *RV* right ventricle, *LV* left ventricle, *IVC* inferior vena cava, *SPAP* systolic pulmonary artery pressure, *VExUS* Venous Excess Ultrasonography Score, * available with transpulmonary thermodilution, ** available with bioreactance monitor

12.7 Monitoring Fluid Responsiveness Prior to SBT

A major challenge in predicting fluid responsiveness in patients close to SBT is the spontaneous breathing itself. Validated tests include PLR, the fluid challenge, and the end-expiratory occlusion test [47]. A diagnostic fluid load is far from ideal, and an occlusion test might not be well tolerated in an awake patient. PLR must be tested against a significant variation in stroke volume, typically 10%. Doppler ultrasound allows estimation of stroke volume by measuring the velocity time integral, LV diastolic properties and filling pressures (E/A and E/E' indexes) [37]. Ultrasound has emerged as a valuable tool which might help in all steps of the proposed algorithm: high risk population screening, determining fluid responsiveness, estimating baseline cardiopulmonary profile, and monitoring the development of lung congestion itself [37].

12.8 Conclusion

Difficulties in weaning a patient from mechanical ventilation are often related to the patient's fluid status at the start of the weaning procedure. Although fluid balances and weight gain are widely used to identify patients at risk, we propose a different, more physiological approach. In this approach, a state of fluid unresponsiveness is seen as a major risk factor for weaning failure. Different techniques exist to assess fluid unresponsiveness in awake patients and diuretic strategies can be used to regain a physiologic state of fluid responsiveness instead of trying to reach an intuitive negative fluid balance or weight loss.

Acknowledgement Funded by FONDECYT-ANID. CHILE. Project number N° 1200248.

References

1. Rivers E, Nguyen B, Havstad S, et al. Early goal-directed therapy in the treatment of severe sepsis and septic shock. N Engl J Med. 2001;345:1368–77.
2. Evans L, Rhodes A, Alhazzani W, et al. Surviving Sepsis Campaign: International Guidelines for Management of Sepsis and Septic Shock 2021. Crit Care Med. 2021;49:e1063–143.
3. Cecconi M, Hofer C, Teboul JL, et al. Fluid challenges in intensive care: the FENICE study. Intensive Care Med. 2015;41:1529–37.
4. Hernández G, Ospina-Tascón GA, Damiani LP, et al. Effect of a resuscitation strategy targeting peripheral perfusion status vs serum lactate levels on 28-day mortality among patients with septic shock: the ANDROMEDA-SHOCK randomized clinical trial. JAMA. 2019;321:654–64.
5. O'Connor ME, Prowle JR. Fluid overload. Crit Care Clin. 2015;31:803–21.
6. Malbrain M, Marik PE, Witters I, et al. Fluid overload, de-resuscitation, and outcomes in critically ill or injured patients: a systematic review with suggestions for clinical practice. Anaesthesiol Intensive Ther. 2014;46:361–80.
7. Malbrain M, Waele DE, Honoré P. Assessment of fluid overload in critically ill patients: role of bioelectrical impedance analysis. In: Vincent JL, editor. Annual update in intensive care and emergency medicine 2018. Heidelberg: Springer; 2018. p. 417–36.
8. Bagshaw SM, Brophy PD, Cruz D, Ronco C. Fluid balance as a biomarker: impact of fluid overload on outcome in critically ill patients with acute kidney injury. Crit Care. 2008;12:169.
9. Cecconi M, Backer D, Antonelli M, et al. Consensus on circulatory shock and hemodynamic monitoring. Task force of the European Society of Intensive Care Medicine. Intensive Care Med. 2014;40:1795–815.
10. Heart N, Lung, and Blood Institute Acute Respiratory Distress Syndrome (ARDS) Clinical Trials Network, Wiedemann HP, Wheeler AP, et al. Comparison of two fluid-management strategies in acute lung injury. N Engl J Med. 2006;354:2564–75.
11. Malbrain ML, Chiumello D, Pelosi P, et al. Incidence and prognosis of intraabdominal hypertension in a mixed population of critically ill patients: a multiple-center epidemiological study. Crit Care Med. 2005;33:315–22.
12. Alsous F, Khamiees M, DeGirolamo A, Amoateng-Adjepong Y, Manthous CA. Negative fluid balance predicts survival in patients with septic shock. Chest. 2000;117:1749–54.
13. Dessap A, Roche-Campo F, Kouatchet A, et al. Natriuretic peptide–driven fluid management during ventilator weaning. Am J Respir Crit Care. 2012;186:1256–63.
14. Fagon JY, Chastre J, Vuagnat A, Trouillet JL, Novara A, Gibert C. Nosocomial pneumonia and mortality among patients in intensive care units. JAMA. 1996;275:866–9.
15. Selvan K, Edriss H, Sigler M, Nugent KM. Complications and resource utilization associated with mechanical ventilation in a medical intensive care unit in 2013. J Intensive Care Med. 2015;32:146–50.
16. Epstein SK, Ciubotaru RL. Independent effects of etiology of failure and time to reintubation on outcome for patients failing extubation. Am J Respir Crit Care Med. 1998;158:489–93.
17. Thille AW, Richard J-CM, Brochard L. The decision to extubate in the intensive care unit. Am J Respir Crit Care. 2013;187:1294–302.
18. Boles J-M, Bion J, Connors A, et al. Weaning from mechanical ventilation. Eur Respir J. 2007;29:1033–56.

19. Esteban A, Ferguson ND, Meade MO, et al. Evolution of mechanical ventilation in response to clinical research. Am J Respir Crit Care. 2008;177:170–7.
20. McConville JF, Kress JP. Weaning patients from the ventilator. N Engl J Med. 2012;367:2233–9.
21. Ely WE, Baker AM, Dunagan DP, et al. Effect on the duration of mechanical ventilation of identifying patients capable of breathing spontaneously. N Engl J Med. 1996;335:1864–9.
22. Girard TD, Kress JP, Fuchs BD, et al. Efficacy and safety of a paired sedation and ventilator weaning protocol for mechanically ventilated patients in intensive care (awakening and breathing controlled trial): a randomised controlled trial. Lancet. 2008;371:126–34.
23. Blackwood B, Alderdice F, Burns K, Cardwell C, Lavery G, O'Halloran P. Use of weaning protocols for reducing duration of mechanical ventilation in critically ill adult patients: Cochrane systematic review and meta-analysis. BMJ. 2011;342:c7237.
24. Dasta JF, McLaughlin TP, Mody SH, Piech CT. Daily cost of an intensive care unit day: the contribution of mechanical ventilation. Crit Care Med. 2005;33:1266–71.
25. Ouellette DR, Patel S, Girard TD, et al. Liberation from mechanical ventilation in critically ill adults: an official American College of Chest Physicians/American Thoracic Society clinical practice guideline: inspiratory pressure augmentation during spontaneous breathing trials, protocols minimizing sedation, and noninvasive ventilation immediately after extubation. Chest. 2017;151:166–80.
26. Béduneau G, Pham T, Schortgen F, et al. Epidemiology of weaning outcome according to a new definition. The WIND study. Am J Respir Crit Care. 2017;195:772–83.
27. Teboul JL. Weaning-induced cardiac dysfunction: where are we today? Intensive Care Med. 2014;40:1069–79.
28. Dres M, Teboul JL, Anguel N, Guerin L, Richard C, Monnet X. Passive leg raising performed before a spontaneous breathing trial predicts weaning-induced cardiac dysfunction. Intensive Care Med. 2015;41:487–94.
29. Pinsky MR. Breathing as exercise: the cardiovascular response to weaning from mechanical ventilation. Intensive Care Med. 2000;26:1164–6.
30. Pinsky MR. Cardiovascular effects of ventilator support and withdrawal. Anesth Analg. 1994;79:567–76.
31. Pinsky MR. Breathing as exercise: the cardiovascular response to weaning from mechanical variation. In: Pinsky MR, Brochard L, Mancebo J, Antonelli M, editors. Applied Physiology in Intensive Care Medicine 2. Berlin: Springer; 2012. p. 323–5.
32. Ferré A, Guillot M, Lichtenstein D, et al. Lung ultrasound allows the diagnosis of weaning-induced pulmonary oedema. Intensive Care Med. 2019;45:1–8.
33. Epstein SK. Decision to extubate. Intensive Care Med. 2002;28:535–46.
34. Lemaire F, Teboul JL, Cinotti L, et al. Acute left ventricular dysfunction during unsuccessful weaning from mechanical ventilation. Anesthesiology. 1988;69:171–9.
35. Liu J, Shen F, Teboul JL, et al. Cardiac dysfunction induced by weaning from mechanical ventilation: incidence, risk factors, and effects of fluid removal. Crit Care. 2016;20:369.
36. Routsi C, Stanopoulos I, Kokkoris S, Sideris A, Zakynthinos S. Weaning failure of cardiovascular origin: how to suspect, detect and treat-a review of the literature. Ann Intensive Care. 2019;9:6.
37. Vignon P. Cardiovascular failure and weaning. Ann Transl Med. 2018;6:354.
38. Silversides JA, Fitzgerald E, Manickavasagam US, et al. Deresuscitation of patients with iatrogenic fluid overload is associated with reduced mortality in critical illness. Crit Care Med. 2018;46:1600.
39. Goldstein S, Bagshaw S, Cecconi M, et al. Pharmacological management of fluid overload. Br J Anaesth. 2014;113:756–63.
40. Malbrain MLNG, Van Regenmortel N, Saugel B, et al. Principles of fluid management and stewardship in septic shock: it is time to consider the four D's and the four phases of fluid therapy. Ann Intensive Care. 2018;8:66.
41. Cordemans C, Laet I, Regenmortel N, et al. Aiming for a negative fluid balance in patients with acute lung injury and increased intra-abdominal pressure: a pilot study looking at the effects of PAL-treatment. Ann Intensive Care. 2012;2:S15.

42. Costanzo M, Saltzberg MT, Jessup M, et al. Ultrafiltration is associated with fewer rehospitalizations than continuous diuretic infusion in patients with decompensated heart failure: results from UNLOAD. J Card Fail. 2010;16:277–84.
43. Bagshaw SM, Gibney RT, Kruger P, Hassan I, McAlister FA, Bellomo R. The effect of low-dose furosemide in critically ill patients with early acute kidney injury: a pilot randomized blinded controlled trial (the SPARK study). J Crit Care. 2017;42:138–46.
44. Douglas IS, Alapat PM, Corl KA, et al. Fluid response evaluation in sepsis hypotension and shock: a randomized clinical trial. Chest. 2020;158:1431–45.
45. Jozwiak M, Monnet X, Teboul JL. Prediction of fluid responsiveness in ventilated patients. Ann Transl Med. 2018;6:352.
46. Arabi YM, Schultz MJ, Salluh JI. Intensive care medicine in 2050: global perspectives. Intensive Care Med. 2017;43:1695–9.
47. Monnet X, Marik PE, Teboul JL. Prediction of fluid responsiveness: an update. Ann Intensive Care. 2016;6:111.

Tidal Volume Challenge Test: Expanding Possibilities

13

S. N. Myatra, N. Prabu, and J.-L. Teboul

13.1 Introduction

The physiological rationale for the administration of fluids in patients with acute circulatory failure is to improve tissue oxygenation by increasing stroke volume and mean arterial pressure. However, giving fluids arbitrarily is not helpful, since only half of the patients with acute circulatory failure respond positively to fluid administration by increasing their stroke volume [1]. Fluid administration is not beneficial if the cardiac output does not increase. Uncorrected hypovolemia may affect tissue oxygenation, leading to organ dysfunction and death [2]. On the other hand, excessive fluid loading is associated with increased complications, duration of intensive care unit (ICU) stay, and mortality, especially in patients with acute respiratory distress syndrome (ARDS) [3, 4]. Therefore it is important to identify which patients will respond positively to fluid loading by increasing their cardiac output (fluid responsiveness) before fluid administration.

Various tests and indices have been proposed to predict fluid responsiveness. Commonly used dynamic indices, such as stroke volume variation (SVV), pulse pressure variation (PVV), respiratory variations in inferior vena cava diameter (ΔIVC), end-expiratory occlusion test, tidal volume challenge, and passive leg

S. N. Myatra (✉)
Department of Anesthesiology, Critical Care and Pain, Tata Memorial Hospital, Homi Bhabha National Institute, Mumbai, India
e-mail: myatrasn@tmc.gov.in

N. Prabu
Department of Critical Care Medicine, St. John's Medical College Hospital, Bengaluru, India

J.-L. Teboul
Service de Médecine Intensive-Réanimation, FHU SEPSIS, Hôpital de Bicêtre, GHU AP-HP, Université Paris-Saclay, Le Kremlin-Bicêtre, France

INSERM-UMR S999 LabEx - LERMIT, Hôpital Marie-Lannelongue, Le Plessis Robinson, France

J.-L. Vincent (ed.), *Annual Update in Intensive Care and Emergency Medicine 2022*, Annual Update in Intensive Care and Emergency Medicine,
https://doi.org/10.1007/978-3-030-93433-0_13

raising (PLR), have proven to be superior and are recommended over the traditionally used static indices, such as central venous pressure (CVP) and pulmonary artery occlusion pressure (PAOP), to predict fluid responsiveness [5–9]. These dynamic tests, other than PLR, depend on heart-lung interactions which have some limitations when used to predict fluid responsiveness. These limitations include mechanical ventilation using low tidal volumes, spontaneous breathing activity, cardiac arrhythmias, low lung compliance, open thorax, increased intraabdominal pressure, or a heart rate to respiratory rate ratio < 3.6; ventilation using low tidal volumes is the most common limiting factor [10].

Among these dynamic tests, the tidal volume challenge is a relatively new test, performed in patients ventilated using low tidal volumes [7]. It is reliable, simple to perform, and can overcome the limitation with the use of low tidal volume ventilation and improve the reliability of other tests using heart-lung interactions to predict fluid responsiveness. In this chapter, we will discuss the current evidence for the use of the tidal volume challenge, its applications, limitations, and prospects.

13.2 Rationale for Developing the Tidal Volume Challenge Test

Of the dynamic indices that depend on heart-lung interactions, PPV and SVV are commonly used in clinical practice and have consistently been shown to be reliable predictors of fluid responsiveness, with PPV having the highest level of evidence [5, 11–13]. Intermittent positive pressure ventilation produces cyclic changes in left ventricular (LV) stroke volume, which is highest during inspiration and lowest during expiration. The magnitude of change in LV stroke volume, or its surrogates, such as pulse pressure, are enhanced when a patient is preload dependent. Therefore, high PPV and SVV values are associated with preload responsiveness and low values with preload unresponsiveness. Values >12–13% for PPV and 10% for SVV have been reported to be highly predictive of volume responsiveness [11–13].

These indices have their advantages and limitations. The major limitations for the use of PPV and SVV are mechanical ventilation using low tidal volume, i.e. ≤6 ml/kg predicted body weight (PBW) [14, 15] and poor lung compliance (Crs <30 ml/cmH_2O) [16]. In clinical practice, mechanical ventilation using low tidal volume is widely used, not only in patients with ARDS but also in patients at risk of ARDS, with septic shock, potential organ donors, and patients undergoing high risk intraabdominal and thoracic surgeries [17, 18].

During ventilation using low tidal volume, the magnitude of change in airway driving pressure may not be sufficient to produce an adequate change in intracardiac pressure. Therefore PPV and SVV may be low even in fluid responders, leading to false negative results [14, 15]. The present wide usage of low tidal volume ventilation, limits the reliability of PPV and SVV and other tests depending on heart-lung interactions to predict fluid responsiveness [10]. To overcome this limitation with the use of PPV and SVV during ventilation using low tidal volume, a new test, the tidal volume challenge, was developed [7].

13.3 Reliability of the Tidal Volume Challenge Test to Predict Fluid Responsiveness

Myatra et al. conducted a prospective study to test the predictive value of the tidal volume challenge to help unmask fluid responders in patients receiving low tidal volume ventilation using volume assist-control mechanical ventilation without spontaneous breathing activity [7]. The tidal volume was transiently increased from 6 ml/kg PBW to 8 ml/kg PBW for 1 min and thereafter reduced back to 6 ml/kg PBW. Fluid responsiveness was defined as an increase in cardiac output >15% to a fluid bolus given after reducing the tidal volume back to 6 ml/kg PBW. As expected, the PPV at 6 ml/kg PBW (PPV_6) could not predict fluid responsiveness, with an area under the receiver operating characteristic curve (AUROC) of 0.69. There was a significant increase in PPV (ΔPPV_{6-8}), following the tidal volume challenge only in fluid responders. The ΔPPV_{6-8} discriminated responders from non-responders with an AUROC of 0.99 (sensitivity 94% and specificity 100%) with a cut-off value of 3.5%. Similar results were also seen using SVV (ΔSVV_{6-8}) with an AUROC of 0.97 (sensitivity 88% and specificity 100%) with a cut-off value of 2.5%. Therefore the changes in PPV and SVV following the tidal volume challenge were found to reliably predict fluid responsiveness in patients ventilated with low tidal volumes [7]. The tidal volume challenge has been subsequently tested in various settings and has become one of the standard tests to predict fluid responsiveness (Table 13.1).

13.4 How to Perform and Interpret the Tidal Volume Challenge Test

The patient should be well sedated and receiving invasive mechanical ventilation using a volume-controlled mode. A hemodynamic monitor that automatically calculates and tracks the dynamic changes of PPV or a monitor that automatically calculates SVV (calibrated or uncalibrated cardiac output monitor) is required to interpret the tidal volume challenge. Assess the patient for the presence of any confounding factor for the use of PPV or SVV. The tidal volume is set at 6 ml/kg PBW. Watch for any fluctuations in hemodynamic parameters; once there is stability, transiently increase the tidal volume from 6 ml/kg PBW to 8 ml/kg PBW for 1 min. Thereafter, reduce the tidal volume back to 6 ml/kg PBW. Note the PPV and SVV values at baseline and after giving the tidal volume challenge. The ΔPPV_{6-8} is then calculated (PPV at tidal volume 8 ml/kg PBW minus PPV at tidal volume 6 ml/kg PBW). The ΔSVV_{6-8} can also be calculated in the same way. A value of $\Delta PPV_{6-8} > 3.5\%$ or $\Delta SVV_{6-8} > 2.5\%$ predicts fluid responsiveness with high accuracy (Fig. 13.1).

For example, in a patient with a PBW of 60 kgs, the tidal volume at 6 ml/kg PBW will be 360 ml and at 8 ml/kg PBW it will be 480 ml. Set the tidal volume at 360 ml initially and then increase it to 480 ml, thus performing a tidal volume challenge for 1 min. After 1 min reduce the tidal volume back to 360 ml. Note the PPV at baseline ($PPV_{6)}$ and after performing the tidal volume challenge (PPV_8). If, for example, the

Table 13.1 Studies testing the reliability of pulse pressure (PPV) and stroke volume (SVV) variation when using a tidal volume challenge to predict fluid responsiveness

Study	Population	Position	AUROC (95% CI) PPV	PPV best cut-off (%)	Sensitivity (%)	Specificity (%)	AUROC (95% CI) SVV	SVV best cut-off (%)	Sensitivity (%)	Specificity (%)	Comments
Myatra et al. (2017) [7]	Critically ill patients	Supine, semi-recumbent	0.99	3.5	94	100	0.97	2.5	88	100	Patients had acute circulatory failure, receiving vasopressors
Taccheri et al. (2021) [20]	Critically ill patients	Supine, semi-recumbent	0.98	≥2	93	100	0.94	≥2	93	73	Patients had acute circulatory failure, receiving vasopressors
Elsayed et al. (2021) [19]	Critically ill patients	Supine, semi-recumbent	0.96	3.5	94	94	–	–	–	–	Patients had acute circulatory failure, receiving vasopressors
Hamzaoui et al. (2021) [21]	Critically ill patients	Supine, semi-recumbent	0.73	2	69	76	–	–	–	–	Mechanically ventilated patients with spontaneous breathing activity Patients had acute circulatory failure, receiving vasopressors
Messina et al. (2019) [22]	Neurosurgical patients	Supine	0.94	13.3[a]	95	76	0.83	12.1[a]	79	95	Normal lungs, not on vasopressors
Messina et al. (2020) [23]	Neurosurgical patients	Prone	0.96	12.2[a]	95	95	0.96	8[a]	95	95	Normal lungs, not on vasopressors

Jun et al. (2019) [25]	Laparoscopic pelvic surgery (robot assisted)	Trendelenburg	0.95	≥2	92	86	0.76	>2	46	100	Normal lungs, not on vasopressors Elevated intra-abdominal pressure Tidal volume challenge done for 3 min
Alvarado Sánchez et al. (2021) Meta-analysis [30]	Critically ill patients	Supine and prone	AUROC – 0.92[b] best cut-off – 3%[b] Sensitivity 0.90 (0.76–0.97)[b] Specificity 0.87 (0.31–0.99)[b]								Meta-analysis of predictors of fluid responsiveness in patients ventilated at low tidal tidal volumes. Two studies included with PVV and SVV Out of all tests, tidal volume challenge had the highest level of evidence

PPV pulse pressure variation, *CI* confidence interval, *AUROC* area under the receiver operating characteristic curve
[a]Percentage change
[b]Values expressed as pooled data (95% CI)

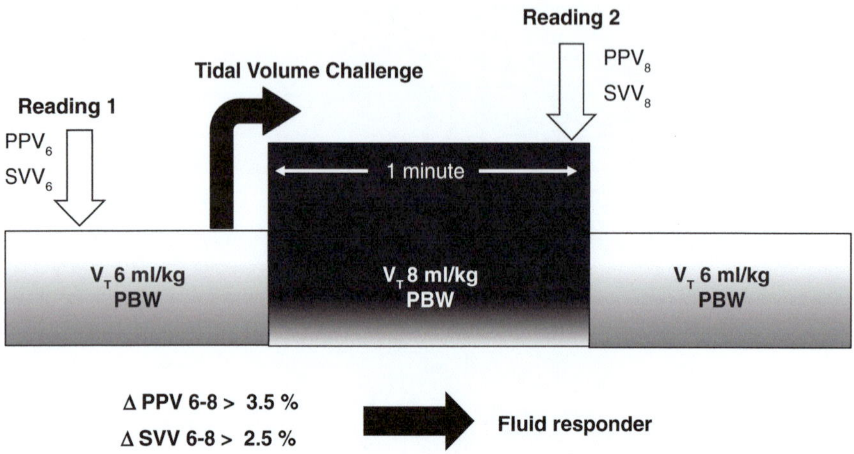

Fig. 13.1 How to perform and interpret the tidal volume challenge test. V_T = tidal volume, PBW = predcted body weight, PPV = pulse pressure variation, SVV = systolic pressure variation, PPV_6 = PPV at V_T 6 ml/kg PBW, SVV_6 = SVV at V_T 6 ml/kg PBW, PPV_8 = PPV at V_T 8 ml/kg PBW, SVV_8 = SVV at V_T 8 ml/kg PBW, ΔPPV_{6-8} = change in PVV after increasing V_T from 6 to 8 ml/kg PBW, ΔSVV_{6-8} = change in SVV after increasing V_T from 6 to 8 ml/kg PBW

PPV_6 = 8% and the PPV_8 = 14%, then the ΔPPV_{6-8} = 14%-8% = 6%. Since ΔPPV_{6-8} is >3.5%, the patient is a fluid-responder.

13.5 Applications of the Tidal Volume Challenge Test

13.5.1 In ICU Patients Mechanically Ventilated Using Low Tidal Volumes

Elsayed et al. compared the ability of the tidal volume challenge using PPV and the PLR test to predict fluid responsiveness in 46 patients with acute circulatory failure ventilated using low tidal volume [19]. Patients were considered as fluid responders if the cardiac output measured by velocity-time integral (VTI) assessment using echocardiography increased ≥15% after volume expansion. Both tidal volume challenge and PLR reliably predicted fluid responsiveness in patients ventilated using low tidal volume. A PPV increase >3.5% with a tidal volume challenge predicted fluid responsiveness with an AUROC of 0.96 (sensitivity 93.8% and specificity 93.9%). The cut-off values for PPV obtained in this study were the same as in the original study by Myatra et al. [7].

Taccheri et al. tested whether changes in PPV, SVV, and respiratory variation of the IVC diameter during a tidal volume challenge and a PLR test could predict fluid responsiveness in 30 critically ill patients receiving low tidal volume ventilation [20]. Changes in PPV ≥ 2 points (absolute change) after a tidal volume challenge reliably predicted fluid responsiveness with an AUROC of 0.98 (sensitivity 93% and specificity 100%). Similarly, changes in SVV ≥ 2 (absolute change) predicted fluid responsiveness with an AUROC of 0.82 (sensitivity 100% and specificity 67%). The cut-off values were lower than those described by Myatra et al. [7]. The effects of the PLR test could be assessed both by changes in PPV and IVC diameter expressed as a percentage.

In the same study, the authors showed that the changes in IVC diameter after tidal volume challenge predicted fluid responsiveness with moderate discrimination (AUROC 0.88). However, the diagnostic cut-off value was 4%, lower than the least significant change in IVC diameter, making the clinical usefulness questionable [20]. The use of tidal volume challenge to improve the reliability of IVC diameter variation to predict fluid responsiveness needs further evaluation.

13.5.2 In Mechanically Ventilated Patients with Spontaneous Breathing Activity

Patients receiving low tidal volume ventilation are not always deeply sedated or receiving neuromuscular blockade; they usually have some spontaneous breathing activity.

Hamzaoui et al. performed a study in 44 critically ill patients receiving controlled mechanical ventilation with persistent spontaneous breathing activity, to evaluate the reliability of PPV after performing a tidal volume challenge and PLR test [21]. All patients had normal respiratory system compliance and were on vasopressor infusions. Transthoracic echocardiography was used to measure the VTI of the LV outflow tract. Patients exhibiting an increase in VTI ≥12% during PLR were defined as preload responders.

As expected, PPV was not reliable in predicting fluid responsiveness in ventilated patients with spontaneous breathing activity. However, an increase in PPV following a tidal volume challenge and the decrease in PPV during PLR helped discriminate preload responders from non-responders with moderate accuracy. The tidal volume challenge predicted fluid responsiveness with an AUROC of 0.73 with a cut-off value of 2% (sensitivity 69% and specificity 76%) [21]. The lower reliability may be because all patients had persistent spontaneous breathing activity compared to the study by Myatra et al. where all patients were deeply sedated and well adapted to the mechanical ventilator [7]. Moreover, the tidal volume may be different for each spontaneous breath, which may affect the reliability of PPV both at baseline and after performing a tidal volume challenge. Nevertheless, these results show that a tidal volume challenge can be used to discriminate preload responders from non-responders with moderate accuracy and better than PPV alone. Although the accuracy is not high, it is acceptable and gives some confidence for using a tidal volume challenge to improve the reliability of PPV to predict fluid responsiveness in patients receiving controlled mechanical ventilation with persistent spontaneous breathing activity, a known limitation for the use of PPV.

13.5.3 In Patients with Normal Lungs Ventilated Using Low Tidal Volumes in the Operating Room

13.5.3.1 In the Supine Position

Patients undergoing surgery are increasingly ventilated using lung protective ventilation [18]. PPV and SVV are unreliable for predicting fluid responsiveness during low tidal volume ventilation [14, 15]. Messina et al. conducted a study in 40 patients undergoing neurosurgery in the supine position in the operating room (OR) to test the ability of a tidal volume challenge and an end-expiratory occlusion test (EEOT) to improve the reliability of PPV and SVV to predict fluid responsiveness in these patients [22]. After induction of anesthesia, patients were recruited if they showed more than 20% reduction in systolic arterial pressure with respect to the values observed before induction of anesthesia. All patients were ventilated with 6 ml/PBW tidal volume. A 250 ml fluid bolus was administered over 10 min to identify fluid responders (increase in stroke volume index ≥10%).

The PPV, SVV, and EEOT performed at 6 ml/kg PBW did not predict fluid responsiveness. An increase in PPV and SVV after a tidal volume challenge predicted fluid responsiveness with an AUROC 0.94 (sensitivity 94.7% and specificity 76.1%) and 0.93 (sensitivity 78.9% and specificity 95.2%), respectively. The cut-off value for PPV and SVV was an increase by 13.3% and 12.1% in the values respectively [22]. Therefore, the changes in PPV and SVV obtained after a tidal volume challenge reliably predict fluid responsiveness in patients with normal lungs ventilated using low tidal volumes in the supine position.

13.5.3.2 In the Prone Position

The reliability of PPV and SVV to predict fluid responsiveness in patients with normal lungs ventilated using low tidal volume in the prone position has not been established. Messina et al. assessed the reliability of PPV, SVV, tidal volume challenge, and EEOT to predict fluid responsiveness during elective spinal surgery in the prone position [23]. PPV, SVV, and EEOT recorded during ventilation using 6 ml/kg PBW and EEOT measured in patients ventilated at 8 ml/kg PBW did not predict fluid responsiveness. The change in PPV after tidal volume challenge predicted fluid responsiveness with an AUROC of 0.96 (95% confidence interval, 0.87-1.00), showing a sensitivity of 95.2% and a specificity of 94.7%. The change in SVV after tidal volume challenge predicted fluid responsiveness with an AUROC of 0.96 (95% confidence interval [CI], 0.89–1.00) with a sensitivity of 95.2% and a specificity of 94.7%. The cut-off value for PPV and SVV was an increase by 12.2% and 8.0% in these indices, respectively [23]. The cut-off values for PPV and SVV were expressed as a percentage increase and these values were lower compared to the study by Myatra et al. [7]. This may be because the patients studied in the OR had normal lungs and were receiving neuromuscular blockade. Nevertheless, both studies have shown that the tidal volume challenge improves the reliability of PPV and SVV in predicting fluid responsiveness in patients with normal lungs, ventilated using low tidal volume both in supine and prone positions during neurosurgery.

Another study in the prone position was conducted by Yonis et al. in 33 ARDS patients with acute circulatory failure, to assess the reliability of the tidal volume challenge used with PPV, EEOT, and the Trendelenburg maneuver to predict fluid responsiveness [24]. Fluid responsiveness was present if cardiac index assessed by transpulmonary thermodilution was ≥15% after fluid administration. Both tidal volume challenge and EEOT predicted fluid responsiveness poorly, but changes in cardiac index during a Trendelenburg maneuver did reliably predict fluid responsiveness in these patients. The median compliance of the respiratory system was 30 (23–39) ml/cmH_2O in these patients. It is worth noting that 42% of the patients had cardiac arrhythmias at baseline, which may explain this poor performance [24]. Further studies in patients with ARDS in the prone position will throw more light on this topic.

13.5.4 During Laparoscopic Surgery Using Pneumoperitoneum in the Trendelenburg Position

The reliability of PPV and SVV to predict fluid responsiveness is questionable while using pneumoperitoneum during laparoscopic surgery in the Trendelenburg position. In addition, these indices are unreliable with the use of low tidal volume ventilation, which is being increasingly used in surgical patients [18]. Jun et al. performed a prospective study in 38 patients undergoing robot-assisted laparoscopic surgery with pneumoperitoneum in the Trendelenburg position using low tidal volume ventilation [25]. The PPV, SVV, and stroke volume index (SVI) were measured at a tidal volume of 6 ml/kg PBW and after performing a tidal volume challenge (increasing the tidal volume to 8 ml/kg PBW). The intraabdominal pressure (IAP) was kept at 15 mmHg. The study was performed when there was no surgical handling or hemodynamic instability. Fluid responsiveness was defined as an increase in SVI ≥15%.

The tidal volume challenge showed excellent predictive capability for fluid responsiveness with PPV >2%, with an AUC of 0.95 [95% CI 0.83–0.99, $p < 0.0001$; sensitivity 92%, specificity 86%] [25]. Previous studies have shown that PPV and SVV values increase with an increase in IAP, especially when the IAP is >20–25 mmHg [26, 27]. However, when the IAP is less than 15 mmHg, PPV values are less affected [26, 28, 29]. The change in SVV after tidal volume challenge showed only a fair ability to predict fluid responsiveness in this study [25]. This discrepancy may be attributed to the fact that pneumoperitoneum can induce significant increases in systemic vascular resistance that affect the trending ability of pressure waveform devices to accurately monitor changes in SVI. Renner et al. reported that increasing IAP to 25 mmHg abolished the ability of SVV, but not PPV, to predict fluid responsiveness [26].

To date there is no easy and reliable way to predict fluid responsiveness in patients with elevated IAP during laparoscopic surgery in the OR. The use of tidal volume challenge has been shown to improve the reliability of PPV in this setting; however, this needs to be further investigated.

13.6 Comparison of Tidal Volume Challenge with Other Tests Used to Predict Fluid Responsiveness

Alvarado Sánchez et al. conducted a systematic review and meta-analysis to evaluate the operative performance of several predictors of fluid responsiveness in critically ill patients mechanically ventilated at low tidal volume (≤8 ml/kg) [30]. A total of 33 studies involving 1352 patients were included in the analysis. The AUROC for predictors of fluid responsiveness were: for tidal volume challenge = 0.92, EEOT = 0.92, SVV = 0.90, PPV = 0.82, ΔIVC = 0.86, and PLR = 0.84. Among all the tests, the tidal volume challenge had excellent performance, with an AUROC of 0.92 with the threshold value of 3% and pooled sensitivity and specificity of 90% and 87%, respectively. Although few studies using tidal volume challenge were included in the meta-analysis, these findings and the positive results seen with the use of tidal volume challenge in subsequent studies, highlight the excellent reliability of this test in predicting fluid responsiveness in patients ventilated using low tidal volume.

13.7 Advantages of the Tidal Volume Challenge

The tidal volume challenge is a simple test that can be easily performed at the bedside without any change in the position of the patient. Since the test is performed by making adjustments on the ventilator and observing hemodynamic changes on the monitor, no patient contact is required, making it applicable for use when minimal patient contact is desirable, as in patients with coronavirus disease 2019 (COVID-19). The test is reliable, accurate, cost-effective, safe to use, not operator dependent, and not requiring any learning curve. The test can be reliably used both in the ICU and in the OR in patients in the supine and prone position. In this regard, it may be helpful in COVID-19 patients with ARDS. When used with PPV it does not require a cardiac output monitor, making it very useful in resource-limited settings.

13.8 Limitations of the Tidal Volume Challenge

The tidal volume challenge may not be able to overcome the other limitations associated with the use of PPV and SVV to predict fluid responsiveness, such as cardiac arrhythmias, open chest, spontaneous breathing, and raised IAP, and needs to be evaluated in these settings. Alternative tests, such as PLR, which do not depend on heart-lung interactions, may be used when applicable.

13.9 Future Directions

The tidal volume challenge is already well established to improve the reliability of PPV and SVV in patients ventilated using low tidal volumes, in various positions, and when there are spontaneous breathing efforts. The reliability of this test in predicting fluid responsiveness in patients with low compliance, as in ARDS, needs to be evaluated. Whether use of a tidal volume challenge will improve the reliability of other tests that work on heart-lung interactions, such as echocardiography-derived parameters (inferior and superior vena cava variability, aortic root velocity variation), ultrasound-derived parameters (carotid peak systolic velocity, internal jugular vein distensibility index, etc.) and plethysmography-derived indices, which have similar limitations for use as PPV and SVV, needs to be studied. The use of tidal volume challenge with PPV and SVV as part of a perioperative goal-directed therapy, across different types of surgery also needs further evaluation.

13.10 Conclusion

The tidal volume challenge is a simple bedside test that can improve the reliability of PPV and SVV to predict fluid responsiveness in patients ventilated using low tidal volume in both in the ICU and OR in various patient positions. The test is useful in resource-limited settings when used with PPV, as it does not require a cardiac output monitor. Whether the tidal volume challenge can improve the reliability of other indices based on heart-lung interactions to predict fluid responsiveness during low tidal volume ventilation needs further investigation.

References

1. Michard F, Teboul JL. Predicting fluid responsiveness in ICU patients: a critical analysis of the evidence. Chest. 2002;121:2000–8.
2. Pinsky MR, Brophy P, Padilla J, Paganini E, Pannu N. Fluid and volume monitoring. Int J Artif Organs. 2008;31:111–26.
3. Wiedemann HP, Wheeler AP, Bernard GR, et al. Comparison of two fluid management strategies in acute lung injury. N Engl J Med. 2006;354:2564–75.
4. Acheampong A, Vincent JL. A positive fluid balance is an independent prognostic factor in patients with sepsis. Crit Care. 2015;19:251.
5. Michard F, Teboul JL. Using heart-lung interactions to assess fluid responsiveness during mechanical ventilation. Crit Care. 2000;4:282–9.
6. Shi R, Monnet X, Teboul JL. Parameters of fluid responsiveness. Curr Opin Crit Care. 2020;26:319–26.
7. Myatra SN, Prabu NR, Divatia JV, Monnet X, Kulkarni AP, Teboul J. The changes in pulse pressure variation or stroke volume variation after a "tidal volume challenge" reliably predict fluid responsiveness during low tidal volume ventilation. Crit Care Med. 2017;45:415–21.
8. Rhodes A, Evans LE, Alhazzani W, et al. Surviving sepsis campaign: international guidelines for Management of Sepsis and Septic Shock: 2016. Intensive Care Med. 2017;43:304–77.
9. Cecconi M, Hernandez G, Dunser M, et al. Fluid administration for acute circulatory dysfunction using basic monitoring: narrative review and expert panel recommendations from an ESICM task force. Intensive Care Med. 2019;45:21–32.
10. Myatra SN, Monnet X, Teboul JL. Use of 'tidal volume challenge' to improve the reliability of pulse pressure variation. Crit Care. 2017;21:60.
11. Marik PE, Cavallazzi R, Vasu T, Hirani A. Dynamic changes in arterial waveform derived variables and fluid responsiveness in mechanically ventilated patients: a systematic review of the literature. Crit Care Med. 2009;37:2642–7.

12. Yang X, Du B. Does pulse pressure variation predict fluid responsiveness in critically ill patients? A systematic review and meta-analysis. Crit Care. 2014;18:650.
13. Hong JQ, He HF, Chen ZY, et al. Comparison of stroke volume variation with pulse pressure variation as a diagnostic indicator of fluid responsiveness in mechanically ventilated critically ill patients. Saudi Med J. 2014;35:261–8.
14. De Backer D, Heenen S, Piagnerelli M, Koch M, Vincent JL. Pulse pressure variations to predict fluid responsiveness: influence of tidal volume. Intensive Care Med. 2005;31:517–23.
15. Lansdorp B, Lemson J, Van Putten MJAM, De Keijzer A, Van Der Hoeven JG, Pickkers P. Dynamic indices do not predict volume responsiveness in routine clinical practice. Br J Anaesth. 2012;108:395–401.
16. Monnet X, Bleibtreu A, Ferré A, et al. Passive leg-raising and end-expiratory occlusion tests perform better than pulse pressure variation in patients with low respiratory system compliance. Crit Care Med. 2012;40:152–7.
17. Serpa Neto A, Cardoso SO, Manetta JA, et al. Association between use of lung-protective ventilation with lower tidal volumes and clinical outcomes among patients without acute respiratory distress syndome: a meta-analysis. JAMA. 2012;308:1651–9.
18. Futier E, Constantin JM, Paugam-Burtz C, et al. A trial of intraoperative low-tidal-volume ventilation in abdominal surgery. N Engl J Med. 2013;369:428–37.
19. Elsayed AI, Selim KA, Zaghla HE, Mowafy HE, Fakher MA. Comparison of changes in PPV using a tidal volume challenge with a passive leg raising test to predict fluid responsiveness in patients ventilated using low tidal volume. Indian J Crit Care Med. 2021;25:685–90.
20. Taccheri T, Gavelli F, Teboul JL, et al. Do changes in pulse pressure variation and inferior vena cava distensibility during passive leg raising and tidal volume challenge detect preload responsiveness in case of low tidal volume ventilation? Crit Care. 2021;110:1–12.
21. Hamzaoui O, Shi R, Carelli S, et al. Changes in pulse pressure variation to assess preload responsiveness in mechanically ventilated patients with spontaneous breathing activity: an observational study. Br J Anaesth. 2021;127:532–8.
22. Messina A, Montagnini C, Cammarota G, et al. Tidal volume challenge to predict fluid responsiveness in the operating room: an observational study. Eur J Anaesthesiol. 2019;36:583–91.
23. Messina A, Montagnini C, Cammarota G, et al. Assessment of fluid responsiveness in prone neurosurgical patients undergoing protective ventilation: role of dynamic indices, tidal volume challenge, and end-expiratory occlusion test. Anesth Analg. 2020;130:752–61.
24. Yonis H, Bitker L, Aublanc M, et al. Change in cardiac output during Trendelenburg maneuver is a reliable predictor of fluid responsiveness in patients with acute respiratory distress syndrome in the prone position. Crit Care. 2017;21:295.
25. Jun JH, Chung RK, Baik HJ, et al. The tidal volume challenge improves the reliability of dynamic preload indices during robot-assisted laparoscopic surgery in the Trendelenburg position with lung-protective ventilation. BMC Anesthesiol. 2019;19:1–11.
26. Renner J, Gruenewald M, Quaden R, et al. Influence of increased intra-abdominal pressure on fluid responsiveness predicted by pulse pressure variation and stroke volume variation in a porcine model. Crit Care Med. 2009;37:650–8.
27. Jacques D, Bendjelid K, Duperret S, Colling J, Piriou V, Viale JP. Pulse pressure variation and stroke volume variation during increased intra-abdominal pressure: an experimental study. Crit Care. 2011;15:R33.
28. Bliacheriene F, Machado SB, Fonseca EB, Otsuke D, Auler JOC, Michard F. Pulse pressure variation as a tool to detect hypovolaemia during pneumoperitoneum. Acta Anaesthesiol Scand. 2007;51:1268–72.
29. Høiseth L, Hoff IE, Myre K, Landsverk SA, Kirkebøen KA. Dynamic variables of fluid responsiveness during pneumoperitoneum and laparoscopic surgery. Acta Anaesthesiol Scand. 2012;56:777–86.
30. Alvarado Sánchez JI, Caicedo Ruiz JD, Diaztagle Fernández JJ, Amaya Zuñiga WF, Ospina-Tascón GA, Cruz Martínez LE. Predictors of fluid responsiveness in critically ill patients mechanically ventilated at low tidal volumes: systematic review and meta-analysis. Ann Intensive Care. 2021;11:28.

Fluid Management in COVID-19 ICU Patients

14

R. Shi, X. Monnet, and J.-L. Teboul

14.1 Introduction

The global pandemic caused by severe acute respiratory syndrome coronavirus 2 (SARS-CoV-2) led to a worldwide medical emergency [1]. Patients with coronavirus disease 2019 (COVID-19) due to infection by SARS-CoV-2 can have a large spectrum of clinical presentations from asymptomatic manifestation to multiple organ failure [1, 2]. In critically ill patients, the respiratory system is often primarily affected [1, 2]. About 30% of patients hospitalized for COVID-19 may develop acute respiratory distress syndrome (ARDS) [3], while other extrapulmonary organs or systems may also be involved during the course of the disease [2]. During the first wave of the pandemic, the prevalence of shock in hospitalized COVID-19 patients was variable. A pooled analysis of five studies from China until March 2020 showed that the incidence of shock was about 6% [4] and it was higher in critically ill patients (up to 35%) [5].

The mechanisms of shock during COVID-19 may be hypovolemic, obstructive, cardiogenic, or distributive [6]. Although these mechanisms are variable, fluid administration remains one of the most important therapies. However, fluid administration is tricky in critically ill patients with COVID-19 and shock. On the one hand, fluid administration should provide adequate tissue perfusion; on the other hand, it might worsen lung edema, especially when vascular permeability is increased, which is the general rule in ARDS [7]. Given the lack of studies on fluid strategy specific to COVID-19, the recommendation of the Surviving Sepsis Campaign (SSC) dedicated to the disease is based on the existing evidence in non-COVID-19 populations with ARDS. The current recommendation is to use a

R. Shi · X. Monnet · J.-L. Teboul (✉)
Service de médecine intensive-réanimation, Hôpital de Bicêtre, AP-HP, Inserm UMR S_999, Université Paris-Saclay, Le Kremlin-Bicêtre, France
e-mail: jean-louis.teboul@aphp.fr

J.-L. Vincent (ed.), *Annual Update in Intensive Care and Emergency Medicine 2022*, Annual Update in Intensive Care and Emergency Medicine,
https://doi.org/10.1007/978-3-030-93433-0_14

conservative over a liberal fluid strategy in COVID-19 with shock [5]. Nevertheless, we do have concerns about this recommendation. In this chapter, we will develop the idea that assessing the benefit/risk ratio of volume expansion is essential in patients with COVID-19 and shock, and that fluid administration should be personalized.

14.2 Why Patients with COVID-19 Can Develop Acute Circulatory Failure?

All the classical shock mechanisms can result in acute circulatory failure during COVID-19, namely hypovolemia, vasoplegia, left or right ventricular failure.

14.2.1 Hypovolemia

A recent international survey (1000 respondents) showed that about 22% of COVID-19 patients hospitalized in the intensive care unit (ICU) were hypovolemic according to echocardiography findings [8]. Hypovolemia during COVID-19 can be secondary to several mechanisms. First, patients may be dehydrated, especially at the time of admission, because of fever, reduced water intake in the previous days, and fluid losses (diarrhea, nausea, etc.) [9], or sometimes due to long-time use of high-flow nasal oxygen therapy. Second, a systemic inflammatory state can occur in COVID-19 patients either due to the response to viral attack or to a secondary bacterial infection. It can result in endothelial dysfunction which, in turn, results in tissue capillary leakage and eventually in absolute hypovolemia [10]. It can also result in increased venous capacitance, which in turn results in relative hypovolemia due to blood volume redistribution toward the unstressed blood volume.

14.2.2 Vasoplegia

In the above-mentioned survey, 56% of the 1000 respondents used vasopressors frequently or very frequently [8]. Vasoplegia can be due to a systemic pro-inflammatory state, occurring either early or more often later if septic shock has developed following nosocomial infection. Secondary nosocomial infections, in particular ventilator-acquired pneumonia (VAP) [11, 12], are frequent in COVID-19 patients and may be more common than in patients with non-COVID pneumonia [13]. Whether dexamethasone and other immunomodulating agents are facilitating factors remains to be proven [13]. Endothelial dysfunction secondary to sepsis could then trigger widespread peripheral vasodilation and lead to hypotension [10]. In addition, systemic vasodilation and hypotension can result from the use of high doses of sedative drugs, which are often required to adapt the patient to the ventilator.

14.2.3 Impaired Left Heart Function

Myocardial injury related to COVID-19 can be generated by multiple mechanisms: direct viral injury through different pathways, such as the downregulation of angiotensin-converting enzyme (ACE)2, cytokine release, microvascular thrombotic injury, etc. [14]. The clinical manifestations may be severe arrhythmia, severe heart failure, and sometimes cardiogenic shock [14]. According to an echocardiography study conducted in 100 hospitalized patients with COVID-19 within 24 h of admission, 10% had left ventricular (LV) systolic dysfunction and 16% LV diastolic dysfunction [15]. Obviously, LV dysfunction may contribute to the severity of shock in addition to other mechanisms, such as hypovolemia and vasoplegia, as in non-COVID-19 septic shock.

14.2.4 Right Ventricular (RV) Dysfunction or Failure

According to a study that systematically assessed left and right cardiac function using echocardiography, the right ventricle is even more often impaired than the left ventricle during COVID-19 [15]. RV dysfunction with or without dilation was found in up to 39% of cases [15]. In COVID-19 ARDS patients, a retrospective study showed that, on day 6 of the ICU stay, RV systolic dysfunction was present in 51% of cases [16]. Impairment of RV function is multifactorial and can be due to increased pulmonary vascular resistance secondary to ARDS (vasoconstrictive inflammatory mediators, hypoxic vasoconstriction, etc.), or to positive pressure ventilation-related pulmonary hypertension (high levels of positive end-expiratory pressure [PEEP] are often required), or to pulmonary embolism. Pulmonary embolism is frequent in COVID-19 patients [17] and in particular in those with ARDS, where its incidence is higher than in patients with non-COVID-19 ARDS [18].

14.3 Consequences of Fluid Therapy in COVID-19 Patients with Shock

Fluid therapy should be considered only in the case of shock and if hypovolemia (absolute or relative) is suspected to be a major contributor to acute circulatory failure.

As in other clinical contexts, the presence of hypovolemia during COVID-19 may lead to low systemic blood flow, which may increase the risk of organ hypoperfusion, and hence of acute kidney injury [19] and other organ failures. Hypovolemia also favors the risk of thrombosis, which is already high in COVID-19 [20]. Indeed, coagulopathy is common and related to the direct effect of SARS-CoV-2 on the endothelial cells resulting in the release of plasminogen activators [20]. Lung microthrombi may contribute to ventilation/perfusion (V/Q) mismatch and subsequent hypoxemia. Microthrombi formation in other organs may also contribute to multiple organ dysfunction or failure. Finally, hypovolemia-induced low cardiac output may worsen hypoxemia through a low mixed venous blood oxygen pressure (PvO_2) effect, in the presence of high pulmonary shunt [21]. If hypovolemia really results in low or inadequate blood flow, all the above-mentioned effects can be pronounced and clinicians should consider their correction by fluid administration. The expected benefits of fluid therapy are thus to prevent or correct the development of multiple organ failure and to decrease the risk of microthrombosis in the lung and in other organs. Moreover, increasing cardiac output may improve arterial oxygenation as a consequence of the increase in PvO_2. Nevertheless, this beneficial effect is uncertain since, at the same time, increasing PvO_2 might also increase the lung venous admixture (or the shunt) [22]. If hypoxic pulmonary vasoconstriction is attenuated as it should be in ARDS [23], the latter effect (increased venous admixture/shunt related to increased PvO_2) would also be attenuated and a substantial improvement in arterial oxygenation can follow a substantial increase in PvO_2 (related to a substantial increase in cardiac output) in the presence of large pulmonary venous admixture or shunt.

On the other hand, COVID-19 is frequently associated with ARDS, which is characterized by alveolar epithelial and endothelial injuries. This results in lung capillary leakage with lung edema, atelectasis and, eventually, in severe V/Q mismatch when hypoxic pulmonary vasoconstriction is markedly attenuated. As a consequence, COVID-19 patients with ARDS often have severe hypoxemia [24]. In such a context, fluid therapy may increase lung edema formation due to capillary leakage and sometimes may also increase the V/Q mismatch due to the increase in cardiac output [22].

14.4 How to Assess the Benefits and the Risks of Fluid Administration in COVID-19 Patients with Shock?

In our point of view, the benefit/risk ratio of fluid therapy should be carefully assessed before any fluid administration in the context of COVID-19 and shock due to the frequent presence of severe ARDS. Such an assessment should be personalized since the benefits as well as the risks may differ among patients and in the same patient at different periods of resuscitation. In this regard, the recommendation of the SSC is questionable as using a conservative over a liberal fluid strategy is suggested [5]. First, "conservative" and "liberal" are unclear words and may mislead therapeutic decisions. Second, this recommendation does not take into consideration individualization of assessment and decisions, which is the key principle of any resuscitation strategy in ICU patients.

To adequately assess the benefit/risk ratio of fluid therapy, one should assess the benefit and the risk and put both in the overall context before deciding. The benefit should be evaluated not only by the presence but also importantly by the degree of fluid responsiveness. There is a lot of evidence that ICU patients can be fluid unresponsive in spite of persisting shock, probably because they have already received fluids and/or they have cardiac dysfunction [25]. There is also a lot of evidence that a positive cumulative fluid balance is associated with poor outcomes in ICU patients, especially in the case of sepsis [26] and ARDS [27]. It is clear that if shock persists in spite of initial resuscitation, prediction of fluid responsiveness makes sense to identify patients who will not benefit from further fluid administration but will rather experience harmful effects. Importantly, the presence of fluid responsiveness is a dynamic phenomenon that can vary over time in the same patient [28]. This suggests that prediction of fluid responsiveness should be tested as often as a therapeutic decision is required. Results from a large multicenter cohort of septic patients showed that the use of fluid responsiveness tests was associated with an improved survival rate [29]. Several tests and indices have been developed during the last decades. International guidelines recommend the use of dynamic over static variables in the general population of critically ill patients as well as in patients with COVID-19 and shock [30].

Most of the dynamic indices or tests of fluid responsiveness are based on the heart-lung interactions in mechanically ventilated patients (Table 14.1) [31]. Pulse pressure variation (PPV) is one of the most investigated variables though it suffers from many limitations in practice [32]. One of them is low tidal volume ventilation [32], which is commonly used in COVID-19 ARDS patients. To overcome this limitation, the tidal volume challenge was proposed in the case of low tidal volume (6 ml/kg) ventilation [33]. Myatra et al. showed that, by transiently increasing tidal volume from 6 to 8 ml/kg for 1 min, an increase in the absolute value of PPV (ΔPPV) ≥3.5% could reliably predict fluid responsiveness [33]. This result was confirmed in a recent study, which showed that an increase in PPV during tidal volume challenge was reliable to predict fluid responsiveness in patients ventilated with low tidal volume for septic shock or ARDS [34]. The tidal volume challenge is particularly helpful in COVID-19 patients with ARDS, who are usually profoundly sedated and well adapted to the ventilator. Importantly, no cardiac output monitoring device is required for performing tidal volume challenge and a simple arterial line is sufficient.

Table 14.1 Summary of tests predicting fluid responsiveness with available monitoring techniques in patients with coronavirus disease 2019 (COIVD-19)

Tests	Main advantages in COVID-19	Available hemodynamic techniques
Passive leg raising	Reversible and no fluid infused Usable in non-intubated patients, in patients with mechanical ventilation regardless of tidal volume, and in patients with or without arrhythmia	Real-time cardiac output monitor, echocardiography
Trendelenburg maneuver	Useful in prone position	Real-time and precise cardiac output monitor
Tidal volume challenge	Useful in case of low tidal volume No requirement for cardiac output monitoring	Arterial catheter to follow the changes in pulse pressure variation
End-expiratory occlusion test	Easy to perform in ventilated patients. Useful in case of low tidal volume and low respiratory system compliance	Real-time and precise cardiac output monitor

The end-expiratory occlusion test (EEOT) is another useful and easy-to-perform fluid responsiveness test. It has been validated even in patients with arrhythmias or low respiratory system compliance [35] and independent of the PEEP levels [36]. By briefly interrupting the ventilator at end-expiration for 15 seconds, an increase in cardiac output ≥5% from baseline allows one to identify fluid responders [37]. A recent meta-analysis including 13 studies showed that the EEOT can predict fluid responsiveness with a summary area under the receiver operating characteristic curve (AUROC) of 0.91 (0.86–0.94) with good sensitivity and specificity and a threshold value of 5% [36]. However, since the EEOT is brief and the threshold value relatively small, a real-time and precise cardiac output monitoring device is required [37].

Passive leg raising (PLR) is another well-established option with a wide range of applications since it can be performed in almost all patients, including those with spontaneous breathing, atrial fibrillation, low lung compliance, or ventilated with a low tidal volume [35, 38]. It mimics a fluid challenge without requiring any fluid. It does not increase the risk of pulmonary edema as the effects on cardiac filling pressure are rapidly reversible [39]. Numerous studies have consistently shown that PLR is a reliable test to predict fluid responsiveness in critically ill patients [38]. Of note, since the effect of PLR on cardiac output is transient, real-time measurement of cardiac output is required [39]. The PLR test was shown to have false negatives in patients with intraabdominal hypertension [40]. In the absence of cardiac output assessment, the decrease in PPV during PLR is helpful as it was shown to be reliable to predict fluid responsiveness [34]. In less sedated mechanically ventilated patients with some spontaneous breathing activity, our group also showed that the decrease in PPV during PLR could be a valuable option as it can predict fluid responsiveness better than PPV alone [41].

Prone position is frequently applied in COVID-19 ARDS patients. In such a condition, a Trendelenburg maneuver, which mobilizes venous blood through a postural maneuver, has been proposed as a reliable fluid responsiveness test [42]. Whether other dynamic parameters or tests (Table 14.1) remain valid during prone position in ARDS requires further research.

The risk of fluid therapy in COVID-19 patients with ARDS is worsening lung edema and hypoxemia. It is important to evaluate this risk before giving fluids in patients with shock even in cases of a positive fluid responsiveness test. The European consensus on management of shock has suggested the use of transpulmonary thermodilution or a pulmonary artery catheter in patients with shock, especially in the case of associated ARDS [43]. In this context, transpulmonary thermodilution systems could be helpful as they provide values of extravascular lung water (EVLW) and pulmonary vascular permeability index (PVPI). The EVLW, which is the amount of fluid accumulated in the alveolar and interstitial lung compartments, is a quantitative measure of lung edema [44]. The PVPI is calculated as the EVLW/pulmonary blood volume ratio [44]. In non-COVID-19 patients with ARDS, the maximal value of EVLW obtained during the patient's stay was shown to be an independent factor associated with mortality [45]. Similar results were found for PVPI [45]. In a recent study, we showed that EVLW and PVPI were also independent predictors of mortality in patients with COVID-19 ARDS [46]. In addition, we showed that compared to patients without COVID-19, ARDS patients with COVID-19 had similar lung mechanics, but higher EVLW and PVPI values from the beginning of the disease [46]. This was associated with worse arterial oxygenation and with more requirement for prone positioning and extracorporeal membrane oxygenation (ECMO) [46]. These findings suggest that COVID-19 ARDS can be associated with severe diffuse alveolar damage and increased permeability pulmonary edema [46]. Importantly, we found a large heterogeneity of EVLW and PVPI values among patients with similar degrees of hypoxemia. For example, in patients with severe ARDS according to the Berlin definition, extremely high values of EVLW and PVPI were measured in some patients and mildly elevated values in others. In the former cases, fluid administration would be very risky even in cases of shock with fluid responsiveness, whereas in the latter cases, careful fluid administration can be attempted [46]. Such heterogeneity confirms that the degree of hypoxemia poorly reflects the severity of lung edema and thus can hardly help in individualizing therapeutic decisions in COVID-19 ARDS.

The pulmonary artery catheter can also be used in patients with shock and ARDS [47]. One of the most valuable variables in this context is the pulmonary artery occlusion pressure (PAOP), a marker of the LV filling pressure. If the PAOP is low, clinicians may be less reluctant to infuse fluids in case of shock, although PAOP as a vascular pressure cannot provide a direct estimation of pulmonary edema. In this regard, no correlation was found between PAOP and EVLW in critically ill patients [48]. Lung ultrasound, a non-invasive method, enables assessment of lung edema using a B-line score, which correlates with EVLW [49]. However, such a score only provides a semi-quantitative assessment of lung edema and no valuable information about capillary permeability can be obtained.

14.5 Summary

Although a conservative fluid strategy is recommended in COVID-19 patients with shock [5] because of the frequently associated ARDS, administration of fluid cannot be totally discarded. The therapeutic decision should be made after a personalized assessment of the benefit/risk ratio of fluid infusion (Fig. 14.1). The benefit can be evaluated using dynamic measures of fluid responsiveness. Not only the presence but mostly the degree of fluid responsiveness is important to consider. For example, an increase in cardiac output by 25% during PLR raises the expectation of an increase in cardiac output after fluid infusion more than double compared to that expected from a PLR-induced increase in cardiac output by 12%, even if fluid responsiveness is present in both cases. The risks of fluid infusion should also be individually evaluated. Indices predicting lung tolerance to fluid infusion such as EVLW and PVPI can be relevant for that purpose.

In addition to the careful assessment of the benefit/risk ratio of fluid infusion, the clinical context is important to consider. For example, for a given favorable benefit/risk ratio, severe circulatory failure in terms of renal dysfunction or hyperlactatemia,

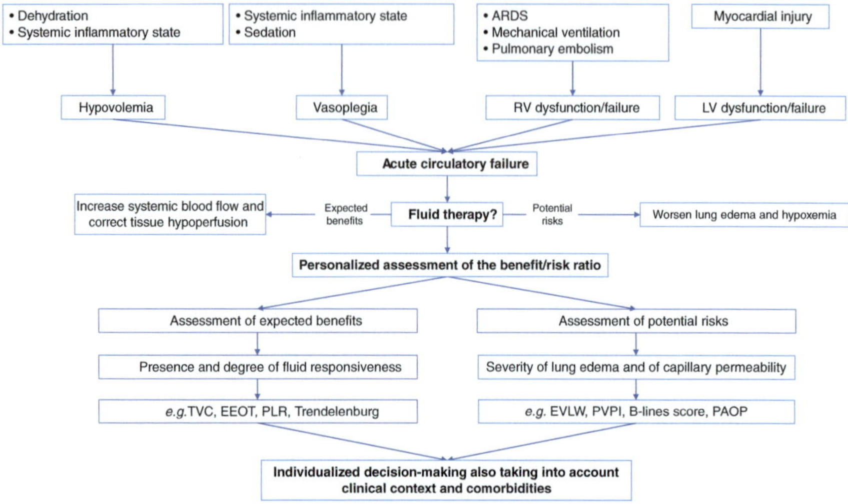

Fig. 14.1 Potential mechanisms of acute circulatory failure in coronavirus disease 2019 (COVID-19) and personalized assessment of benefit and risk for fluid administration. *ARDS* acute respiratory distress syndrome, *EEOT* end-expiratory occlusion test, *EVLW* extravascular lung water, *LV* left ventricular, *PAOP* pulmonary artery occlusion pressure, *PLR* passive leg raising, *PVPI* pulmonary vascular permeability index, *RV* right ventricular, *TVC* tidal volume challenge

would encourage clinicians to consider fluid therapy. Presence of LV systolic or diastolic dysfunction is also an important factor that could refrain or limit administration of fluids even in the case of a favorable benefit/risk ratio. Performance of echocardiography is of utmost importance to evaluate the cardiac function in this context as well as in all other shock states [43].

14.6 Conclusion

No general recommendation on fluid therapy can be made in COVID-19 patients with shock. An individual and careful assessment of the benefit/risk ratio of fluid infusion is necessary.

References

1. Yang X, Yu Y, Xu J, et al. Clinical course and outcomes of critically ill patients with SARS-CoV-2 pneumonia in Wuhan, China: a single-centered, retrospective, observational study. Lancet Respir Med. 2020;8:475–81.
2. Wiersinga WJ, Rhodes A, Cheng AC, Peacock SJ, Prescott HC. Pathophysiology, transmission, diagnosis, and treatment of coronavirus disease 2019 (COVID-19): a review. JAMA. 2020;324:782–93.
3. Tzotzos SJ, Fischer B, Fischer H, Zeitlinger M. Incidence of ARDS and outcomes in hospitalized patients with COVID-19: a global literature survey. Crit Care. 2020;24:516.

4. Desai R, Singh S, Parekh T, et al. COVID-19 and shock: a cautionary tale for elderly patients from a pooled analysis. Ann Emerg Med. 2020;75:789–91.
5. Alhazzani W, Møller MH, Arabi YM, et al. Surviving sepsis campaign: guidelines on the management of critically ill adults with coronavirus disease 2019 (COVID-19). Intensive Care Med. 2020;46:854–87.
6. Fox S, Vashisht R, Siuba M, Dugar S. Evaluation and management of shock in patients with COVID-19. Cleve Clin J Med. 2020; Jul 17. https://doi.org/10.3949/ccjm.87a.ccc052. Epub ahead of print.
7. Vignon P, Evrard B, Asfar P, et al. Fluid administration and monitoring in ARDS: which management? Intensive Care Med. 2020;46:2252–64.
8. Michard F, Malbrain ML, Martin GS, et al. Haemodynamic monitoring and management in COVID-19 intensive care patients: an international survey. Anaesth Crit Care Pain Med. 2020;39:563–9.
9. Boockvar KS, Mak W, Burack OR, et al. Co-occurring dehydration and cognitive impairment during COVID-19 in long-term care patients. J Am Med Dir Assoc. 2021;22:2270–1.
10. Sinha P, Matthay MA, Calfee CS. Is a "cytokine storm" relevant to COVID-19? JAMA Intern Med. 2020;180:1152–4.
11. Contou D, Claudinon A, Pajot O, et al. Bacterial and viral co-infections in patients with severe SARS-CoV-2 pneumonia admitted to a French ICU. Ann Intensive Care. 2020;10:119.
12. Grasselli G, Scaravilli V, Mangioni D, et al. Hospital-acquired infections in critically ill patients with COVID-19. Chest. 2021;160:454–65.
13. Llitjos JF, Bredin S, Lascarrou JB, et al. Increased susceptibility to intensive care unit acquired pneumonia in severe COVID-19 patients: a multicentre retrospective cohort study. Ann Intensive Care. 2021;11:20.
14. Hendren NS, Drazner MH, Bozkurt B, Cooper LT Jr. Description and proposed management of the acute COVID-19 cardiovascular syndrome. Circulation. 2020;141:1903–14.
15. Szekely Y, Lichter Y, Taieb P, et al. Spectrum of cardiac manifestations in COVID-19: a systematic echocardiographic study. Circulation. 2020;142:342–53.
16. Chotalia M, Ali M, Alderman JE, et al. Right ventricular dysfunction and its association with mortality in coronavirus disease 2019 acute respiratory distress syndrome. Crit Care Med. 2021;49:1757–68.
17. Poissy J, Goutay J, Caplan M, et al. Pulmonary embolism in patients with COVID-19: awareness of an increased prevalence. Circulation. 2020;142:184–6.
18. Helms J, Tacquard C, Severac F, et al. High risk of thrombosis in patients with severe SARS-CoV-2 infection: a multicenter prospective cohort study. Intensive Care Med. 2020;46:1089–98.
19. Selby NM, Forni LG, Laing CM, et al. Covid-19 and acute kidney injury in hospital: summary of NICE guidelines. BMJ. 2020;369:m1963.
20. Iba T, Levy JH, Connors JM, Warkentin TE, Thachil J, Levi M. The unique characteristics of COVID-19 coagulopathy. Crit Care. 2020;24:360.
21. Dantzker DR. The influence of cardiovascular function on gas exchange. Clin Chest Med. 1983;4:149–59.
22. Lynch JP, Mhyre JG, Dantzker DR. Influence of cardiac output on intrapulmonary shunt. J Appl Physiol Respir Environ Exerc Physiol. 1979;46:315–21.
23. Gierhardt M, Pak O, Walmrath D, et al. Impairment of hypoxic pulmonary vasoconstriction in acute respiratory distress syndrome. Eur Respir Rev. 2021;30:210059.
24. Santamarina MG, Boisier D, Contreras R, Baque M, Volpacchio M, Beddings I. COVID-19: a hypothesis regarding the ventilation-perfusion mismatch. Crit Care. 2020;24:395.
25. Michard F, Teboul JL. Predicting fluid responsiveness in ICU patients: a critical analysis of the evidence. Chest. 2002;121:2000–8.
26. Vincent JL, Sakr Y, Sprung CL, et al. Sepsis in European intensive care units: results of the SOAP study. Crit Care Med. 2006;34:344–53.
27. Sakr Y, Vincent JL, Reinhart K, et al. High tidal volume and positive fluid balance are associated with worse outcome in acute lung injury. Chest. 2005;128:3098–108.

28. Kattan E, Ospina-Tascón GA, Teboul JL, et al. Systematic assessment of fluid responsiveness during early septic shock resuscitation: secondary analysis of the ANDROMEDA-SHOCK trial. Crit Care. 2020;24:23.
29. Dubin A, Loudet C, Kanoore Edul VS, et al. Characteristics of resuscitation, and association between use of dynamic tests of fluid responsiveness and outcomes in septic patients: results of a multicenter prospective cohort study in Argentina. Ann Intensive Care. 2020;10:40.
30. Evans L, Rhodes A, Alhazzani W, et al. Surviving sepsis campaign: international guidelines for Management of Sepsis and Septic Shock 2021. Intensive Care Med. 2021;47:1181–247.
31. Jozwiak M, Monnet X, Teboul JL. Prediction of fluid responsiveness in ventilated patients. Ann Transl Med. 2018;6:352.
32. Michard F, Chemla D, Teboul JL. Applicability of pulse pressure variation: how many shades of grey? Crit Care. 2015;19:144.
33. Myatra SN, Prabu NR, Divatia JV, Monnet X, Kulkarni AP, Teboul JL. The changes in pulse pressure variation or stroke volume variation after a "tidal volume challenge" reliably predict fluid responsiveness during low tidal volume ventilation. Crit Care Med. 2017;45:415–21.
34. Taccheri T, Gavelli F, Teboul JL, Shi R, Monnet X. Do changes in pulse pressure variation and inferior vena cava distensibility during passive leg raising and tidal volume challenge detect preload responsiveness in case of low tidal volume ventilation? Crit Care. 2021;25:110.
35. Monnet X, Bleibtreu A, Ferré A, et al. Passive leg-raising and end-expiratory occlusion tests perform better than pulse pressure variation in patients with low respiratory system compliance. Crit Care Med. 2012;40:152–7.
36. Gavelli F, Shi R, Teboul JL, Azzolina D, Monnet X. The end-expiratory occlusion test for detecting preload responsiveness: a systematic review and meta-analysis. Ann Intensive Care. 2020;10:65.
37. Gavelli F, Teboul JL, Monnet X. The end-expiratory occlusion test: please, let me hold your breath! Crit Care. 2019;23:274.
38. Monnet X, Marik P, Teboul JL. Passive leg raising for predicting fluid responsiveness: a systematic review and meta-analysis. Intensive Care Med. 2016;42:1935–47.
39. Monnet X, Teboul JL. Passive leg raising: five rules, not a drop of fluid! Crit Care. 2015;19:18.
40. Beurton A, Teboul JL, Girotto V, et al. Intra-abdominal hypertension is responsible for false negatives to the passive leg raising test. Crit Care Med. 2019;47:e639–e47.
41. Hamzaoui O, Shi R, Carelli S, et al. Changes in pulse pressure variation to assess preload responsiveness in mechanically ventilated patients with spontaneous breathing activity: an observational study. Br J Anaesth. 2021;127:532–8.
42. Yonis H, Bitker L, Aublanc M, et al. Change in cardiac output during Trendelenburg maneuver is a reliable predictor of fluid responsiveness in patients with acute respiratory distress syndrome in the prone position under protective ventilation. Crit Care. 2017;21:295.
43. Cecconi M, De Backer D, Antonelli M, et al. Consensus on circulatory shock and hemodynamic monitoring. Task force of the European Society of Intensive Care Medicine. Intensive Care Med. 2014;40:1795–815.
44. Monnet X, Teboul JL. Transpulmonary thermodilution: advantages and limits. Crit Care. 2017;21:147.
45. Jozwiak M, Silva S, Persichini R, et al. Extravascular lung water is an independent prognostic factor in patients with acute respiratory distress syndrome. Crit Care Med. 2013;41:472–80.
46. Shi R, Lai C, Teboul JL, et al. COVID-19 ARDS is characterized by higher extravascular lung water than non-COVID-19 ARDS: the PiCCOVID study. Crit Care. 2021;25:186.
47. Richard C, Warszawski J, Anguel N, et al. Early use of the pulmonary artery catheter and outcomes in patients with shock and acute respiratory distress syndrome: a randomized controlled trial. JAMA. 2003;290:2713–20.
48. Boussat S, Jacques T, Levy B, et al. Intravascular volume monitoring and extravascular lung water in septic patients with pulmonary edema. Intensive Care Med. 2002;28:712–8.
49. Enghard P, Rademacher S, Nee J, et al. Simplified lung ultrasound protocol shows excellent prediction of extravascular lung water in ventilated intensive care patients. Crit Care. 2015;19:36.

Electrolytes in the ICU 15

A. Reintam Blaser, A. R. H. van Zanten, and A. M. E. de Man

15.1 Introduction

Electrolytes are chemical compounds in solutions that are ionizable, forming either positively (cations) or negatively (anions) charged ions. Electrolytes are of paramount importance for maintaining homeostasis, including acid-base balance and osmolality. Interplay of different electrolytes is important, but has been studied scarcely in critically ill. Yet, electrolyte abnormalities are common in patients admitted to the intensive care unit (ICU) due to severe illness, major fluid shifts, and treatments causing rapid and relevant changes in electrolytes. However, clear

A. Reintam Blaser (✉)
Department of Anaesthesiology and Intensive Care, University of Tartu, Tartu, Estonia

Department of Intensive Care Medicine, Lucerne Cantonal Hospital, Lucerne, Switzerland
e-mail: annika.reintam.blaser@ut.ee

A. R. H. van Zanten
Department of Intensive Care Medicine and Research, Gelderse Vallei Hospital, Ede, The Netherlands

Division of Human Nutrition and Health, Wageningen University and Research, HELIX, Wageningen, The Netherlands

A. M. E. de Man
Department of Intensive Care, Amsterdam UMC, Location VUmc, Amsterdam, The Netherlands

Amsterdam Cardiovascular Science, Amsterdam, The Netherlands

Amsterdam Infection and Immunity Institute, Amsterdam, The Netherlands

Amsterdam Medical Data Science, Amsterdam, The Netherlands

J.-L. Vincent (ed.), *Annual Update in Intensive Care and Emergency Medicine 2022*, Annual Update in Intensive Care and Emergency Medicine,
https://doi.org/10.1007/978-3-030-93433-0_15

cut-offs for electrolyte levels that lead to adverse outcome are largely lacking. Accordingly, clear guidance for management of electrolyte abnormalities in critically ill is not available for most electrolytes. Therefore, knowledge of physiology and pathophysiology is essential to understand and manage electrolyte disturbances in critical illness.

In the current chapter, we summarize the physiology and pathophysiology of electrolyte changes, with the focus of interplay between different electrolytes. Acid-base balance is beyond the focus of this review. However, bicarbonate will be addressed from the aspect of the interplay with other electrolytes. Additionally, we review the evidence on the management of electrolyte disturbances in patients admitted to the ICU.

15.2 Physiology and Pathophysiology

Intra- and extracellular levels, common reference values for serum measurements, and main role in homeostasis for each electrolyte are presented in Table 15.1.

Table 15.1 Electrolyte composition of body fluids and role in homeostasis [1]

	Average intracellular concentration (mmol/l)	Average extracellular concentration (mmol/l)	Average reference value for serum measurement (mmol/l)[a]	Main role in homeostasis
Cations				
Sodium [3]	10	140	135–145	Serum osmolality
Potassium [3]	155	4	3.5–5.0	Intracellular osmolality, action potential of cell membranes
Magnesium [2]	10	1	0.63–1.02	Transmembrane electrolyte flux, co-factor for phosphate in energy metabolism, calcium antagonist
Calcium (ionized) [2]	<0.01	1	1.12–1.30	Cell-to-cell communication and adhesion, contractility, and conduction
Anions				
Bicarbonate [5]	10	28	22–28	Acid-base balance
Chloride [21]	3	102	98–107	Serum osmolality, acid-base balance
Phosphate [2]	105	1	0.87–1.45	ATP-synthesis, energy metabolism

[a]Reference values may differ slightly between laboratories

15.2.1 Sodium: Regulator of Osmolality

15.2.1.1 Physiology

The most important role for sodium is as the major osmotically active substance of the extracellular fluid. Serum sodium concentration is maintained within the normal range by water intake, antidiuretic hormone excretion, renal sodium excretion and adrenal aldosterone excretion [1].

15.2.1.2 Pathophysiology

Hyponatremia may occur in patients with decreased, normal, or increased total body sodium concentrations. Assessment of serum osmolality and fluid volume is necessary to elucidate the underlying causes, which can be numerous (such as gastrointestinal or renal losses, syndrome of inappropriate antidiuretic hormone secretion [SIADH], liver cirrhosis, heart failure, hypercortisolism) [2]. Symptoms of hyponatremia are related to the rate and severity of decline in sodium concentrations, and mostly start to occur below 125 mmol/l. Typical symptoms are headache, lethargy, disorientation, nausea, confusion, seizures, and coma [1, 2].

Hypernatremia is always associated with hyperosmolality. The main reasons for ICU-acquired hypernatremia are superfluous administration of saline solutions (e.g., NaCl 0.9% = Na 154 mmol/l), gastrointestinal fluid loss, and concomitant renal dysfunction with reduced urinary concentration capability (9). In addition, aggressive deresuscitation with loop-diuretics frequently leads to hypernatremia. Symptoms mostly arise from sodium levels >155 mmol/l and include irritability, drowsiness, confusion, and coma [1]. Rapid changes in sodium levels may lead to symptoms more frequently and at lower absolute levels. Conversely, chronic hypernatremia is often well tolerated.

Sodium levels are the main regulator of serum osmolality, with sodium levels decreasing in response to increased osmolality from other osmotically active substances (e.g., glucose). Sodium abnormalities are often accompanied by chloride abnormalities.

15.2.2 Potassium: Determinant of Excitability

15.2.2.1 Physiology

Potassium is the main intracellular osmotic provider. Other important physiological functions are: regulation of the electrical action potential across the cell membranes, cellular metabolism, glycogen and protein synthesis [2]. High intracellular potassium levels are maintained by the Na^+/K^+/ATPase pump, affected by insulin, glucagon, catecholamines, aldosterone, acid-base status, plasma osmolality, and intracellular potassium levels [2].

15.2.2.2 Pathophysiology

Hypokalemia in critically ill patients commonly occurs due to potassium shifting to the intracellular compartment induced by correction of acidosis or as a refeeding mechanism. As the normal range is very narrow, and potassium levels are highly dependent on acid-base balance and glucose metabolism and control, life-threatening hypokalemia may rapidly occur. Other common causes are decreased intake or increased losses by the kidney and gastrointestinal tract [1]. Typical symptoms associated with hypokalemia are vomiting, muscle weakness, rhabdomyolysis, and cardiac arrhythmias, such as ventricular tachycardia/fibrillation or *torsade de pointes*.

Hyperkalemia in the ICU is most commonly caused by renal insufficiency, extensive cell destruction, and/or transcellular shift from intra- to extracellular. In addition, pseudohyperkalemia may arise from sampling errors. Clinical manifestations include paresthesias, weakness, paralysis, bradycardia, electrocardiogram (EKG)-alterations (elevated T wave, prolonged PR interval, widened QRS complex, idioventricular rhythms, and eventually even asystole).

15.2.3 Magnesium: Membrane Stabilizer

15.2.3.1 Physiology

Magnesium is, second to potassium, the most important intracellular cation. Since most magnesium is present intracellularly, plasma magnesium concentrations do not reflect the total magnesium pool well. The key role of magnesium is to serve as cofactor for phosphate transfer reactions in cell replication and energy metabolism. Moreover, it is crucial for muscle contractility and neuronal transmission [1, 3]. Magnesium levels are mostly kept within normal ranges by absorption in the gastrointestinal tract (inhibited by high protein, phosphate, and fat intake) and renal elimination (regulated by parathyroid hormone [PTH], calcitonin, glucagon, vasopressin, acid-base status, potassium, and magnesium concentrations).

15.2.3.2 Pathophysiology

Hypomagnesemia is commonly caused by diuretics, refeeding syndrome, diarrhea, and/or vomiting. Symptoms mostly do not correlate with magnesium plasma concentrations, but are rare with levels >0.5 mmol/l. Clinical signs are weakness, muscle cramps, tachyarrhythmias, EKG-alterations, tremors, confusion, and convulsions.

Hypermagnesemia is usually iatrogenic by excessive administration of magnesium salts, especially with concomitant renal insufficiency. Clinical features are hypotension, respiratory depression, hyporeflexia, confusion, and cardiac arrhythmias (bradycardia, total AV-block, asystole).

15.2.4 Calcium: Conduction and Contraction

15.2.4.1 Physiology

Calcium is essential for clotting, cell membrane permeability, contractility, and neuromuscular conduction. Calcium levels are primarily kept within normal ranges by PTH, calcitonin, and vitamin D [1, 3].

15.2.4.2 Pathophysiology

Hypocalcemia may be caused by vitamin D deficiency, renal insufficiency, hyperphosphatemia, and massive blood transfusions (citrate effect) [3]. The hallmark sign of hypocalcemia is tetany. Other symptoms are cramps, convulsions, mental alterations, hypotension, and cardiac arrhythmias.

Hypercalcemia is linked to specific underlying conditions such as malignancy or hyperparathyroidism, but drugs and immobilization can also contribute [3]. Clinical features are nausea, vomiting, pancreatitis, lethargy, obstipation, mental alterations, polyuria, polydipsia, metastatic calcifications, renal failure, cardiac arrhythmias, and coma [3].

15.2.5 Phosphate: Cellular Energy

15.2.5.1 Physiology

Phosphate is the principal intracellular anion, being important for cell membrane and bone composition, nerve conduction, muscle function, ATP-synthesis, glucose utilization, glycolysis, and 2,3-diphosphoglycerate (2,3-DPG) synthesis and numerous biochemical reactions [2]. Phosphate is kept within the normal range predominantly by the kidneys and to a lesser extent by gastrointestinal absorption and bone resorption/deposition under the influence of calcitriol, vitamin D, and PTH.

15.2.5.2 Pathophysiology

Hypophosphatemia may be caused by increased cellular uptake (refeeding, insulin, alkalosis), malnutrition, or renal replacement therapy (RRT). Clinical features are paresthesias, seizures, muscle weakness, acute respiratory failure, and arrhythmias [1, 2].

Hyperphosphatemia is most commonly caused by renal insufficiency. Other causes can be excessive oral or intravenous administration of phosphate or phosphate containing laxative, especially in combination with impaired renal function or rhabdomyolysis [2]. Clinically, hyperphosphatemia can lead to calcium-phosphate precipitation, resulting in hypocalcemia (manifesting as tetany) and nephrocalcinosis (due to deposits of calcium-phosphate crystals) [2, 4].

15.2.6 Bicarbonate: A Buffer

15.2.6.1 Physiology

Bicarbonate (HCO_3^-) is the second most abundant extracellular anion. Its most essential function is as a buffer. It is generated out of the end products of aerobic metabolism (CO_2 and $H_2O \leftrightarrow HCO_3^-$ and H^+). Bicarbonate is transported in the blood and in the lungs converted to and exhaled as CO_2.

15.2.6.2 Pathophysiology

In metabolic acidosis, pH is <7.35, HCO_3^- is <22 mmol/l, while total venous CO_2 is <30 mmol/l [5]. Metabolic acidosis can be caused by exogenous acids (salicylate, methanol, and ethylene glycol) or endogenous acids (ketoacids and lactic acid), decreased renal acid excretion, gastrointestinal (diarrhea) or renal losses. Symptoms are highly dependent on the underlying cause. Mild acidemia is asymptomatic, more severe can lead to hyperventilation, cardiac dysfunction with hypotension and shock, ventricular arrhythmias, and coma.

In metabolic alkalosis pH is >7.45, HCO_3^- is >28 mmol/l and total venous CO_2 is >30 mmol/l (in simple acid-base disorders; in mixed this can be different) [5]. Administration of sodium bicarbonate, gastrointestinal (gastric fluid by vomiting or nasogastric suction) or renal losses, renal production of new HCO_3^- (primary hyperaldosteronism, loop or thiazide diuretics), all can lead to metabolic alkalosis [5]. Symptoms are mostly caused by concomitant hypokalemia, hypophosphatemia, hypocalcemia, hypovolemia, and hypoventilation. Mild to moderate metabolic alkalosis (HCO_3^- up to 40 mmol/l) is usually well tolerated. HCO_3^- >45 mmol/l can result in tetany, seizures, cardiac arrhythmias, and delirium [5].

15.2.7 Chloride: A Strong Ion

15.2.7.1 Physiology

Chloride is the principal extracellular anion. Its key functions are maintaining osmolarity, acid-base balance, electro-neutrality of body fluids, and muscular activity [6]. Chloride concentrations are kept within the normal range by the gastrointestinal tract and kidney (99% is reabsorbed) [6].

15.2.7.2 Pathophysiology

Hypochloremia may occur due to gastrointestinal losses of chloride (vomiting, nasogastric drainage) and renal (chloruretic drugs,), water gain (congestive heart failure, SIADH, hypotonic solutions) or sodium exceeding chloride gain (e.g., administration of sodium bicarbonate). Clinical signs are mostly those of the concomitant metabolic alkalosis: cardiac arrhythmias, confusion, and neuromuscular irritability [6].

Hyperchloremia in the ICU is often caused by administration of chloride-rich fluids.

Symptoms are difficult to specify since it is difficult to attribute these solely to increased chloride concentrations [6].

15.3 Interplay between Electrolytes

Homeostasis of different electrolytes is closely related (Table 15.2). Although too complex to fully describe, several relevant interactions will be discussed.

Table 15.2 Interplay of electrolyte abnormalities

	Sodium	Potassium	Magnesium	Calcium	Bicarbonate	Chloride	Phosphate
Sodium ↑		↓	↓	↑	↑	↑	↓
Potassium ↑	↑		↑ ↓	↑ ↓	↓		
Magnesium ↑		↑		↑ ↓			
Calcium ↑	↑ ↓	↓	↓		↓	↑ ↓	↑ ↓
Bicarbonate ↑	↑ ↓	↓	↓	↓		↓	↓
Chloride ↑	↑	↑	↓	↓	↓		↓
Phosphate ↑	↑	↑	↑	↓	↓	↑	

	Sodium	Potassium	Magnesium	Calcium	Bicarbonate	Chloride	Phosphate
Sodium ↓		↑ ↓	↑ ↓	↑ ↓	↑ ↓	↑ ↓	↑ ↓
Potassium ↓	↓		↓	↑ ↓	↑		↑ ↓
Magnesium ↓	↓	↓		↓	↓		
Calcium ↓	↑ ↓	↑ ↓	↓		↑	↑ ↓	↑ ↓
Bicarbonate ↓	↑ ↓	↑	↓	↑		↑	↑
Chloride ↓	↓	↓			↑		
Phosphate ↓	↑ ↓	↓	↓	↑ ↓	↑		

Interplay between electrolytes is very complex and a change in one electrolyte can lead to different changes in another depending on the mechanism of the initial change, concomitant conditions and other dyselectrolytemias. Uncertain areas are marked in gray. If a field is blank, no data are available.

15.3.1 Sodium and Potassium

Sodium and potassium concentrations are strongly interrelated. The Na^+/K^+ ATPase membrane pump, ubiquitously present in all cells, plays an essential role in sodium and potassium homeostasis by active transport of potassium from the extracellular to the intracellular fluid and sodium in the opposite direction. This generates a concentration gradient across the cell membrane, maintaining the potential of the cell membrane. Insulin, adrenergic catecholamines, and aldosterone can all stimulate Na^+/K^+ ATPase pumps. Aldosterone secretion is stimulated by hyponatremia and hyperkalemia [3].

Serum sodium concentration is directly proportional to the total amount of exchangeable Na^+ and K^+. Administration of potassium can therefore increase serum sodium concentration by three different mechanisms. First, intracellular K^+ uptake leads to equivalent extracellular sodium movement. Second, parallel K^+-Cl^- intracellular uptake increases intracellular osmolality, subsequently reducing extracellular free water. Third, intracellular K^+-uptake can lead to an equivalent extracellular H^+-movement. H^+ will be buffered, but intracellular K^+ increase will raise intracellular osmolality and, due to free water shift, increase extracellular serum Na^+ [7].

15.3.2 Magnesium and Potassium

It is hard to treat hypokalemia with coexisting hypomagnesemia. Magnesium deficiency probably decreases Na-K-ATPase activity, reducing cellular uptake of K^+. Moreover, release of the magnesium-mediated inhibition of renal outer medullary potassium channel (ROMK) increases potassium secretion in the distal nephron [8].

Therefore, correction of magnesium deficiency is essential to enable correction of hypokalemia [2].

Conversely, hypokalemia may lead to hypomagnesemia by reduction of magnesium reabsorption in the thick ascending loop of Henle and the distal convoluted tubule [9].

15.3.3 Calcium and Potassium

Hypercalcemia can lead to hypokalemia. Hypercalcemia can increase urinary sodium excretion, increasing sodium delivery to the distal tubule and augmenting sodium-potassium exchange with subsequent potassium loss. In patients with hypercalcemia, the increase of filtered calcium in the loop of Henle can decrease magnesium reabsorption and thus serum magnesium concentrations [10].

15.3.4 Calcium, Phosphate, and Magnesium

Calcium, phosphate, and magnesium homeostasis are closely related. Hyperphosphatemia can lead to hypocalcemia by precipitating calcium-phosphate crystals in bone and extraskeletal tissue (leading to organ damage), reducing vitamin D production, and interfering with PTH-mediated bone resorption [11].

Hypomagnesemia can also induce hypocalcemia. Magnesium deficiency probably leads to hypocalcemia due to reduced PTH secretion and refractoriness of bone and renal tubules to PTH [12]. Remarkably, severe hypermagnesemia can also occasionally lead to hypocalcemia by suppressing PTH secretion due to impaired sensitivity of calcium-sensing receptors.

Furthermore, phosphate depletion can decrease magnesium uptake and thus result in hypomagnesemia, as was suggested in animal studies. The underlying mechanism remains to be elucidated [9].

15.3.5 Acid-Base and Potassium

Acidosis promotes hyperkalemia, whereas alkalosis promotes hypokalemia. Mineral (hyperchloremic normal gap) metabolic acidosis causes more severe hyperkalemia than organic (high anion gap) metabolic acidosis. An increase in extracellular hydrogen ion (H^+) with mineral acidosis will decrease the rate of Na^+/H^+ exchange by the Na^+/H^+ exchanger and the cotransport of Na^+ and HCO_3^- into the cell. The intracellular Na^+ concentration will decline and reduce Na^+/K^+ ATPase activity, decreasing intracellular K^+. The lower extracellular HCO_3^- concentration will increase movement of Cl^- into the cell by Cl^-/HCO_3^- exchange, stimulating K^+ efflux by K^+/Cl^- cotransport. In organic acidosis, movement of organic anions and H^+ into the cell reduces intracellular pH, promoting inward Na^+ movement through Na^+/H^+ exchange and cotransport of Na^+ and HCO_3^-. The increase in intracellular

Na^+ preserves Na^+-K^+ ATPase activity, so the extracellular K^+ concentration remains unchanged [13]. In metabolic alkalosis, extracellular potassium will decrease because of increased Na^+/K^+ ATPase activity and stimulated renal K^+ secretion. Hypokalemia directly induces metabolic alkalosis. It stimulates intracellular movement of hydrogen ions into the cell, leading to bicarbonate reabsorption. Hypokalemia also activates the H^+-K^+ ATPase exchanger in the collecting duct, which enhances distal H^+ secretion [14].

15.3.6 Acid-Base and Magnesium

Metabolic acidosis can promote magnesium deficiency. It can increase the serum ionized magnesium concentration and therefore the magnesium load for renal excretion. Furthermore, metabolic acidosis may impair cellular magnesium uptake [9].

15.3.7 Acid-Base and Calcium

The acid-base status of patients affects serum ionized calcium concentrations, as it influences the binding between calcium and serum proteins. Alkalemia increases calcium binding to albumin, decreasing serum ionized calcium concentration, whereas acidemia increases ionized calcium [3].

15.3.8 Acid-Base and Phosphate

Both acute respiratory alkalosis and metabolic alkalosis can induce hypophosphatemia, with respiratory alkalosis resulting in a more substantial decrease in serum phosphate. Respiratory alkalosis stimulates the glycolytic pathway, which activates intracellular phosphate entry, thus leading to hypophosphatemia. Respiratory alkalosis increases muscular phosphate uptake and makes the kidney refractory to the phosphaturic effect of PTH [15]. In chronic respiratory alkalosis, this resistance of the kidney to PTH can lead to hyperphosphatemia and hypocalcemia [16]. Metabolic acidosis decreases glycolysis rate and cellular uptake of phosphate, leading to hyperphosphatemia [11].

15.3.9 Acid-Base and Chloride

Hypochloremia can lead to metabolic alkalosis. When serum chloride concentration decreases, due to gastrointestinal or renal loss, reabsorption of bicarbonate is stimulated proportionally, and results in metabolic alkalosis. Acidosis due to renal or gastrointestinal loss is often associated with hyperchloremia [6], whereas hyperchloremia itself leads to hyperchloremic acidosis.

15.4 Evidence of Electrolyte Abnormalities in ICU Patients

Electrolyte levels outside of the reference ranges are often seen in ICU patients [17] (Table 15.3). Nevertheless, data on their prevalence, effect on outcome, and guidance on management is scarce. International guidelines for management are only available for hyponatremia [18]. Diverse electrolyte disorders occur for various reasons and at different time points during the patient's ICU stay. Not rarely, patients experience both 'hypo' and 'hyper' situations concerning the same electrolyte during the same admission. Some electrolyte abnormalities may be a cause for ICU admission (e.g., hyponatremia), whereas some manifest later during the patient's ICU stay (e.g., hypernatremia, hyperchloremia, hypophosphatemia), often in response to treatments applied (diuretics, feeding, correction of acidosis or levels of other electrolytes).

To study the impact of electrolyte abnormalities on outcome is difficult as an individual patient often may switch between two distinct abnormalities during the ICU stay. Prevalence of concomitant electrolyte disorders in the ICU has not been specifically addressed in the literature.

15.4.1 Sodium

Hyponatremia (mostly mild) is a common feature at ICU admission present in 11-33% of patients [2, 17, 19]. Fewer, but still a considerable proportion of patients (11-16%), develop hyponatremia during their ICU stay [17, 19].

By contrast, hypernatremia is less prevalent on ICU admission (<10%) and becomes more frequent during the ICU stay (up to 30% of patients) [17, 19, 20].

Both hypo- and hypernatremia have been independently associated with increased hospital mortality [17]. Additionally, sodium fluctuations were associated with increased risk of death in surgical ICU patients [20].

15.4.2 Chloride

Hypochloremia is less common than hyponatremia, occurring in less than 10% of ICU patients, whereas hyperchloremia is very common (up to 45%) [17, 21].

Hyperchloremia appears to be associated with adverse outcome, but the mechanisms are not completely clear [21]. Chloride is important in homeostasis as a strong ion involved in acid-base balance. Hyperchloremia-associated metabolic acidosis may impair outcome via hemodynamic instability or coagulopathy.

15.4.3 Potassium

Abnormal serum potassium levels occur in around half of the patients admitted to the ICU [22, 23]. On ICU admission, hypokalemia has been reported in 17% and hyperkalemia in 12% of mixed ICU patients [17], whereas as many as two thirds of

Table 15.3 Prevalence and management of dyselectrolytemias in the ICU

Condition and range (mmol/l) [ref]	Prevalence	Management	Pitfalls and consequences of correction
Hypo-Na [3] Mild 130–134 Moderate 125–129 Severe <125	11–33% at admission, up to 16% during stay	3% NaCl if severe or moderate symptoms. Otherwise, based on the mechanism	Correction max. 10 mmol/24 h and 1–2 mmol/h. Overcorrection may lead to demyelination (not clear whether re-lowering after overcorrection is helpful)
Hyper-Na [17] Mild 146–150 Moderate 151–155 Severe >155	<10% at admission, up to 30% during stay	Hypotonic fluids if severe symptoms, isotonic fluids if hypotension	Overcorrection may lead to cerebral edema. Chronic conditions should be corrected, especially slowly
Hypo-K [3] Mild 3.0–3.4 Moderate 2.5–2.9 Severe <2.5	17% at admission 24% during ICU stay	Correct to normal (needed daily dosage may in some cases be several hundreds of mmol)	Overcorrection in case of concomitant worsening of renal function and/or development of acidosis. Correction with potassium phosphate may lead to hyper-Pi
Hyper-K [3] Mild 5.1–6.0 Moderate 6.1–7.0 Severe >7.0	12% at admission 21% during ICU stay	(1) i.v. calcium; (2) shifting with i.v. glucose + insulin ± salbutamol inhalation; (3) potassium binders; (4) hemodialysis	Overcorrection may occur with concomitant treatment/resolving of acidosis
Hypo-Mg [2] Mild to Moderate 0.41–0.62 Severe <0.41	20–50%	Correct to normal (target not clear), up to 6 g within 8-12 h is considered safe	Prediction of change with replacement is not easily predictable
Hyper-Mg [2] Mild 1.03–1.65 Moderate 1.65–5.14 Severe >5.14	7–12%	(1) Ca-gluconate, (2) furosemide, (3) dialysis if very severe	
Hypo-Ca [2] Mild-moderate 0.9–1.1 Severe <0.9	>50%	No specific guidance for supplementation	Prediction of change with replacement is not easily predictable
Hyper-Ca [4] Mild 1.4–2.0 Moderate 2.0–2.5 Severe >2.5	2–15%	If severe: (1) restoration of extracellular volume, (2) furosemide; (3) calcitonin	Phosphate lowers calcium but may increase the risk of renal damage. Bisphosphonates may be used if the cause is excessive bone resorption
Hypo-Pi [2] Mild 0.74–0.87 Moderate 0.48–0.73 Severe <0.48	10–30%	Correct to normal (no evidence on targets), i.v. phosphate up to 45 mmol/24 h is considered safe	Prediction of change with replacement is not easily predictable. Overcorrection may quickly occur, especially with concomitant impairment of renal function

(continued)

Table 15.3 (continued)

Condition and range (mmol/l) [ref]	Prevalence	Management	Pitfalls and consequences of correction
Hyper-Pi [2, 49] Mild-moderate 1.45–2.10 Severe >2.10	20–45%	Dialysis if very severe (cut-off unclear)	Treatment of concomitant hypocalcemia may aggravate building of calcium phosphate depositions in the kidneys
Hypo-Cl <98 [21]	7–9%	No specific guidance available	Changes usually occur concomitantly with sodium correction
Hyper-Cl [21] Moderate 107–110 Severe >110	17–45%		

Classification of mild/moderate/severe is based on provided references. Uniform specific classifications for severity and management recommendations for ICU patients are not available. *Na* sodium, *K* potassium, *Mg* magnesium, *Ca* calcium, *Pi* phosphate, *Cl* chloride, *i.v.* intravenous

patients with severe trauma were reported to present with hypokalemia at admission [24].

A U-shaped relationship between serum potassium levels and in-hospital mortality as well as an independent association between individual potassium variability and outcome has been reported [22, 25].

With correction of acidosis or manifestation of refeeding syndrome, the levels of magnesium and phosphate commonly decrease concomitantly with potassium levels.

15.4.4 Magnesium

Hypomagnesemia is present in 20-50% of patients on ICU admission, and hypermagnesemia in 7–12% [17, 26].

Two meta-analyses have shown associations between hypomagnesemia with higher mortality, need for mechanical ventilation, and length of ICU stay [27, 28], and hypermagnesemia was reported to impact mortality in a large cohort study [29]. However, a recent large study showed that neither hypo- nor hypermagnesemia on ICU admission was associated with mortality, but ICU-acquired hypermagnesemia was [26]. Hypomagnesemia may cause secondary hypokalemia and hypocalcemia.

15.4.5 Phosphate

The prevalence of hypophosphatemia in ICU patients has been reported as 10–30% [17, 30], and of hyperphosphatemia 20–45% [17, 30], but most of the studies had retrospective designs and did not measure phosphate in all concomitant patients. Moreover, as clinical features are variable (e.g., arrhythmias, neurological disturbances, muscle weakness) and may be attributed to different conditions present in critically ill patients, it is difficult to draw firm conclusions on the importance of phosphate disturbances. A recent meta-analysis demonstrated an association of hypophosphatemia with ICU length of stay [31]. The causality of this relationship remains unclear; in our opinion, it should rather to be interpreted that hypophosphatemia occurs more often in patients staying longer in the ICU. This hypothesis is further supported by a study reporting the prevalence of hypophosphatemia as >50% in patients with aneurysmal subarachnoid hemorrhage [32]. A meta-analysis did not confirm associations of hypophosphatemia with increased mortality [31]. Accordingly, the conviction that hypophosphatemia impairs outcome originates mainly from case series and the personal clinical experience of the authors of this manuscript. Additionally, a randomized controlled trial on refeeding syndrome demonstrated that nutrient reduction was able to improve outcomes despite serum electrolyte levels being successfully corrected in both groups, supporting the hypothesis that refeeding syndrome (diagnosed based on development of hypophosphatemia) itself affects outcome [33]. Possibly, the magnitude of change in phosphate level reflecting the magnitude of the refeeding mechanism may be more important than the absolute value of measured phosphate.

Hypophosphatemia often occurs along with hypokalemia, whereas hyperphosphatemia itself causes hypocalcemia that can lead to hypotension.

15.4.6 Calcium

More than half of ICU patients have hypocalcemia during their ICU stay, whereas hypercalcemia is less common (2–15%) [17, 34].

Serum calcium levels and/or their change were shown to have a U-shaped association with mortality [34]. Calcium levels are in a close interplay with phosphate and magnesium. Hyperphosphatemia caused by renal insufficiency or overcorrection of phosphate levels is one important cause of hypocalcemia in critically ill patients.

15.5 Management

Aggressive correction of any electrolyte abnormalities is common practice in the ICU. Sometimes this is required (e.g., severe hypokalemia), but can sometimes be harmful (e.g., hypo- or hypernatremia). Specific evidence-based treatment targets are lacking for nearly all electrolytes during critical illness. Overcorrection of electrolyte levels is probably common, but respective evidence is lacking. Importantly, when correction is undertaken, concomitant changes in other electrolytes need to be understood, anticipated, and monitored. All available recommendations (Table 15.3) are not specifically for critically ill patients, and focus mostly on correction of severe symptoms, which may not be obvious in critically ill patients due to their severe condition/underlying disease.

15.5.1 Sodium and Chloride

The key factor of correction of sodium levels is to prevent permanent neurological injury and reduce symptoms while avoiding osmotic injury caused by rapid correction of sodium. A specific management strategy needs to be chosen based on the pathophysiological mechanism, requiring careful differential diagnosis.

International guidelines are available for correction of hyponatremia [18], advocating administration of 3% NaCl for active correction of hyponatremia with severe or moderate symptoms without suggesting a clear cut-off for serum Na^+. Correction limits of max 10 mmol/24 h for the first day and max 8 mmol/24 h for the next days have been proposed without solid underlying evidence (recommendation level 2D), but re-lowering of sodium if correction happens faster than these limits was recommended (1D (!)). Obviously, evidence is very weak, and the optimal rate of correction (including the rate in the first hours, during later phases, and in acute and chronic hyponatremia) is controversial, as is the rationale for re-lowering of sodium if correction was faster than these arbitrarily set limits [35]. In our own clinical experience, suggested fast correction with 3% NaCl often leads to overcorrection, whereas a careful start with 0.9% NaCl or Ringer's solution with frequent monitoring may provide more smooth correction and avoid overcorrection. Importantly, Ringer's solution is still significantly hyperosmotic for a patient with very low sodium values.

Hypernatremia is addressed in Dutch guidelines [36], suggesting immediate treatment with hypotonic fluids for acute or severely symptomatic hypernatremia, and preferring isotonic fluids in case of hypotension. Acute hypernatremia may be corrected fast initially (1–2 mmol/l/h) with maximum limits of 8–10 mmol/24 h thereafter, whereas rapid correction should be avoided in chronic hypernatremia [36]. Increased 28-day mortality has been demonstrated in patients with persisting hypo- or hypernatremia on day 3 [37]. Chloride is usually corrected together with sodium with application of hyper- or hypotonic solutions.

15.5.2 Low Potassium, Phosphate, and Magnesium

Hypokalemia needs to be corrected fast, arbitrarily to at least >3.0 mmol/l. Hypokalemia due to correction of acidosis or refeeding should be anticipated and managed in a timely manner. Serum potassium levels of less than 3.5 mmol/l were associated with ventricular arrhythmia and mortality in patients with acute myocardial infarction [38], indicating that even mild hypokalemia in patients with concomitant triggering factors for arrhythmias [39] may be life-threatening. One before-and-after study demonstrated that integrating potassium control with computerized glucose control reduced potassium variability and prevalence of abnormal values [22]. Correction of hypokalemia to normal levels has been associated with improved short-term survival [25].

Hypophosphatemia and hypomagnesemia need to be anticipated and looked for/detected in parallel with hypokalemia if the mechanism of hypokalemia is K^+ shift. However, recommendations for clear treatment targets for phosphate and magnesium are not available. Intravenous administration of phosphate up to 45 mmol [40] and of magnesium up to 6 g within 8–12 h [41] is generally considered safe. Importantly, as these electrolytes are mainly intracellular, increase in serum levels in response is dependent on intracellular levels and an effect of a certain dosage on serum level cannot be well predicted. Correction of serum magnesium near to the upper normal level for 3 days increased lactate clearance in septic patients in one small randomized controlled trial [42], whereas a loading-dose of 7.5 g in 8 hours improved insulin resistance indices in critically ill patients with stress-induced hyperglycemia in another [43].

15.5.3 High Potassium, Phosphate, and Magnesium

Hyperkalemia management guidelines from the Renal Association [44] recommend the following steps for management of severe hyperkalemia (defined as >6.5 mmol/l): (1) administration of intravenous calcium salts (1C); (2) shifting K^+ into cells with insulin-glucose infusion (1B) and with inhalation of salbutamol as an additive option (1B), but not supporting routine use of sodium bicarbonate infusion for shifting (2C); (3) removing K^+ from the body by administration of potassium binders (1B), but not supporting cation-exchange resin for severe but rather as an option for moderate hyperkalemia. There is no clear recommendation for the initiation of RRT.

Rapid increase in extracellular phosphate concentrations in patients with tumor lysis syndrome, acute kidney injury, or receiving phosphate-containing bowel preparation solutions or enemas may lead to acute phosphate nephropathy with calcium phosphate depositions in the kidneys [45]. Data on the management of hyperphosphatemia in the ICU are scarce; one study showed better control of phosphate levels with continuous vs. intermittent RRT [46]. In critically ill patients with acute kidney injury receiving continuous enteral nutrition, a reduced effect of phosphate binders is expected and more frequent dosing could be considered [45]. In case of severe hypermagnesemia, intravenous administration of calcium gluconate has been suggested [47].

15.5.4 Calcium

There is no solid evidence that calcium supplementation (with the aim of correction to normal) is successful or that it may improve outcomes [48]. Hypercalcemia is often associated with hypovolemia, requiring restoration of blood volume. The other therapeutic options are limited to serious cases and include loop diuretics and calcitonin to increase urinary calcium excretion.

15.6 Conclusion

Electrolyte abnormalities are commonly encountered in critically ill patients. Most occur during the ICU stay rather than being a reason for ICU admission. A U-shaped association with mortality has been observed for several electrolytes and higher variability from 'hypo' to 'hyper' appears to be associated with impaired outcome. Many electrolyte abnormalities are induced by the interplay of other electrolyte disturbances or may be due to correction of these. Overcorrection may occur easily due to the narrow normal ranges and may lead to iatrogenic electrolyte abnormalities as a consequence. Rate of correction may also impact on outcome for some electrolyte abnormalities.

Triggers and targets for correction of electrolyte levels are lacking for most electrolytes during critical illness. Whether correction is always necessary and improves outcome warrants further research, as there is a paucity of data in ICU patients.

References

1. Bersten A, Handy J. Oh's intensive care manual. Oxford: Elsevier; 2018.
2. Kraft MD, Btaiche IF, Sacks GS, Kudsk KA. Treatment of electrolyte disorders in adult patients in the intensive care unit. Am J Health Syst Pharm. 2005;62:1663–82.
3. Berardi RTM, Lenci E, Pecci F, Morgese F, Rinaldi S. Electrolyte disorders in cancer patients: a systematic review. J Cancer Metastasis Treat. 2019;5:79.
4. Chang WT, Radin B, McCurdy MT. Calcium, magnesium, and phosphate abnormalities in the emergency department. Emerg Med Clin North Am. 2014;32:349–66.
5. Tinawi M. Pathophysiology, evaluation, and management of metabolic alkalosis. Cureus. 2021;13:e12841.
6. Berend K, van Hulsteijn LH, Gans RO. Chloride: the queen of electrolytes? Eur J Intern Med. 2012;23:203–11.
7. Pham PM, Pham PA, Pham SV, Pham PT, Pham PT, Pham PC. Correction of hyponatremia and osmotic demyelinating syndrome: have we neglected to think intracellularly? Clin Exp Nephrol. 2015;19:489–95.
8. Huang CL, Kuo E. Mechanism of hypokalemia in magnesium deficiency. J Am Soc Nephrol. 2007;18:2649–52.
9. Pham PC, Pham PM, Pham SV, Miller JM, Pham PT. Hypomagnesemia in patients with type 2 diabetes. Clin J Am Soc Nephrol. 2007;2:366–73.
10. Na D, Tao G, Shu-Ying L, Qin-Yi W, et al. Association between hypomagnesemia and severity of primary hyperparathyroidism: a retrospective study. BMC Endocr Disord. 2021;21:170.
11. Wadsworth RL, Siddique S. Phosphate homeostasis in critical care. BJA Education. 2016;16:305–9.
12. Martin KJ, Gonzalez EA, Slatopolsky E. Clinical consequences and management of hypomagnesemia. J Am Soc Nephrol. 2009;20:2291–5.
13. Palmer BF, Clegg DJ. Physiology and pathophysiology of potassium homeostasis: core curriculum. Am J Kidney Dis. 2019;2019:74682–95.
14. Kapoor M, Chan GZ. Fluid and electrolyte abnormalities. Crit Care Clin. 2001;17:503–29.
15. Amanzadeh J, Reilly RF Jr. Hypophosphatemia: an evidence-based approach to its clinical consequences and management. Nat Clin Pract Nephrol. 2006;2:136–48.
16. Pham PC, Konanur Ventakaram R, Pham J, et al. Severe hyperphosphatemia in a patient with mild acute kidney injury. Case Rep Med. 2021;2021:9962624.
17. Reintam Blaser A, van Zanten ARH. Electrolyte disorders during the initiation of nutrition therapy in the ICU. Curr Opin Clin Nutr Metab Care. 2021;24:151–8.

18. Spasovski G, Vanholder R, Allolio B, et al. Clinical practice guideline on diagnosis and treatment of hyponatraemia. Intensive Care Med. 2014;40:320–31.
19. Sim JK, Ko RE, Na SJ, et al. Intensive care unit-acquired hyponatremia in critically ill medical patients. J Transl Med. 2020;18:268.
20. Sakr Y, Rother S, Ferreira AM, et al. Fluctuations in serum sodium level are associated with an increased risk of death in surgical ICU patients. Crit Care Med. 2013;41:133–42.
21. Van Regenmortel N, Verbrugghe W, Van den Wyngaert T, Jorens PG. Impact of chloride and strong ion difference on ICU and hospital mortality in a mixed intensive care population. Ann Intensive Care. 2016;6:91.
22. Hessels L, Hoekstra M, Mijzen LJ, et al. The relationship between serum potassium, potassium variability and in-hospital mortality in critically ill patients and a before-after analysis on the impact of computer-assisted potassium control. Crit Care. 2015;19:4.
23. Tongyoo S, Viarasilpa T, Permpikul C. Serum potassium levels and outcomes in critically ill patients in the medical intensive care unit. J Int Med Res. 2018;46:1254–62.
24. Safavi M, Honarmand A, Mehrizi MK, et al. Hypokalemia at the time of admission to the intensive care unit (iCU) increases the need for mechanical ventilation and time of ventilation in critically ill trauma patients. Adv Biomed Res. 2017;6:50.
25. Krogager ML, Søgaard P, Torp-Pedersen C, et al. Impact of plasma potassium normalization on short-term mortality in patients with hypertension and hypokalemia or low normal potassium. BMC Cardiovasc Disord. 2020;20:386.
26. Laupland KB, Tabah A, Jacobs N, Ramanan M. Determinants of serum magnesium abnormalities and outcome among admissions to the intensive care unit. Anaesth Crit Care Pain Med. 2020;39:793–7.
27. Jiang P, Lv Q, Lai T, Xu F. Does hypomagnesemia impact on the outcome of patients admitted to the intensive care unit? A systematic review and meta- analysis. Shock. 2017;47:288–95.
28. Upala S, Jaruvongvanich V, Wijarnpreecha K, Sanguankeo A. Hypomagnesemia and mortality in patients admitted to intensive care unit: a systematic review and meta-analysis. QJM. 2016;109:453–9.
29. Broman M, Hansson F, Klarin B. Analysis of hypo- and hypermagnesemia in an intensive care unit cohort. Acta Anaesthesiol Scand. 2018;62:648–57.
30. Sin JCK, Laupland KB, Ramanan M, Tabah A. Phosphate abnormalities and outcomes among admissions to the intensive care unit: a retrospective multicentre cohort study. J Crit Care. 2021;64:154–9.
31. Sin JCK, King L, Ballard E, Llewellyn S, Laupland KB, Tabah A. Hypophosphatemia and outcomes in ICU: a systematic review and meta-analysis. J Intensive Care Med. 2021;36:1025–35.
32. Erritzøe-Jervild M, Wesierski J, Romano S, et al. Hypophosphataemia is common in patients with aneurysmal subarachnoid haemorrhage. Acta Anaesthesiol Scand. 2021;65:1431–8.
33. Doig GS, Simpson F, Heighes PT, et al. Restricted versus continued standard caloric intake during the management of refeeding syndrome in critically ill adults: a randomized, parallel-group, multicentre, single blind controlled trial. Lancet Respir Med. 2015;3:943–52.
34. Thongprayoon C, Cheungpasitporn W, Hansrivijit P, et al. Impact of changes in serum calcium levels on in-hospital mortality. Medicina (Kaunas). 2020;56:106.
35. Sterns RH. Treatment of severe hyponatremia. Clin J Am Soc Nephrol. 2018;13:641–9.
36. Hoorn EJ, Tuut MK, Hoorntje SJ, van Saase JL, Zietse R, Geers AB. Dutch guideline for the management of electrolyte disorders - 2012 revision. Neth J Med. 2013;71:153–65.
37. Darmon M, Pichon M, Schwebel C, et al. Influence of early dysnatremia correction on survival of critically ill patients. Shock. 2014;41:394–9.
38. Colombo MG, Kirchberger I, Amann U, Dinser L, Meisinger C. Association of serum potassium concentration with mortality and ventricular arrhythmias in patients with acute myocardial infarction: a systematic review and meta-analysis. Eur J Prev Cardiol. 2018;25:576–95.
39. Osadchii OE. Mechanisms of hypokalemia-induced ventricular arrhythmogenicity. Fundam Clin Pharmacol. 2010;24:547–59.
40. Geerse DA, Bindels AJ, Kuiper MA, Roos AN, Spronk PE, Schultz MJ. Treatment of hypophosphatemia in the intensive care unit: a review. Crit Care. 2010;14:R147.

41. Velissaris D, Karamouzos V, Pierrakos C, Aretha D, Karanikolas M. Hypomagnesemia in critically ill sepsis patients. J Clin Med Res. 2015;7:911–8.
42. Noormandi A, Khalili H, Mohammadi M, Abdollahi A. Effect of magnesium supplementation on lactate clearance in critically ill patients with severe sepsis: a randomized clinical trial. Eur J Clin Pharmacol. 2020;76:175–84.
43. Heidary Z, Khalili H, Mohammadi M, Beigmohammadi MT, Abdollahi A. Effect of magnesium loading dose on insulin resistance in patients with stress-induced hyperglycemia: a randomized clinical trial. J Intensive Care Med. 2020;35:687–93.
44. Renal Association Clinical Practice Guidelines – Treatment of Acute Hyperkalaemia in Adults – July 2020. Available at: https://ukkidney.org/sites/renal.org/files/RENAL%20ASSOCIATION%20HYPERKALAEMIA%20GUIDELINE%202020.pdf Accessed 21 Nov 2021.
45. Leaf DE, Christov M. Dysregulated mineral metabolism in AKI. Semin Nephrol. 2019;39:41–56.
46. Tan HK, Bellomo R, M'Pisi DA, Ronco C. Phosphatemic control during acute renal failure: intermittent hemodialysis versus continuous hemodiafiltration. Int J Artif Organs. 2001;24:186–91.
47. Swaminathan R. Magnesium metabolism and its disorders. Clin Biochem Rev. 2003;24:47–66.
48. Forsythe RM, Wessel CB, Billiar TR, Angus DC, Rosengart MR. Parenteral calcium for intensive care unit patients. Cochrane Database Syst Rev. 2008;4:CD006163.
49. Rodriguez-Benot A, Martin-Malo A, Alvarez-Lara MA, Rodriguez M, Aljama P. Mild hyperphosphatemia and mortality in hemodialysis patients. Am J Kidney Dis. 2005;46:68–77.

Part V

Renal Failure

16 Hemodynamic Instability During Continuous Renal Replacement Therapy: Is It All About Fluid?

S. M. T. Nasser, N. Boyer, and L. G. Forni

16.1 Introduction

The use of renal replacement therapies (RRT) remains the mainstay of treatment for patients with severe acute kidney injury (AKI) and encompasses intermittent hemodialysis (IHD), prolonged intermittent therapies, and continuous renal replacement therapies (CRRT) among others. Common to all these techniques is hemodynamic instability related to RRT, manifest predominantly by a drop in blood pressure. Much of our understanding behind hemodynamic instability related to RRT is derived from studies on patients undergoing IHD where solute clearance, based on diffusion across the dialysis membrane, is driven by a concentration gradient between blood and dialysate. Fluid removal is achieved through ultrafiltration whereby water under hydrostatic pressure passes through the semipermeable membrane. The total amount of solute transported per unit of time (clearance), depends on the molecular weight of the molecule, membrane characteristics, dialysate flow,

S. M. T. Nasser · N. Boyer
Department of Critical Care, Royal Surrey Hospital, Guildford, Surrey, UK

SPACeR Group (Surrey Peri-Operative, Anaesthesia & Critical Care Collaborative Research Group), Royal Surrey Hospital, Guildford, Surrey, UK

L. G. Forni (✉)
Department of Critical Care, Royal Surrey Hospital, Guildford, Surrey, UK

SPACeR Group (Surrey Peri-Operative, Anaesthesia & Critical Care Collaborative Research Group), Royal Surrey Hospital, Guildford, Surrey, UK

Department of Clinical & Experimental Medicine, Faculty of Health Sciences, University of Surrey, Guildford, UK
e-mail: luiforni@nhs.net

J.-L. Vincent (ed.), *Annual Update in Intensive Care and Emergency Medicine 2022*, Annual Update in Intensive Care and Emergency Medicine, https://doi.org/10.1007/978-3-030-93433-0_16

and blood flow [1]. Given fluid is not replaced in IHD, the consequence of rapid fluid removal may be responsible for any observed hemodynamic instability.

CRRT describes a variety of blood purification techniques that differ according to the mechanism of solute transport, the type of membrane used, as well as the presence or absence of dialysate solution. Although ultrafiltration is again employed to remove plasma water, where required, the process of convection is relatively inefficient. This necessitates higher ultrafiltration rates and as a consequence, replacement of fluid [2]. The overall effect is slower (net) fluid removal in convective CRRT, which has been preferred by some in intensive care, with the expectation that this would limit hemodynamic instability related to RRT in the critically ill. Despite this, the evidence that CRRT is associated with less hemodynamic instability has been mixed. In a meta-analysis of 9 randomized controlled trials (RCTs), CRRT was found to be associated with a lower burden of hemodynamic instability than intermittent RRT (OR = 0.66; 95% CI 0.45–0.96, p = 0.03). However, two of the largest studies included in the analysis excluded patients with hemodynamic instability. No significant difference was seen in relation to mortality or recovery to RRT independence [3]. A subsequent Cochrane meta-analysis comparing CRRT and IHD showed no significant difference in ICU or in-hospital mortality, hemodynamic instability, hypotensive episodes, or vasopressor requirement, while showing significantly higher mean arterial pressures during therapy with CRRT than with IHD [3, 4].

16.2 Defining Hemodynamic Instability Related to RRT

The incidence of reported hemodynamic instability related to RRT varies considerably. For example, in CRRT, rates of hemodynamic instability of up to 43% have been reported whilst in IHD, rates of over 70% are described [5–8]. One of the explanations behind such disparity is the lack of consensus as to a definition for hemodynamic instability related to RRT particularly in the critically ill. In 2005, the Kidney Disease Outcomes Quality Initiative (KDIGO) originally defined intradialytic hypotension as a ≥20 mmHg drop in systolic blood pressure (SBP) or a >10 mmHg drop in mean arterial blood pressure (MAP) and, crucially, in the presence of symptoms related to intradialytic hypotension [9]. More recently a refinement to the definition has been suggested, to include any symptomatic decrease in SBP or a nadir intradialytic SBP of <90 mmHg, which should prompt reassessment of blood pressure and volume management [10]. Although applicable to the outpatient setting, such definitions are not relevant to patients treated with RRT on the ICU for several reasons. First, the recorded SBP of the patient is dependent on many other factors including the underlying condition causing the AKI, such as sepsis, as well as interventions such as the use of vasopressors or the effect of mechanical ventilation. Second, in most cases the patient will not be able to reliably report symptoms of hemodynamic instability. In terms of defining hemodynamic instability related to RRT in the critically ill, a pragmatic approach may be an observed drop in SBP on commencing RRT or the necessity for an intervention to prevent a hypotensive episode.

16.3 Consequences of Hemodynamic Instability Related to RRT

What is clear from the available evidence is that the development of hemodynamic instability related to RRT is associated with significant morbidity and mortality, either through direct cardiovascular ischemia or through repeated kidney insult, precipitating worse long-term renal recovery [11]. For example, the association between intradialytic hypotension and 2-year at-risk mortality showed that a nadir of 90 SBP in ≥30% of IHD sessions was most strongly associated with mortality, with an adjusted odds ratio of 1.56 (CI 1.09–2.31) [12]. However, there is little evidence from the critical care literature although hemodynamic instability related to RRT is associated with increased hospital mortality [11].

16.4 Potential Mechanisms of Hemodynamic Instability Related to RRT

When considering the mechanisms behind hemodynamic instability related to RRT in the ICU it is apparent that this phenomenon may be related to the application of the RRT technique itself or the response of the individual patient to the extracorporeal circuit. Hence part of this may be modifiable, such as ultrafiltration rate or temperature of dialysate applied, whereas the individual response may be unpredictable (Fig. 16.1).

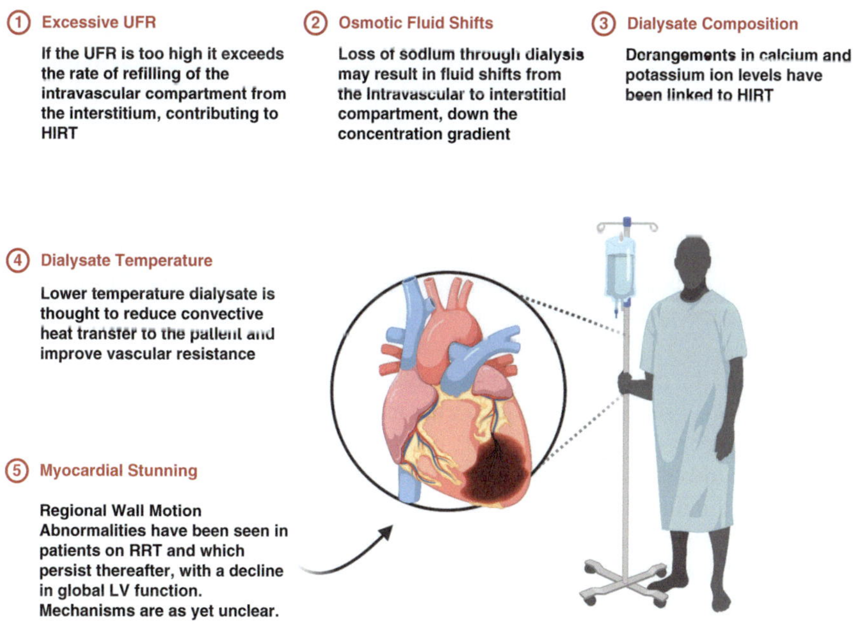

Fig. 16.1 Outline of major mechanisms contributing to hemodynamic instability related to renal replacement therapy (HIRT). *UFR* ultrafiltration rate, *RRT* renal replacement therapy, *LV* left ventricular. (Figure created with BioRender.com)

16.4.1 RRT Related Mechanisms of Hemodynamic Instability

Perhaps the most discussed aspect of RRT leading to hemodynamic instability is that of ultrafiltration rate and fluid removal. In terms of intradialytic hypotension complicating end-stage renal disease, debate has traditionally focused on the role of the circulating blood volume. Simplistically, dialysis may be viewed as the consequence of the rate of ultrafiltrate extraction exceeding that of the refilling rate from the interstitial compartment to the intravascular compartment with resulting reduction in circulating volume and subsequently, cardiac preload. In keeping with this paradigm, the ultrafiltration rate has been shown to exhibit a dose-dependent relationship with both intradialytic hypotension and mortality, with ultrafiltration rate of 12.37 ml/h/kg of body weight the best discriminatory point for predicting 2-year survival [13]. However, to what extent do these factors play a role in CRRT? Critically unwell patients may require renal support for different indications including correction of acidosis, refractory pulmonary edema or fluid overload and, given the diversity of etiologies that can lead to such indications, it cannot be assumed that all hemodynamic instability related to RRT is due to over-zealous ultrafiltration. However, it is likely these mechanisms are also applicable to hemodynamic instability in CRRT to some extent. Although CRRT may result in a lower rate of fluid removal, the threshold at which (net) fluid removal exceeds the interstitial-intravascular re-filling rate may be lower, resulting in preload depletion and higher frequency of hemodynamic instability in CRRT at a lower fluid removal rate than in the outpatient hemodialysis setting. Given that paradoxical intravascular volume depletion with extensive tissue edema is a common finding in the critically ill, this may go unrecognized, leading to volume depletion with a reduction in cardiac preload. Indeed, one study on 42 critically ill patients addressed the relationship between preload dependency and hemodynamic instability in CRRT demonstrating that hemodynamic instability was associated with preload-dependence in 131 of 243 episodes (54%; CI 95% 48–60%) [14]. Preload dependence was assessed by postural assessment every 4 h and during every episode of hemodynamic instability, defined by a decrease in SBP. Interestingly, multivariate analysis found no CRRT-related factor associated with the development of hemodynamic instability, but pre-CRRT initiation preload dependence was strongly associated with hemodynamic instability.

As well as the rate of fluid removal potentially driving hemodynamic instability related to RRT, osmotic fluid shifts during treatment may also be relevant. Again, studies have concentrated on patients on IHD where rapid electrolyte (sodium) clearance in the intravascular space results in loss of fluid to the intravascular compartment and intradialytic hypotension, as evidenced by individuals with a higher calculated plasma osmolarity at the initiation of hemodialysis being at highest risk of intradialytic hypotension [15]. The role of small solutes, sodium in particular, as an important factor in driving osmotic shifts that trigger hemodynamic instability, has been supported by two RCTs, finding that sodium profiling was effective in decreasing the frequency of hypotensive episodes in patients undergoing sustained low-efficiency dialysis (SLED) or IHD [16, 17]. Similarly, oncotic pressure may also play a prominent role in hemodynamic instability related to RRT, especially given that critical illness is associated strongly with loss of plasma proteins, albumin in particular [18]. Indeed, in critically ill patients, hypoalbuminemia has been considered as a risk factor for intradialytic hypotension although this may be confounded by a low albumin reflecting the severity of illness and being an independent predictor of mortality. However, one recent randomized, crossover trial has shown less intradialytic hypotension frequency and severity with administration of 100 ml 25% albumin over 100 ml 0.9% saline in hospitalized, hypoalbuminemic patients at initiation of hemodialysis, a finding replicated in a recent, small, single center, pilot RCT, again comparing albumin 25% with 0.9% saline when initiating SLED [19, 20].

As well as manipulation of the ultrafiltration rate, the composition and the temperature of the dialysate may play a role in the development of hemodynamic instability related to RRT. Cooler dialysate fluid has been hypothesized to result in less convective transfer of heat to the blood, resulting in higher peripheral resistance, and a subsequently higher preload as well as afterload. A systematic review of 22 randomized, crossover studies found that reduction in dialysate fluid temperature resulted in a significant improvement in both frequency and severity of hemodynamic instability related to RRT [21]. A more recent meta-analysis also concluded that lower dialysate temperature reduced the frequency of intradialytic hypotension (mean 70%; CI 49–89%) and raised intradialytic MAP (mean 12 mmHg; CI 8–16 mmHg), but that high quality, multicenter RCTs are needed for greater confidence as to the exact degree of benefit in reducing hemodynamic instability related to RRT [22].

Regarding dialysate fluid composition, this may also play a role in terms of regulating vascular tone where significant electrolytic shifts due to large differences between serum and dialysate electrolyte concentrations have been the subject of scrutiny as possible reasons for hemodynamic instability related to RRT. For example, a higher dialysate calcium concentration was associated with a higher intradialytic MAP in an albeit small, prospective, cross-over study [23]. This is of less relevance to the CRRT population, particularly where citrate-based anticoagulation is being performed, given strict adherence to protocols to ensure ionized calcium levels are maintained in the circulation. This is relevant as relative hypocalcemia may result in cardiac rhythm disturbances, myocardial stunning and hypotension [24]. Similarly, potassium levels may be of relevance given the observation that a rapid decrease in potassium serum concentration as a result of a significant serum–dialysate potassium concentration gradient, has been associated with lower blood pressure correlating to a lower peripheral vascular resistance [25]. However, to-date there have been no studies assessing the relationship between potassium dialysate concentration and hemodynamic instability related to RRT in critically ill patients [26].

16.4.2 Patient Related Factors Associated with Hemodynamic Instability Related to RRT

The response of an individual to the application of RRT also plays a significant role in determining hemodynamic instability, not least the response of the cardiovascular system. For example, the theoretical mechanism of cooler dialysate increasing systemic vascular resistance and decreasing the frequency if intradialytic hypotension has been challenged, with reduction of myocardial stunning proposed as an alternative mechanism [27]. Recent evidence has demonstrated that reduced regional wall motion abnormalities (RWMAs), were associated with increased intradialytic SBP, higher total peripheral resistance, and lower cardiac output in a crossover study of 11 patients receiving dialysate fluid tailored to individual body temperature [28]. These results are further evidenced by results showing that cooling dialysis at 0.5 °C below body temperature (between group-difference 1.2 °C ± 0.3 °C) for 12 months post-initiation of hemodialysis was associated with slower progression of hemodialysis-associated cardiomyopathy [29]. In the chronic hemodialysis population, two or more RWMAs occurring during dialysis were strongly associated with adverse patient outcomes, in a dose-dependent manner [30]. Such RWMAs have also been seen in acute patients with single organ AKI who did not require inotropic or ventilatory support, with a median sequential organ failure assessment (SOFA) score of 6 (interquartile range [IQR] 2) on the day of the study [31]. RRT was commenced within the first 48 h of hospital admission. All patients developed two or more new RWMAs during dialysis, with a median of 5 (IQR 4–6) affected left ventricular (LV) segments. These changes persisted after dialysis (median number of RWMAs 4, IQR 3–6) with a decline in global LV contractility falling from a normal pre-dialysis level of -17.8 ± 3.7% to an abnormal level during dialysis (-15.3 ± 2.3%, p = 0.03) and remaining low in the post-dialysis period (-14.8 ± 2.8%, p = 0.002) (Fig. 16.2). Interestingly, high-sensitivity troponin-T values were significantly higher 6 h after dialysis; 56 μg/l (IQR 394 μg/l) versus 39 μg/l (IQR 216 μg/l), p = 0.003. Of note these changes occurred on a backdrop of only modest ultrafiltration (mean ultrafiltration rate 5 ± 3 ml/h/kg, mean ultrafiltration volume 1.4 ± 1 l) and although no significant change in MAP was observed, this masked individual variation given that seven patients had an episode of intradialytic hypotension [31]. A similar study in 11 critically ill patients found that CRRT also resulted in significant myocardial stunning and, interestingly, no change in blood pressure, heart rate, dose of vasoactive medication or lactate was seen. However, only four patients survived off RRT during the study [32]. It may be hypothesized that these acutely observed areas of RWMA develop fixed segmental systolic dysfunction deficits, which are observed in some end-stage renal disease patients [33].

Hemodynamic instability can start minutes after commencement of RRT, before significant ultrafiltration or osmotic shifts have occurred and is strongly associated with in-hospital mortality [34]. It follows that some other mechanism(s) must play a significant role and interest has turned to the effect of RRT on the microcirculation.

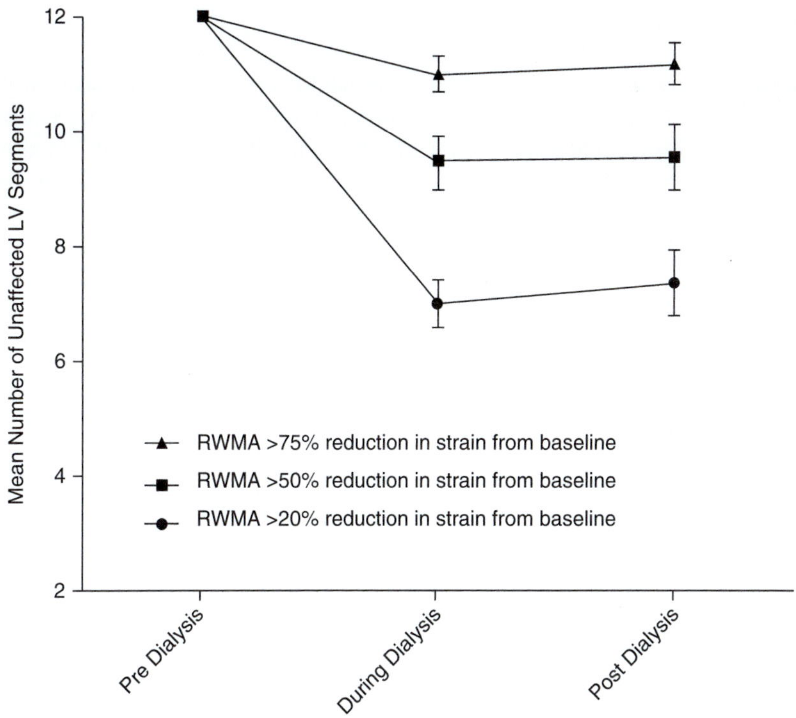

Fig. 16.2 The number of unaffected left ventricular (LV) segments during dialysis, demonstrating the onset of regional LV dysfunction. All patients experienced new regional wall motion abnormalities (RWMAs) during dialysis using the pre-defined definition of ≥20% reduction in segmental longitudinal strain. At 50% threshold, results were broadly similar with 9 out of the 11 patients demonstrating two or more new RWMAs. (Reproduced from [31] and distributed under the terms of the Creative Commons Attribution-NonCommercial 4.0 International License)

Shunting of blood volume from the microcirculation to the macrocirculation is observed in patients on hemodialysis post-ultrafiltration, resulting in volume depletion in the microcirculation and slowing of blood velocity [35, 36]. Furthermore, in critically ill patients receiving SLED, a significant reduction in circulating levels of the nitric oxide (NO) metabolites, nitrate and nitrite, and cGMP, a signaling marker of bioactive NO was observed, with levels of nitrate and nitrite returning to baseline levels before the commencement of the second SLED session [37]. These findings accord with previous studies demonstrating decreased NO production in patients on hemodialysis [38]. Of note, IHD is known to increase levels of cell-free hemoglobin, a highly efficient scavenger of NO, with sequestration of free NO by more than 70% as observed in chronic hemodialysis patients, at the same time as observed impairment of vascular function [39]. The degree to which this mechanism contributes to hemodynamic instability in patients on hemodialysis or CRRT needs further characterization, especially in light of the essential role endothelial-derived and hemoglobin-bound NO play in maintaining microcirculatory blood flow [40].

16.5 Conclusion

The mechanisms behind the hemodynamic instability observed in patients undergoing RRT clearly go beyond simple volume removal and, although minimizing osmotic and oncotic fluid shifts and use of a judicious ultrafiltration rates in those at highest risk identified through assessment of preload dependence may be relevant, strong evidence for this in the CRRT setting is missing. More recently, it has been observed that RWMAs and myocardial stunning seen in RRT may be of relevance in determining outcomes. In this regard, it has been shown that critically ill patients who tolerate more intensive ultrafiltration have an improved outcome at 1 year and perhaps in this group the effects on myocardial performance are less profound [41]. Therefore, mitigating hemodynamic instability to allow more ultrafiltration may be of relevance, particularly in the context of significant fluid overload where reduction in ultrafiltration rate may not always be the appropriate course of action. What is clear is that we have much to learn with regard to hemodynamic instability related to RRT, no matter how it is defined, and reducing its incidence may well translate into improved outcomes for our patients.

References

1. Pannu N, Gibney RN. Renal replacement therapy in the intensive care unit. Ther Clin Risk Manag. 2005;1:141–50.
2. Forni LG, Hilton PJ. Continuous hemofiltration in the treatment of acute renal failure. N Engl J Med. 1997;336:1303–9.
3. Bagshaw SM, Berthiaume LR, Delaney A, Bellomo R. Continuous versus intermittent renal replacement therapy for critically ill patients with acute kidney injury: a meta-analysis. Crit Care Med. 2008;36:610–7.
4. Rabindranath KS, Adams J, MacLeod AM, Muirhead N. Intermittent versus continuous renal replacement therapy for acute renal failure in adults. Cochrane Database Syst Rev. 2007:CD003773.
5. Tonelli M, Astephen P, Andreou P, Beed S, Lundrigan P, Jindal K. Blood volume monitoring in intermittent hemodialysis for acute renal failure. Kidney Int. 2002;62:1075–80.
6. Bitker L, Bayle F, Yonis H, et al. Prevalence and risk factors of hypotension associated with preload-dependence during intermittent hemodialysis in critically ill patients. Crit Care. 2016;20:44.
7. Uchino S, Bellomo R, Morimatsu H, et al. Continuous renal replacement therapy: a worldwide practice survey. The beginning and ending supportive therapy for the kidney (B.E.S.T. kidney) investigators. Intensive Care Med. 2007;33:1563–70.
8. Akhoundi A, Singh B, Vela M, et al. Incidence of adverse events during continuous renal replacement therapy. Blood Purif. 2015;39:333–9.
9. Workgroup KD. K/DOQI clinical practice guidelines for cardiovascular disease in dialysis patients. Am J Kidney Dis. 2005;45:S1–S153.
10. Flythe JE, Chang TI, Gallagher MP, et al. Blood pressure and volume management in dialysis: conclusions from a kidney disease: improving global outcomes (KDIGO) controversies conference. Kidney Int. 2020;97:861–76.
11. Silversides JA, Pinto R, Kuint R, et al. Fluid balance, intradialytic hypotension, and outcomes in critically ill patients undergoing renal replacement therapy: a cohort study. Crit Care. 2014;18:1–10.

12. Flythe JE, Xue H, Lynch KE, Curhan GC, Brunelli SM. Association of mortality risk with various definitions of intradialytic hypotension. J Am Soc Nephrol. 2015;26:724–34.
13. Assimon MM, Wenger JB, Wang L, Flythe JE. Ultrafiltration rate and mortality in maintenance hemodialysis patients. Am J Kidney Dis. 2016;68:911–22.
14. Chazot G, Bitker L, Mezidi M, et al. Prevalence and risk factors of hemodynamic instability associated with preload-dependence during continuous renal replacement therapy in a prospective observational cohort of critically ill patients. Ann Intensive Care. 2021;11:1–12.
15. Mc Causland FR, Waikar SS. Association of predialysis calculated plasma osmolarity with intradialytic blood pressure decline. Am J Kidney Dis. 2015;66:499–506.
16. Lima EQ, Silva RG, Donadi EL, Fernandes AB, Zanon JR, Pinto KR, Burdmann EA. Prevention of intradialytic hypotension in patients with acute kidney injury submitted to sustained low-efficiency dialysis. Ren Fail. 2012;34:1238–43.
17. Paganini E, Sandy D, Moreno L, Kozlowski L, Sakai K. The effect of sodium and ultrafiltration modelling on plasma volume changes and haemodynamic stability in intensive care patients receiving haemodialysis for acute renal failure: a prospective, stratified, randomized, cross-over study. Nephrol Dial Transplant. 1996;11(Suppl 8):32–7.
18. Nicholson J, Wolmarans M, Park G. The role of albumin in critical illness. Br J Anaesth. 2000;85:599–610.
19. Macedo E, Karl B, Lee E, Mehta RL. A randomized trial of albumin infusion to prevent intradialytic hypotension in hospitalized hypoalbuminemic patients. Crit Care. 2021;25:1–8.
20. Clark E, McIntyre L, Watpool I, et al. Intravenous albumin for the prevention of hemodynamic instability during sustained low-efficiency dialysis. A randomized controlled feasibility trial (the SAFER-SLED study). Ann Intensive Care. 2021;11:174.
21. Selby NM, McIntyre CW. A systematic review of the clinical effects of reducing dialysate fluid temperature. Nephrol Dial Transplant. 2006;21:1883–98.
22. Mustafa RA, Bdair F, Akl EA, et al. Effect of lowering the dialysate temperature in chronic hemodialysis: a systematic review and meta-analysis. Clin J Am Soc Nephrol. 2016;11:442–57.
23. Sherman RA, Bialy GB, GazinskiL B, Bernholc AS, Eisinger RP. The effect of dialysate calcium levels on blood pressure during hemodialysis. Am J Kidney Dis. 1986;8:244–7.
24. Langote A, Ahearn M, Zimmerman D. Dialysate calcium concentration, mineral metabolism disorders, and cardiovascular disease: deciding the hemodialysis bath. Am J Kidney Dis. 2015;66:348–58.
25. Gabutti L, Salvadé I, Lucchini B, Soldini D, Burnier M. Haemodynamic consequences of changing potassium concentrations in haemodialysis fluids. BMC Nephrol. 2011;12:1–8.
26. Douvris A, Zeid K, Hiremath S, et al. Mechanisms for hemodynamic instability related to renal replacement therapy: a narrative review. Intensive Care Med. 2019;45:1333–46.
27. Selby NM, Burton JO, Chesterton LJ, McIntyre CW. Dialysis-induced regional left ventricular dysfunction is ameliorated by cooling the dialysate. Clin J Am Soc Nephrol. 2006;1:1216–25.
28. Jefferies HJ, Burton JO, McIntyre CW. Individualised dialysate temperature improves intradialytic haemodynamics and abrogates haemodialysis-induced myocardial stunning, without compromising tolerability. Blood Purif. 2011;32:63–8.
29. Odudu A, Eldehni MT, McCann GP, McIntyre CW. Randomized controlled trial of individualized dialysate cooling for cardiac protection in hemodialysis patients. Clin J Am Soc Nephrol. 2015;10:1408–17.
30. Assa S, Hummel YM, Voors AA, Kuipers J, Westerhuis R, de Jong PE, Franssen CF. Hemodialysis-induced regional left ventricular systolic dysfunction: prevalence, patient and dialysis treatment-related factors, and prognostic significance. Clin J Am Soc Nephrol. 2012;7:1615–23.
31. Mahmoud H, Forni LG, McIntyre CW, Selby NM. Myocardial stunning occurs during intermittent haemodialysis for acute kidney injury. Intensive Care Med. 2017;43:942–4.
32. Slessarev M, Salerno F, Ball IM, McIntyre CW. Continuous renal replacement therapy is associated with acute cardiac stunning in critically ill patients. Hemodial Int. 2019;23:325–32.

33. Burton JO, Jefferies HJ, Selby NM, McIntyre CW. Hemodialysis-induced repetitive myocardial injury results in global and segmental reduction in systolic cardiac function. Clin J Am Soc Nephrol. 2009;4:1925–31.
34. Schortgen FDR, Soubrier N, Delclaux C, et al. Hemodynamic tolerance of intermittent hemodialysis in critically ill patients: usefulness of practice guidelines. Am J Respir Crit Care Med. 2000;162:197–202.
35. Mitra S, Chamney P, Greenwood R, Farrington K. The relationship between systemic and whole-body hematocrit is not constant during ultrafiltration on hemodialysis. J Am Soc Nephrol. 2004;15:463–9.
36. Pierro ML, Kainerstorfer JM, Civiletto A, Weiner DE, Sassaroli A, Hallacoglu B, Fantini S. Reduced speed of microvascular blood flow in hemodialysis patients versus healthy controls: a coherent hemodynamics spectroscopy study. J Biomed Opt. 2014;19:026005.
37. Martinez AH, Diez GR, Ferraris V, et al. Removal of nitrate and nitrite by hemodialysis in end-stage renal disease and by sustained low-efficiency dialysis in acute kidney injury. Nitric Oxide. 2020;98:33–40.
38. Bryan NS, Torregrossa AC, Mian AI, Berkson DL, Westby CM, Moncrief JW. Acute effects of hemodialysis on nitrite and nitrate: potential cardiovascular implications in dialysis patients. Free Radic Biol Med. 2013;58:46–51.
39. Meyer C, Heiss C, Drexhage C, et al. Hemodialysis-induced release of hemoglobin limits nitric oxide bioavailability and impairs vascular function. J Am Coll Cardiol. 2010;55:454–9.
40. Premont RT, Reynolds JD, Zhang R, Stamler JS. Role of nitric oxide carried by hemoglobin in cardiovascular physiology: developments on a three-gas respiratory cycle. Circ Res. 2020;126:129–58.
41. Murugan R, Balakumar V, Kerti SJ, et al. Net ultrafiltration intensity and mortality in critically ill patients with fluid overload. Crit Care. 2018;22:223.

How to Prolong Filter Life During Continuous Renal Replacement Therapy?

17

Y. Tsujimoto and T. Fujii

17.1 Introduction

Renal replacement therapy (RRT), now also called kidney replacement therapy [1], is an essential intervention in critical care. Epidemiological studies have reported around 40% of patients in the intensive care unit (ICU) have acute kidney injury (AKI) [2–4]. However, effective strategies to prevent or treat AKI have yet to be established. Thus, RRT remains the mainstay of supportive measures for critically ill patients with AKI. It has been reported that 17–24% of critically ill patients with AKI receive some form of RRT during the ICU stay [2–4].

Continuous renal replacement therapy (CRRT), which runs slowly but continuously over 24 h, is more likely to be used than intermittent RRT in the ICU. Its mild impact on hemodynamics and solute clearance rate is preferred for critically ill patients. However, CRRT requires some measure(s) to prevent the filter from clotting due to the nature of the extracorporeal circuit. Filter clotting causes downtime of the therapy, leading to undertreatment, which may not be sufficiently recognized in clinical settings.

A recent randomized controlled trial (RCT) [5] added evidence on the choice of anticoagulation strategies to prolong filter life in critically ill patients with AKI. The

Y. Tsujimoto
Health Promotion and Human Behavior, Kyoto University Graduate School of Medicine, Kyoto, Japan

Scientific Research Works Peer Support Group (SRWS-PSG), Osaka, Japan

T. Fujii (✉)
Health Promotion and Human Behavior, Kyoto University Graduate School of Medicine, Kyoto, Japan

Intensive Care Unit, Jikei University Hospital, Tokyo, Japan
e-mail: tofujii-tky@umin.net

J.-L. Vincent (ed.), *Annual Update in Intensive Care and Emergency Medicine 2022*, Annual Update in Intensive Care and Emergency Medicine,
https://doi.org/10.1007/978-3-030-93433-0_17

trial compared regional citrate administration with systemic heparin administration to find that regional citrate could increase filter life span by 11 h.

Attempts that are made in the ICU to prevent filters from clotting are not limited to anticoagulation therapies. Choices of the modality, blood flow, filter, and catheters potentially affect filter life [6, 7]. Clinical research related to AKI or RRT in the ICU has revealed variations across countries or facilities in the prescription of RRT [3, 4, 8–10]. The variations imply much uncertainty in the prescription of RRT to improve clinical practice.

This state-of-the-art chapter summarizes the latest best available evidence for pharmacological and non-pharmacological interventions to prevent filters from clotting during CRRT in the ICU, focusing on recent clinical trials and observational studies.

17.2 Pharmacological Interventions to Prolong Filter Life

Pharmacological approaches include intravenous anticoagulants, oral anticoagulants, and antiplatelet agents. Regional citrate anticoagulation and systemic heparin are commonly used to maintain adequate patency of the extracorporeal circuit during CRRT. A major downside of the pharmacological approach is bleeding. Critically ill patients are commonly at high risk of bleeding due to coagulation abnormalities, including thrombocytopenia, prolonged prothrombin time (PT), and activated partial thromboplastin time (APTT). For such patients, clinicians may prescribe CRRT without anticoagulants for filter clotting prevention, concerned that the bleeding risk exceeds the benefits of the drug in providing an extended circuit life. In fact, a recent large multinational clinical trial of CRRT reported that 24% of patients did not receive any anticoagulants during CRRT [9].

However, the evidence to support the practice, i.e., no anticoagulation for CRRT in patients at high risk of bleeding, is scarce. Only small and inconclusive trials have examined the effects of pharmacological interventions, including systemic heparin, regional heparin with protamine reversal, and nafamostat mesylate, on filter life and bleeding events compared with no anticoagulation (Table 17.1) [11–13].

17.2.1 Regional Citrate Anticoagulation Versus Systemic Heparin, Low Molecular Weight Heparin, or Regional Heparin with Protamine Reversal

The Kidney Disease: Improving Global Outcomes (KDIGO) guidelines suggest using regional citrate anticoagulation for CRRT based on a low certainty of evidence [14]. The mechanism of action of regional anticoagulation with citrate is that citrate chelates calcium and acts as a local anticoagulant when administered pre-filter, reducing the risk of bleeding compared to systemic anticoagulation. However, citrate poses a risk of hypocalcemia, metabolic acidosis, or metabolic alkalosis if partially metabolized and accumulated.

Table 17.1 Pharmacological interventions investigated in randomized clinical trials for preventing clotting during continuous renal replacement therapy. Adapted from a Cochrane systematic review [6] and the RICH trial [5]

Intervention	Number of trials	Total number of participants in the trials
Anticoagulants		
Regional citrate anticoagulation	14	1697
Systemic heparin infusion	24	1837
Low molecular weight heparin	11	584
Regional heparin with protamine reversal	6	441
Nafamostat mesylate	2	133
Direct thrombin inhibitors (hirudin and bivalirudin)	3	53
Antiplatelet agents		
Prostaglandin I2 inhibitors (epoprostenol and iloprost)	5	154
Prostaglandin E1 inhibitors (Alprostadil)	1	54
Glycoprotein IIb/IIIa antagonists (tirofiban)	1	40
Placebo or no pharmacological intervention	3	177

An observational study from Germany (n = 1059) reported that citrate accumulated in 2% of patients in the first 48 h of continuous venovenous hemodialysis (CVVHD) in the ICU [15]. In addition, the study explored the predictability of lactate clearance for citrate accumulation and reported a threshold of 24.3% at 12 h of CRRT. The finding suggested regional citrate anticoagulation can be used safely with close monitoring of lactate clearance. A Cochrane review published in 2020 summarized the evidence from RCTs. Regional citrate anticoagulation probably decreases major bleeding events with no difference in successful prevention of clotting compared with systemic heparin [6].

The RICH trial was the largest so far, enrolling 596 patients, to compare the effects of regional citrate anticoagulation with those of systemic heparin anticoagulation on filter life and mortality [5]. The trial was terminated after the first interim analysis for the early proof of the superiority of regional citrate anticoagulation on filter life and futility in effects on mortality at 90 days. With the available data, anticoagulation with regional citrate significantly prolonged filter life (mean difference, 11.2 h [95%CI, 8.2–14.3]) and reduced bleeding complications (odds ratio, 0.27 [95%CI, 0.15–0.49]).

Regional citrate anticoagulation was compared with systemic low molecular weight heparin (LMWH) in two trials (n = 268 in total) [6]. The larger trial (n = 215) using nadroparin reported similar filter life in the two groups (median, 27 h vs. 26 h); however, adverse events that required discontinuation of study anticoagulant occurred more frequently with nadroparin (2% vs. 19%) [16]. Three trials compared regional anticoagulation with regional heparin accompanied by protamine reversal (n = 252 in total) [6]. The largest trial (n = 212) found longer filter life with regional citrate anticoagulation (median, 39.2 h vs. 22.8 h) [17]. The two largest RCTs in these two comparisons showed superiority of regional citrate anticoagulation over the comparator in terms of filter life and adverse events. Unfortunately, no trial has been conducted to compare regional citrate anticoagulation with other anticoagulation strategies [6].

17.2.2 Systemic Heparin Versus Regional Heparin with Protamine Reversal, Low Molecular Weight Heparin, Thrombin Antagonists, or Antiplatelet Agents

KDIGO guidelines recommend using either unfractionated or low molecular weight heparin, rather than other anticoagulants during CRRT in patients with contraindications for citrate, such as liver failure or shock representing a risk of citrate accumulation [14]. Alternatives include nafamostat mesylate, thrombin antagonists (e.g., hirudin or bivalirudin), and antiplatelet agents (e.g., epoprostenol, iloprost, alprostadil, or tirofiban).

A recent large multinational RCT showed that less than 3% of patients undergoing CRRT received such alternative anticoagulation strategies [9]. In addition, the recent Cochrane systematic review found no convincing evidence to indicate the superiority or inferiority of systemic heparin, regional heparin with protamine reversal, LMWH, or other alternative anticoagulants [6].

17.2.3 Implications for Clinicians and Future Research on Pharmacological Interventions

- Benefits from any pharmacological intervention compared to no pharmacological intervention are uncertain, particularly in patients at high risk of bleeding.
- If there is no contraindication, regional citrate anticoagulation is the first choice as a pharmacological strategy to maintain filter patency.
- Clinical research is needed to investigate which/whether anticoagulants should be used for patients at high risk of bleeding or patients with contraindication/s to regional citrate anticoagulation.

17.3 Non-pharmacological Interventions to Prolong Filter Life

Non-pharmacological interventions to prolong filter life during CRRT include the strategic selection of modalities, blood flow rates, catheter sites and types, and filters. However, the effects of those non-pharmacological interventions in patients undergoing CRRT have not been well studied compared with pharmacological interventions. Only a few randomized trials have been conducted so far (Table 17.2); furthermore, most studies were conducted more than a decade ago [7]. The clinical

Table 17.2 Non-pharmacological interventions investigated in randomized clinical trials for preventing clotting during continuous renal replacement therapy. Adapted from a Cochrane systematic review [7]

Interventions	Number of trials	Number of participants in the trials
Modes		
CVVH, CVVHD, or CVVHDF	10	520
Pre-dilution or post-dilution	2	48
Blood flow		
Higher blood flow or standard blood flow	2	134
Catheter types		
Long or short catheter	1	100
Surface-modified double-lumen catheter	1	236
Filter types		
AN69ST	3	76
More and shorter hollow fiber	1	6
Flat plate fiber[a]	1	38
Filter with a larger membrane surface area[a]	1	38
Others		
Single- or double-site infusion anticoagulation[a]	1	38

[a] From one study embedding three comparisons. *CVVH* continuous venovenous hemofiltration, *CVVHD* continuous venovenous hemodialysis, *CVVHDF* continuous venovenous hemodiafiltration, *AN69ST* polyethylenimine-treated AN69 membrane

practice in this field has changed dramatically, as exemplified by the widespread use of regional citrate. However, some evidence, including "no evidence of effect", may inform clinicians in decisions on the use of non-pharmacological interventions and is, therefore, summarized here with some recent observational findings.

17.3.1 Modes of Continuous Renal Replacement Therapy

Standard modes of CRRT include continuous venovenous hemofiltration (CVVH), CVVHD, and continuous venovenous hemodiafiltration (CVVHDF). Theoretically, CVVH has a better clearance of medium-sized solutes than CVVHD, but in practice it has been suggested that CVVHD provides equivalent clearance [18].

Although many studies have compared different modes of CRRT to each other for solute clearance or mortality, filter life was seldom measured as an outcome [7]. Limited available evidence (n = 77 in total) shows that CVVHD or CVVHDF might prolong filter life compared with CVVH [18, 19]. However, a single-center observational study published in 2021 (n = 284) reported no difference in filter life between CVVHD and CVVHDF (median, 16.4 h vs. 16.8 h) [20].

When CVVH or CVVHDF is used, replacement fluid can be infused before and/or after the filter: pre-dilution and/or post-dilution. The effect of pre-dilution on filter life was compared with post-dilution in two very small RCTs (n = 47 in total)

[7]. The pooled effect reported in the recent Cochrane systematic review implied that pre-dilution filtration might improve filter lifespan compared with the post-dilution technique [7]. Pre-dilution CRRT aims to decrease hemoconcentration; however, excessive hemodilution reduces solute clearance. To this end, replacement fluid may be split between pre- and post-filter, or blood flow rate may be kept high at at least 200 ml/min [21].

17.3.2 Blood Flow Rate

The blood flow rate of CRRT is variably prescribed from 80 to >300 ml/min worldwide [22, 23]. Expert consensus recommends a blood flow rate of >200 ml/min [24]. However, evidence from two RCTs (n = 499 in total) found that a higher blood flow rate may make little or no difference to circuit lifespan compared with a standard blood flow rate [7]. In addition, a recent observational study suggested that low blood flow did not independently affect filter life [20].

17.3.3 Vascular Access and Catheter Types

KDIGO guidelines [14] recommend using uncuffed, non-tunneled dialysis catheters, rather than tunneled catheters for initiating CRRT, based on a small RCT [25]. The RCT (n = 34) showed less dysfunction, fewer infectious or thrombotic complications, and more prolonged catheter survival with tunneled catheters [25]. However, tunneled catheters required increased insertion time and resulted in more femoral hematomas. The uncertainty of the findings due to the small sample size and uncommon catheter insertion procedure for CRRT settings precluded the recommendation of tunneled catheters [14]. A RCT comparing the functionalities of tunneled and non-tunneled catheters as the initial catheter for CRRT was registered (ClinicalTrials.gov Identifier: NCT03496935); however, the trial status is unclear.

The guidelines recommend using the right jugular vein, then the femoral vein, the left jugular vein, and the subclavian vein in this order when inserting catheters [14], based on observational studies. Catheters in the right jugular vein have fewer complication of stenosis or thrombosis as they have a straight course into the superior vena cava and the least contact with the vessel wall. By contrast, a catheter inserted through the subclavian or the left jugular vein has one or more angulations, which increases the risk of contact with blood vessels. An RCT (n = 750) that included patients having CRRT or intermittent hemodialysis showed little difference between femoral or jugular catheter placement in catheter survival and complications except in patients with a high body mass index [26].

Several types of catheters have also been studied [7]. Compared with short catheters targeting tip placement in the superior vena cava, long catheters arriving in the right atrium may prolong the filter life [27]. A surface-modified double-lumen catheter compared with a standard double-lumen catheter may also extend filter life [28].

17.3.4 Types of Filters

Many filters have been examined for effects on clinical outcomes; however, most evidence is of very low certainty [7]. Polyethylenimine-coated AN69 membranes (AN69ST), in which unfractionated heparin is bound onto the polymers, have been suggested to reduce the need for anticoagulation during CRRT [29, 30]. However, the AN69ST membrane has yet to be proven to provide longer filter life than other membranes in randomized studies (n = 56 in total) [7]. Furthermore, a small RCT suggested that citrate would provide better regional anticoagulation than AN69ST membranes in patients at high risk of bleeding [31]. As such, AN69ST should not be used to extend filter life at this stage. Two RCTs are currently underway to determine the impact of AN69ST on filter life (ClinicalTrials.gov Identifiers: NCT03426943 and NCT01779635).

For the other types of filter, including filters with more and shorter fibers, hollow fibers, or flat plate fibers, and filters with large membrane areas, there is no reliable evidence regarding their impact on filter life [7].

17.3.5 Implications for Clinicians and Future Research on Non-pharmacological Interventions

- Convection predominant modes may shorten the filter life; however, the evidence is uncertain.
- Keeping blood flow rates greater than 200 ml/min appears not to prolong filter life.
- Jugular access does not have evident superiority over femoral access in terms of filter life.
- There is insufficient evidence on the effects of non-pharmacological interventions on preventing filter clotting during CRRT to be able to make recommendations for routine practice. In particular, up to-date evidence is lacking.

17.4 Conclusion

The recent RICH trial [5] confirmed evidence that regional citrate anticoagulation provides longer filter life than systemic heparin anticoagulation during CRRT in critically ill patients. The effects of other anticoagulants, even compared with no anticoagulation, are uncertain. Non-pharmacological interventions have not been investigated sufficiently. With the widespread use of regional citrate anticoagulation over the last decade, high quality pragmatic trials investigating second line anticoagulation and non-pharmacological interventions in current ICU settings are warranted.

Acknowledgments This work was supported by Grant-in-Aid for Early-Career Scientists (JSPS KAKENHI 21K16580) to TF.

References

1. Levey AS, Eckardt KU, Dorman NM, et al. Nomenclature for kidney function and disease: report of a kidney disease: improving global outcomes (KDIGO) consensus conference. Kidney Int. 2020;97:1117–29.
2. Nisula S, Kaukonen KM, Vaara ST, et al. Incidence, risk factors and 90-day mortality of patients with acute kidney injury in Finnish intensive care units: the FINNAKI study. Intensive Care Med. 2013;39:420–8.
3. Hoste EA, Bagshaw SM, Bellomo R, et al. Epidemiology of acute kidney injury in critically ill patients: the multinational AKI-EPI study. Intensive Care Med. 2015;41:1411–23.
4. Fujii T, Uchino S, Doi K, Sato T, Kawamura T, et al. Diagnosis, management, and prognosis of patients with acute kidney injury in Japanese intensive care units: the JAKID study. J Crit Care. 2018;47:185–91.
5. Zarbock A, Kullmar M, Kindgen-Milles D, et al. Effect of regional citrate anticoagulation vs systemic heparin anticoagulation during continuous kidney replacement therapy on dialysis filter life span and mortality among critically ill patients with acute kidney injury: a randomized clinical trial. JAMA. 2020;324:1629–39.
6. Tsujimoto H, Tsujimoto Y, Nakata Y, Fujii T, Takahashi S, Akazawa M, Kataoka Y. Pharmacological interventions for preventing clotting of extracorporeal circuits during continuous renal replacement therapy. Cochrane Database Syst Rev. 2020;3:CD012467.
7. Tsujimoto Y, Miki S, Shimada H, Tsujimoto H, Yasuda H, Kataoka Y, Fujii T. Non-pharmacological interventions for preventing clotting of extracorporeal circuits during continuous renal replacement therapy. Cochrane Database Syst Rev. 2021;9:CD013330.
8. Schneider AG, Bellomo R, Bagshaw SM, et al. Choice of renal replacement therapy modality and dialysis dependence after acute kidney injury: a systematic review and meta-analysis. Intensive Care Med. 2013;39:987–97.
9. Bagshaw SM, Wald R, Adhikari NKJ, et al. Timing of initiation of renal-replacement therapy in acute kidney injury. N Engl J Med. 2020;383:240–51.
10. Gaudry S, Hajage D, Schortgen F, et al. Initiation strategies for renal-replacement therapy in the intensive care unit. N Engl J Med. 2016;375:122–33.
11. Choi JY, Kang YJ, Jang HM, et al. Nafamostat mesilate as an anticoagulant during continuous renal replacement therapy in patients with high bleeding risk: a randomized clinical trial. Medicine (Baltimore). 2015;94:e2392.
12. Bellomo R, Teede H, Boyce N. Anticoagulant regimens in acute continuous hemodiafiltration: a comparative study. Intensive Care Med. 1993;19:329–32.
13. Lee YK, Lee HW, Choi KH, Kim BS. Ability of nafamostat mesilate to prolong filter patency during continuous renal replacement therapy in patients at high risk of bleeding: a randomized controlled study. PLoS One. 2014;9:e108737.
14. KDIGO AKI Work Group. KDIGO clinical practice guideline for acute kidney injury. Kidney Int Suppl. 2012;2:1–138.
15. Khadzhynov D, Dahlinger A, Schelter C, et al. Hyperlactatemia, lactate kinetics and prediction of citrate accumulation in critically ill patients undergoing continuous renal replacement therapy with regional citrate anticoagulation. Crit Care Med. 2017;45:e941–6.
16. Oudemans-van Straaten HM, Bosman RJ, Koopmans M, et al. Citrate anticoagulation for continuous venovenous hemofiltration. Crit Care Med. 2009;37:545–52.
17. Gattas DJ, Rajbhandari D, Bradford C, Buhr H, Lo S, Bellomo R. A randomized controlled trial of regional citrate versus regional heparin anticoagulation for continuous renal replacement therapy in critically ill adults. Crit Care Med. 2015;43:1622–9.
18. Ricci Z, Ronco C, Bachetoni A, et al. Solute removal during continuous renal replacement therapy in critically ill patients: convection versus diffusion. Crit Care. 2006;10:R67.
19. Saudan P, Niederberger M, De Seigneux S, et al. Adding a dialysis dose to continuous hemofiltration increases survival in patients with acute renal failure. Kidney Int. 2006;70:1312–7.

20. Sansom B, Sriram S, Presneill J, Bellomo R. Low blood flow continuous veno-venous haemodialysis compared with higher blood flow continuous veno-venous haemodiafiltration: effect on alarm rates, filter life, and azotaemic control. Blood Purif. 2021;May 19:1–8. https://doi.org/10.1159/000516146. Epub ahead of print.
21. Clark WR, Turk JE, Kraus MA, Gao D. Dose determinants in continuous renal replacement therapy. Artif Organs. 2003;27:815–20.
22. Fealy N, Aitken L, Toit E, Baldwin I. Continuous renal replacement therapy: current practice in Australian and New Zealand intensive care units. Crit Care Resusc. 2015;17:83–91.
23. Uchino S, Bellomo R, Morimatsu H, et al. Continuous renal replacement therapy: a worldwide practice survey. The beginning and ending supportive therapy for the kidney (B.E.S.T. kidney) investigators. Intensive Care Med. 2007;33:1563–70.
24. Ronco C, Ricci Z, De Backer D, et al. Renal replacement therapy in acute kidney injury: controversy and consensus. Crit Care. 2015;19:146.
25. Klouche K, Amigues L, Deleuze S, Beraud JJ, Canaud B. Complications, effects on dialysis dose, and survival of tunneled femoral dialysis catheters in acute renal failure. Am J Kidney Dis. 2007;49:99–108.
26. Parienti J-J, Thirion M, Mégarbane B, et al. Femoral vs jugular venous catheterization and risk of nosocomial events in adults requiring acute renal replacement therapy: a randomized controlled trial. JAMA. 2008;299:2413–22.
27. Morgan D, Ho K, Murray C, Davies H, Louw J. A randomized trial of catheters of different lengths to achieve right atrium versus superior vena cava placement for continuous renal replacement therapy. Am J Kidney Dis. 2012;60:272–9.
28. Meier P, Meier R, Turini P, Friolet R, Blanc E. Prolonged catheter survival in patients with acute kidney injury on continuous renal replacement therapy using a less thrombogenic micropatterned polymer modification. Nephrol Dial Transplant. 2011;26:628–35.
29. Chanard J, Lavaud S, Maheut H, Kazes I, Vitry F, Rieu P. The clinical evaluation of low-dose heparin in haemodialysis: a prospective study using the heparin-coated AN69 ST membrane. Nephrol Dial Transplant. 2008;23:2003–9.
30. Kessler M, Gangemi C, Gutierrez Martones A, et al. Heparin-grafted dialysis membrane allows minimal systemic anticoagulation in regular hemodialysis patients: a prospective proof-of-concept study. Hemodial Int. 2013;17:282 93.
31. Evenepoel P, Dejagere T, Verhamme P, Claes K, Kuypers D, Bammens B, Vanrenterghem Y. Heparin-coated polyacrylonitrile membrane versus regional citrate anticoagulation: a prospective randomized study of 2 anticoagulation strategies in patients at risk of bleeding. Am J Kidney Dis. 2007;49:642–9.

Prevention of Acute Kidney Injury After Cardiac Surgery

18

M. Ostermann, K. Weerapolchai, and N. Lumlertgul

18.1 Introduction

Patients undergoing cardiac surgery are at high risk of acute kidney injury (AKI). There are several contributing factors, including hemodynamic instability, inflammation, iron release, and exposure to nephrotoxic agents [1]. In its most severe form, AKI is associated with a longer stay in the intensive care unit (ICU) and in hospital, risk of non-renal organ dysfunction, high healthcare costs, and reduced chances of survival [1, 2]. Survivors are at risk of premature chronic kidney disease, even if renal function initially recovers. In this chapter, we summarize current perioperative strategies to prevent the development or progression of AKI after cardiac surgery and outline areas of uncertainties.

M. Ostermann (✉)
Department of Critical Care, King's College London, Guy's & St Thomas' NHS Foundation Trust, London, UK
e-mail: Marlies.Ostermann@gstt.nhs.uk

K. Weerapolchai
Division of Urology, Royal Thai Navy Hospital, Bangkok, Thailand

N. Lumlertgul
Department of Critical Care, King's College London, Guy's & St Thomas' NHS Foundation Trust, London, UK

Division of Nephrology, Department of Internal Medicine and Excellence Center in Critical Care Nephrology, King Chulalongkorn Memorial Hospital, Bangkok, Thailand

J.-L. Vincent (ed.), *Annual Update in Intensive Care and Emergency Medicine 2022*, Annual Update in Intensive Care and Emergency Medicine,
https://doi.org/10.1007/978-3-030-93433-0_18

18.2 Preoperative Measures

Pharmacologic and non-pharmacologic measures have been investigated to prevent AKI after cardiac surgery. However, most studies are relatively small and limited by differences in inclusion criteria, and application of heterogeneous definitions of AKI.

18.2.1 Pharmacological Interventions

18.2.1.1 Angiotensin Converting Enzyme Inhibitors and Angiotensin Receptor Blockers

The evidence for management of angiotensin converting enzyme inhibitors (ACEIs) and angiotensin receptor blockers (ARBs) preoperatively is limited to observational studies with conflicting results. Most studies reported a higher risk of intraoperative hypotension in patients who had received ACEIs/ARBs preoperatively, although, in some studies, an association with postoperative AKI was also noted [3, 4]. For this reason, it is currently recommended that ACEIs and ARBs should be withheld during the perioperative period [1].

18.2.1.2 Statins

Systemic inflammation during cardiac surgery contributes to AKI and death postoperatively. Statins are effective at attenuating inflammation and oxidative stress. However, there is no evidence that they reduce the risk of AKI after cardiac surgery [5]. In fact, the STICS (Statin Therapy in Cardiac Surgery) trial randomized 1922 patients to either perioperative rosuvastatin or placebo and reported a significantly higher AKI incidence in the statin group [6]. Thus, starting a statin in statin-naïve patients pre-cardiac surgery to prevent AKI is not recommended.

18.2.1.3 Corticosteroids

The rationale for exploring the role of corticosteroids to prevent AKI after cardiac surgery is based on their ability to inhibit pro-inflammatory cytokines and upregulate antiinflammatory cytokines. Two large randomized controlled trials (RCTs), 'Dexamethasone in Cardiac Surgery' (DECS) and 'Steroids in Cardiac Surgery' (SICS), and a subsequent large meta-analysis concluded that steroids did not protect against AKI after cardiac surgery [7–9]. However, need for renal replacement therapy (RRT) was not explored as a separate outcome. In a follow-up analysis of the DECS trial, the investigators reported a reduced incidence of AKI requiring RRT in patients treated with dexamethasone [10]. Further research is necessary to confirm these findings.

18.2.1.4 Albumin

A single-center RCT in patients undergoing off-pump cardiac surgery showed that correction of hypoalbuminemia (<4 g/dl) by administering albumin 20% immediately before surgery was associated with increased urine output during surgery and a reduced risk of postoperative AKI [11].

18.2.1.5 N-acetylcysteine

N-acetylcysteine (NAC) is a precursor of intracellular glutathione, an antioxidant, and reduces pro-inflammatory cytokines and oxygen free-radical production, and ameliorates ischemia–reperfusion injury. Although it may theoretically reduce postoperative complications after cardiac surgery, two recent meta-analyses concluded that there was no role for NAC in preventing cardiac surgery associated AKI [12, 13].

18.2.1.6 Erythropoietin

A porcine model demonstrated that exogenous erythropoietin (EPO) was protective against ischemia–reperfusion injury via immunomodulatory effects. The role of EPO in patients undergoing cardiac surgery remains uncertain. While clinical trials and a meta-analysis concluded that exogenous EPO did not reduce the risk of AKI, a subgroup analysis suggested that the effect may be dose-dependent [14]. Low-dose EPO (200–300 IU/kg) but not high-dose EPO (400–500 IU/kg) before anesthesia was protective against AKI after cardiac surgery. Further research will be necessary to explore the exact role of EPO in this setting.

18.2.1.7 Sodium Bicarbonate

There are theoretical benefits with sodium bicarbonate therapy, but studies have failed to show any evidence that sodium bicarbonate administration reduces the risk of AKI after cardiac surgery; instead, it may be associated with prolonged mechanical ventilation and longer stay in the ICU [15, 16].

18.2.1.8 Avoidance of Nephrotoxic Exposure

Cardiac surgery should be delayed until 24–72 h after the administration of contrast provided the clinical condition allows [1]. Non-steroidal anti-inflammatory drugs should be avoided perioperatively. If aminoglycosides are necessary, they should be used for as short a period as possible.

18.2.1.9 New Drugs

QPI-1002 is a synthetic small interfering ribonucleic acid (si-RNA) designed to temporarily downregulate the expression of the pro-apoptotic gene *p53* via activation of the RNA interference (RNAi) pathway. It was hypothesized that inhibition of p53 may provide time for renal tubular epithelial cells to repair before apoptosis. Although a phase I study in patients at risk of AKI after on-pump cardiac surgery showed that QPI-1002 was safe and well-tolerated [17], a subsequent larger multicenter phase 3 trial was negative (ClinicalTrials.gov Identifier: NCT03510897).

18.3 Intraoperative Strategies

A number of intraoperative measures have been studied to either protect the kidneys or to optimize renal blood flow and oxygen delivery during surgery, including surgical and anesthetic techniques, hemodynamic management, and fluid therapy.

18.3.1 Surgical Techniques

Cardiopulmonary bypass (CPB) and systemic inflammation may contribute to the development of AKI. A large multicenter RCT compared off-pump with on-pump coronary artery bypass graft (CABG) surgery in 4752 patients [17]. There was no difference in the incidence of severe AKI; new renal failure requiring dialysis was 1.3% in both groups after 1 year with a 5-year incidence of 1.7% in the off-pump and 1.9% in the on-pump group. Similar results were seen in other multicenter RCTs comparing off-pump and on-pump CABG surgery [18].

18.3.2 Bypass Related Factors

18.3.2.1 Biocompatible Coatings

Heparin-bonded or phosphorylcholine coated circuits have been proposed as "more physiological surface" equipment. Studies investigating their role showed improved outcomes, such as reduced requirement for blood transfusions and shorter length of stay in hospital, but also less postoperative creatinine elevations [19]. Recent European guidelines recommend biocompatible coatings with class IIa evidence [20].

18.3.2.2 Minimally Invasive Extracorporeal Circulation

The concept of minimally invasive extracorporeal circulation (MiECC) includes the routine use of heparin-coated circuits, a small priming volume, a closed system, a centrifugal pump, and no venous reservoir. A retrospective propensity score matched analysis showed that MiECC was associated with a lower incidence of AKI post-CABG surgery [21]. However, a subsequent small RCT comparing miniaturized CPB with conventional CPB surgery in 68 patients showed no difference in the incidence of AKI [22]. The exact reasons for this discrepancy are not clear but may be related to the fact that non-invasive techniques, such as minimal priming volumes and heparin coated circuits, have already been adopted in routine clinical practice.

18.3.2.3 Leukocyte Depletion

Experimental data show that neutrophils and leukocytes accumulate in kidneys following ischemia-reperfusion mediated injury. Leukocyte depletion filters have been proposed to attenuate inflammation and to prevent AKI. Interestingly, a meta-analysis including 6 trials and 374 patients found that leukocyte depletion filters indeed reduced the incidence of worsening kidney function [23]. However, the trials included in the analysis were small with varying definitions of AKI. A subsequent Cochrane review found no benefit with leukocyte depletion filters [24] and the most recent European CPB guidelines do not recommend the routine use of leukodepletion [20].

18.3.2.4 Intra-aortic Balloon Pump

There is an association between the use of intra-aortic balloon pump (IABP) during CPB in selected high-risk patients and improved whole-body perfusion, less endothelial activation, less AKI, and reduced need for RRT [25]. However, concern exists that IABP may also significantly lower aortic pressure in the distal portion of the aorta and in fact impair renal perfusion. Therefore, it should only be used in carefully selected patients.

18.3.3 Cardiac Anesthesia

18.3.3.1 Remote Ischemic Preconditioning

Remote ischemic preconditioning is a technique that involves repetitive brief periods of ischemia by inflating a blood pressure cuff on the upper arm or thigh for several minutes followed by release for reperfusion. It is proposed that these ischemia-reperfusion processes stimulate the release and activation of anti-inflammatory cytokines, neural autonomic pathways, and humoral signaling pathways, thus preventing distal organ dysfunction. The role of remote ischemic preconditioning in preventing cardiac surgery-associated AKI is controversial. Although experimental data and results from small RCTs support the application of remote ischemic preconditioning, large multicenter RCTs found no difference in the incidence of postoperative AKI [26–28]. However, these results do not exclude the possibility that remote ischemic preconditioning is beneficial in specific patient groups.

18.3.3.2 Volatile Versus Intravenous Anesthesia

Experimental data suggest that volatile anesthetics have renal protective effects. Propofol may also protect the kidneys, as demonstrated in a small RCT in patients undergoing valve surgery [29]. A meta-analysis comparing volatile and intravenous anesthesia did not show any difference in postoperative AKI [30]. Thus, a potential renal protective effect by either volatile or intravenous anesthetics as suggested by experimental data, has not been consistently shown in clinical practice.

Dexmedetomidine is an alpha-2-adrenoreceptor agonist with sedative, analgesic, and sympathicolytic effects. Immediately after induction or before CPB, administration of dexmedetomidine might attenuate inflammatory cytokines and renal ischemia. A meta-analysis of 9 RCTs including 1308 patients reported a significantly reduced incidence of AKI after cardiac surgery, in particular in patients older than 60 years [31]. Larger high-quality trials are required to confirm this finding.

18.3.4 Intraoperative Fluid and Hemodynamic Management

Goal-directed therapy is a strategy to increase cardiac output by using fluids and/or inotropes to improve oxygen delivery to organs and tissues. It has been shown to be associated with a lower incidence of AKI after cardiac surgery and was included as a class I recommendation in recent European guidelines [20].

18.3.4.1 Fluids

Type and volume of fluid are associated with risk of AKI. A single center, prospective cohort study indicated that a higher positive fluid balance was associated with a higher need for RRT following cardiac surgery [32]. Similarly, a large retrospective analysis demonstrated an association between a positive fluid balance and AKI post cardiac surgery [33]. Whether there is a role for active fluid restriction in cardiac surgery has not been investigated.

The type of fluid may also impact the risk of postoperative AKI. A large RCT in 600 patients undergoing off-pump CABG surgery showed that the use of balanced crystalloid solutions was associated with a significantly decreased incidence of stage 1 AKI postoperatively [34].

18.3.4.2 Hemodynamic Management

Hemodynamic management during CPB is crucial to maintain an adequate perfusion pressure in the kidneys. A trial comparing a high mean arterial blood pressure (MAP) target (70–80 mmHg) with a low MAP target (40–50 mmHg) during CPB showed that significantly more patients randomized to the high MAP target doubled their creatinine levels [35]. In contrast, a study in 410 patients undergoing cardiac surgery with CPB demonstrated that blood pressure excursions below the lower limit of the cerebral autoregulation threshold were associated with AKI [36]. The mean lower limit of cerebral autoregulation is 66 mmHg but individual values vary between 40 and 90 mmHg. The recent European guidelines recommend MAP targets between 50 and 80 mmHg during CPB but individualized blood pressure management may be most effective [20].

Oxygen delivery (DO_2) during CPB has been shown to be directly associated with postoperative AKI. A large multicenter RCT compared a goal-directed perfusion strategy aimed at maintaining a high normal DO_2 target >280 ml/min/m^2 with conventional perfusion and demonstrated that patients receiving goal-directed perfusion during CPB had a significantly lower incidence of postoperative AKI [37].

18.3.4.3 Blood Products

Preoperative anemia is associated with AKI and mortality after cardiac surgery, but transfusion of at least two units of packed red blood cells (RBCs) during surgery is also considered a risk factor for AKI after cardiac surgery. Two large RCTs in which patients were randomized to a liberal versus restrictive RBC transfusion strategy intraoperatively and postoperatively (hemoglobin trigger <9.5 g/dl versus <7.5 g/dl) showed no difference in postoperative AKI [38, 39]. Therefore, blood transfusion beyond traditional transfusion triggers is not considered an effective strategy to protect kidney function.

18.3.5 Mechanical Ventilation

Need for mechanical ventilation is a common risk factor for AKI during critical illness, in particular in patients with acute respiratory failure. The contributing mechanisms include hemodynamic, neurohormonal, and immune-mediated processes. Mechanical ventilation strategies during CPB were investigated in a meta-analysis and semi-quantitative review of 16 RCTs, including a total of 814 patients [40]. Whilst continuous positive airway pressure (CPAP) and vital capacity maneuvers during CPB improved oxygenation variables after CPB, there was no sustained benefit and AKI was not included as an outcome variable. Whether particular ventilation strategies during cardiac surgery (pre- and post-CPB) protect kidney function more than others remains unclear. Until further research results are available, it is recommended to monitor tidal volumes and ventilation pressures and to apply lung protective ventilation strategies whenever possible to reduce the impact on lung and kidney function [41].

18.3.6 Intraoperative Drugs

There are no specific pharmacological interventions to prevent cardiac surgery-associated AKI. Many drugs, including dopamine, diuretics, mannitol, and natriuretic peptides, have been studied. Although they may increase urine output, none are routinely used due to limited and conflicting data and, in some cases, evidence of harm [1].

Furosemide: Prophylactic administration of furosemide has not been shown to reduce postoperative AKI after cardiac surgery in small RCTs and therefore cannot be recommended as a strategy to protect kidney function [42].

Mannitol: Perioperative mannitol was investigated in two small RCTs in 50 patients with established renal dysfunction and 40 patients with normal preoperative kidney function [43, 44]. There were no beneficial renal effects.

Atrial natriuretic peptide: Meta-analyses of studies performed in patients undergoing cardiovascular surgery showed that there was a reduced need for RRT with administration of low-dose atrial natriuretic peptide (ANP) [45]. In high doses, ANP was associated with more adverse events. However, most studies on ANP were underpowered and considered of low or moderate quality. Therefore, ANP is not currently recommended for treatment of AKI [1].

Fenoldopam: Fenoldopam has been studied in several trials. Although meta-analyses have suggested a decrease in RRT with fenoldopam in patients with AKI after cardiac surgery, a multicenter RCT including 667 patients with AKI after cardiac surgery was stopped for futility after an interim analysis [46]: fenoldopam infusion, compared with placebo, did not reduce the need for RRT but caused more harm, in particular hypotension.

18.4 Postoperative Strategies

The 2012 Kidney Disease: Improving Global Outcomes (KDIGO) guideline recommends optimization of fluid status and hemodynamics, consideration of early functional hemodynamic monitoring, avoidance of hyperglycemia and radiocontrast agents, and discontinuation of nephrotoxic medications to prevent or mitigate AKI [47]. Two RCTs investigated whether the implementation of the KDIGO recommendations impacted the occurrence of AKI in high-risk cardiac surgery patients [48, 49]. In both studies, the urinary cell cycle arrest biomarkers tissue inhibitor of metalloproteinase-2 (TIMP-2) and insulin growth factor binding protein 7 (IGFBP7) were measured 4 h after cardiac surgery to identify patients with early kidney injury. The first RCT was a single center study of 276 patients and showed that, in patients with a positive urinary cell cycle arrest result after surgery, adherence to the KDIGO recommendations resulted in a significantly lower incidence and reduced severity of AKI compared to usual care [49]. However, there were no significant differences in any other secondary outcomes including all-cause mortality, requirement for RRT, or length of stay in ICU or hospital. The second RCT was a multinational study with a similar design [48]. It showed a significant reduction in stage 2–3 AKI in the intervention group but no significant difference in overall rates of AKI or any of the secondary outcomes including mortality, renal recovery, length of stay in ICU or hospital, or persistent renal dysfunction at day 90. Outcomes beyond 90 days, including the risk of premature chronic kidney disease, were not explored.

The guidelines for perioperative care in cardiac surgery by the Enhanced Recovery After Surgery Society recommend the routine use of urinary cell cycle arrest biomarkers after cardiac surgery to identify patients for intensified management to prevent AKI [50].

18.5 Conclusion

Perioperative strategies to prevent or mitigate cardiac surgery-associated AKI are limited to general supportive measures (Fig. 18.1). Current evidence supports a multi-modal risk-stratification approach including goal-directed perfusion, use of biocompatible coatings during CPB, perioperative goal-directed therapy, the use of fluids with restricted chloride content, and biomarker-guided management of high-risk patients based on the KDIGO recommendations. If AKI occurs, transfer of information to all caregivers, medication reconciliation, and patient education are essential to reduce the risk of long-term complications.

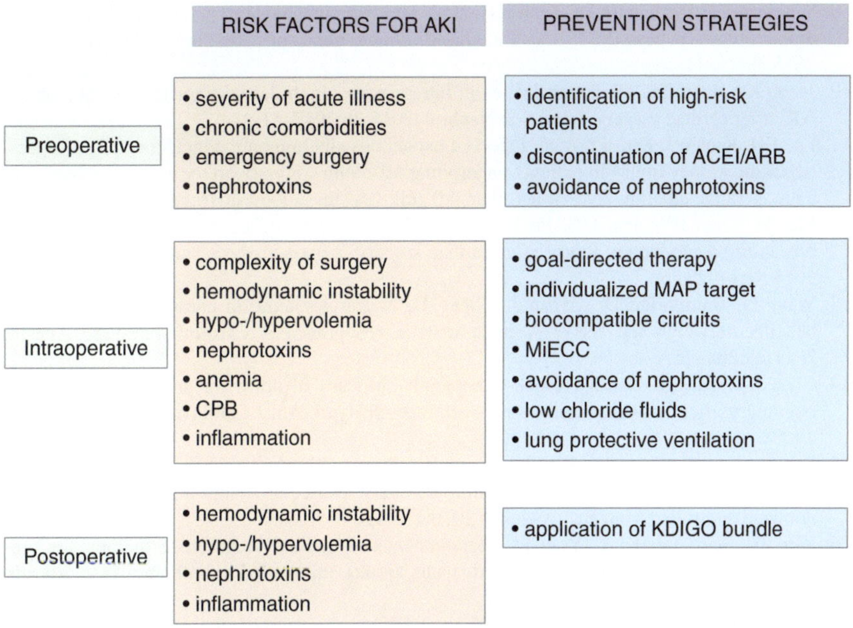

Fig. 18.1 Risk factors for acute kidney injury (AKI) after cardiac surgery and perioperative strategies to prevent it. *ACEI* angiotensin converting enzyme inhibitor, *ARB* angiotensin receptor blocker, *CPB* cardiopulmonary bypass, *KDIGO* Kidney Disease: Improving Global Outcomes, *MAP* mean arterial pressure, *MiECC* minimally invasive extracorporeal circulation

References

1. Nadim MK, Forni LG, Bihorac A, et al. Cardiac and vascular surgery-associated acute kidney injury: the 20th international consensus conference of the ADQI (Acute Disease Quality Initiative) Group. J Am Heart Assoc. 2018;7:e008834.
2. Ostermann M, Cennamo A, Meersch M, Kunst G. A narrative review of the impact of surgery and anaesthesia on acute kidney injury. Anaesthesia. 2020;75(Suppl 1):e121–33.
3. Ling Q, Gu Y, Chen J, Chen Y, Shi Y, Zhao G, Zhu Q. Consequences of continuing renin angiotensin aldosterone system antagonists in the preoperative period: a systematic review and meta-analysis. BMC Anesthesiol. 2018;18:26.
4. Coca SG, Garg AX, Swaminathan M, et al. Preoperative angiotensin-converting enzyme inhibitors and angiotensin receptor blocker use and acute kidney injury in patients undergoing cardiac surgery. Nephrol Dial Transplant. 2013;28:2787–99.
5. Putzu A, de Carvalho ESC, de Almeida JP, Belletti A, Cassina T, Landoni G, Hajjar LA. Perioperative statin therapy in cardiac and non-cardiac surgery: a systematic review and meta-analysis of randomized controlled trials. Ann Intensive Care. 2018;8:95.
6. Zheng Z, Jayaram R, Jiang L, et al. Perioperative rosuvastatin in cardiac surgery. N Engl J Med. 2016;374:1744–53.
7. Dieleman JM, Nierich AP, Rosseel PM, et al. Intraoperative high-dose dexamethasone for cardiac surgery: a randomized controlled trial. JAMA. 2012;308:1761–7.
8. Dvirnik N, Belley-Cote EP, Hanif H, et al. Steroids in cardiac surgery: a systematic review and meta-analysis. Br J Anaesth. 2018;120:657–67.

9. Whitlock RP, Devereaux PJ, Teoh KH, et al. Methylprednisolone in patients undergoing cardiopulmonary bypass (SIRS): a randomised, double-blind, placebo-controlled trial. Lancet. 2015;386:1243–53.
10. Jacob KA, Leaf DE, Dieleman JM, et al. Intraoperative high-dose dexamethasone and severe AKI after cardiac surgery. J Am Soc Nephrol. 2015;26:2947–51.
11. Lee EH, Kim WJ, Kim JY, et al. Effect of exogenous albumin on the incidence of postoperative acute kidney injury in patients undergoing off-pump coronary artery bypass surgery with a preoperative albumin level of less than 4.0 g/dl. Anesthesiology. 2016;124:1001–11.
12. Mei M, Zhao HW, Pan QG, Pu YM, Tang MZ, Shen BB. Efficacy of N-acetylcysteine in preventing acute kidney injury after cardiac surgery: a meta-analysis study. J Investig Surg. 2018;31:14–23.
13. Wang G, Bainbridge D, Martin J, Cheng D. N-acetylcysteine in cardiac surgery: do the benefits outweigh the risks? A meta-analytic reappraisal. J Cardiothorac Vasc Anesth. 2011;25:268–75.
14. Chen X, Huang T, Cao X, Xu G. Comparative efficacy of drugs for preventing acute kidney injury after cardiac surgery: a network meta-analysis. Am J Cardiovasc Drugs. 2018;18:49–58.
15. Soh S, Song JW, Shim JK, Kim JH, Kwak YL. Sodium bicarbonate does not prevent postoperative acute kidney injury after off-pump coronary revascularization: a double-blinded randomized controlled trial. Br J Anaesth. 2016;117:450–7.
16. Kim JH, Kim HJ, Kim JY, et al. Meta-analysis of sodium bicarbonate therapy for prevention of cardiac surgery-associated acute kidney injury. J Cardiothorac Vasc Anesth. 2015;29:1248–56.
17. Lamy A, Devereaux PJ, Prabhakaran DT, et al. Five-year outcomes after off-pump or on-pump coronary-artery bypass grafting. N Engl J Med. 2016;375:2359–68.
18. Diegeler A, Börgermann J, Kappert U, et al. Off-pump versus on-pump coronary-artery bypass grafting in elderly patients. N Engl J Med. 2013;368:1189–98.
19. Mangoush O, Purkayastha S, Haj-Yahia S, et al. Heparin-bonded circuits versus nonheparin-bonded circuits: an evaluation of their effect on clinical outcomes. Eur J Cardiothorac Surg. 2007;31:1058–69.
20. Kunst G, Milojevic M, Boer C, et al. 2019 EACTS/EACTA/EBCP guidelines on cardiopulmonary bypass in adult cardiac surgery. Br J Anaesth. 2019;123:713–57.
21. Benedetto U, Luciani R, Goracci M, et al. Miniaturized cardiopulmonary bypass and acute kidney injury in coronary artery bypass graft surgery. Ann Thorac Surg. 2009;88:529–35.
22. Chew ST, Ng RR, Liu W, Goh SG, Caleb MG, Ti LK. Miniaturized versus conventional cardiopulmonary bypass and acute kidney injury after cardiac surgery. Perfusion. 2016;31:60–7.
23. Scrascia G, Guida P, Rotunno C, de Luca Tupputi Schinosa L, Paparella D. Anti-inflammatory strategies to reduce acute kidney injury in cardiac surgery patients: a meta-analysis of randomized controlled trials. Artif Organs. 2014;38:101–12.
24. Spencer S, Tang A, Khoshbin E. Leukodepletion for patients undergoing heart valve surgery. Cochrane Database Syst Rev. 2013:CD009507.
25. Wang J, Yu W, Gao M, Gu C, Yu Y. Preoperative prophylactic intraaortic balloon pump reduces the incidence of postoperative acute kidney injury and short-term death of high-risk patients undergoing coronary artery bypass grafting: a meta-analysis of 17 studies. Ann Thorac Surg. 2016;101:2007–19.
26. Hausenloy DJ, Candilio L, Evans R, et al. Remote ischemic preconditioning and outcomes of cardiac surgery. N Engl J Med. 2015;373:1408–17.
27. Meybohm P, Bein B, Brosteanu O, et al. A multicenter trial of remote ischemic preconditioning for heart surgery. N Engl J Med. 2015;373:1397–407.
28. Zarbock A, Kellum JA, Schmidt C, et al. Effect of early vs delayed initiation of renal replacement therapy on mortality in critically ill patients with acute kidney injury: the ELAIN randomized clinical trial. JAMA. 2016;315:2190–9.
29. Yoo YC, Shim JK, Song Y, Yang SY, Kwak Y. Anesthetics influence the incidence of acute kidney injury following valvular heart surgery. Kidney Int. 2014;86:414–22.

30. Bonanni A, Signori A, Alicino C, et al. Volatile anesthetics versus propofol for cardiac surgery with cardiopulmonary bypass: meta-analysis of randomized trials. Anesthesiology. 2020;132:1429–46.
31. Peng K, Li D, Applegate RL II, Lubarsky DA, Ji FH, Liu H. Effect of dexmedetomidine on cardiac surgery-associated acute kidney injury: a meta-analysis with trial sequential analysis of randomized controlled trials. J Cardiothorac Vasc Anesth. 2020;34:603–13.
32. Haase-Fielitz A, Haase M, Bellomo R, et al. Perioperative hemodynamic instability and fluid overload are associated with increasing acute kidney injury severity and worse outcome after cardiac surgery. Blood Purif. 2017;43:298–308.
33. Shen Y, Zhang W, Cheng X, Ying M. Association between postoperative fluid balance and acute kidney injury in patients after cardiac surgery: a retrospective cohort study. J Crit Care. 2018;44:273–7.
34. Bhaskaran K, Arumugam G, Vinay Kumar PV. A prospective, randomized, comparison study on effect of perioperative use of chloride liberal intravenous fluids versus chloride restricted intravenous fluids on postoperative acute kidney injury in patients undergoing off-pump coronary artery bypass grafting surgeries. Ann Cardiac Anaesth. 2018;21:413–8.
35. Vedel AG, Holmgaard F, Rasmussen LS, et al. High-target versus low-target blood pressure management during cardiopulmonary bypass to prevent cerebral injury in cardiac surgery patients: a randomized controlled trial. Circulation. 2018;137:1770–80.
36. Ono M, Arnaoutakis GJ, Fine DM, et al. Blood pressure excursions below the cerebral autoregulation threshold during cardiac surgery are associated with acute kidney injury. Crit Care Med. 2013;41:464–71.
37. Ranucci M, Romitti F, Isgrò G, et al. Oxygen delivery during cardiopulmonary bypass and acute renal failure after coronary operations. Ann Thorac Surg. 2005;80:2213–20.
38. Mazer CD, Whitlock RP, Fergusson DA, et al. Restrictive or liberal red-cell transfusion for cardiac surgery. N Engl J Med. 2017;377:2133–44.
39. Reeves BC, Pike K, Rogers CA, et al. A multicentre randomised controlled trial of transfusion indication threshold reduction on transfusion rates, morbidity and health-care resource use following cardiac surgery (TITRe2). Health Technol Assess. 2016;20:1–260.
40. Schreiber JU, Lancé MD, de Korte M, Artmann T, Aleksic I, Kranke P. The effect of different lung-protective strategies in patients during cardiopulmonary bypass: a meta-analysis and semiquantitative review of randomized trials. J Cardiothorac Vasc Anesth. 2012;26:448–54.
41. Joannidis M, Forni LG, Klein SJ, et al. Lung-kidney interactions in critically ill patients: consensus report of the Acute Disease Quality Initiative (ADQI) 21 Workgroup. Intensive Care Med. 2020;46:654–72.
42. Fakhari S, Bavil FM, Bilehjani E, Abolhasani S, Mirinazhad M, Naghipour B. Prophylactic furosemide infusion decreasing early major postoperative renal dysfunction in on-pump adult cardiac surgery: a randomized clinical trial. Res Rep Urol. 2017;9:5–13.
43. Smith MN, Best D, Sheppard SV, Smith DC. The effect of mannitol on renal function after cardiopulmonary bypass in patients with established renal dysfunction. Anaesthesia. 2008;63:701–4.
44. Yallop KG, Sheppard SV, Smith DC. The effect of mannitol on renal function following cardio-pulmonary bypass in patients with normal pre-operative creatinine. Anaesthesia. 2008;63:576–82.
45. Nigwekar SU, Navaneethan SD, Parikh CR, Hix JK. Atrial natriuretic peptide for preventing and treating acute kidney injury. Cochrane Database Syst Rev. 2009:CD006028.
46. Bove T, Zangrillo A, Guarracino F, et al. Effect of fenoldopam on use of renal replacement therapy among patients with acute kidney injury after cardiac surgery: a randomized clinical trial. JAMA. 2014;312:2244–53.
47. Kellum JA, Lameire N. Diagnosis, evaluation, and management of acute kidney injury: a KDIGO summary (part 1). Crit Care. 2013;17:204.
48. Zarbock A, Küllmar M, Ostermann M, et al. Prevention of cardiac surgery-associated acute kidney injury by implementing the KDIGO guidelines in high-risk patients identified by biomarkers: the PrevAKI-multicenter randomized controlled trial. Anesth Analg. 2021;133:292–302.

49. Meersch M, Schmidt C, Hoffmeier A, et al. Prevention of cardiac surgery-associated AKI by implementing the KDIGO guidelines in high risk patients identified by biomarkers: the PrevAKI randomized controlled trial. Intensive Care Med. 2017;43:1551–61.
50. Engelman DT, Ben Ali W, Williams JB, et al. Guidelines for perioperative care in cardiac surgery: enhanced recovery after surgery society recommendations. JAMA Surg. 2019;154:755–66.

Part VI

Circulatory Shock

Contrast-Enhanced Renal Ultrasound for Assessment of Renal Perfusion in Critically Ill Patients

19

J. Watchorn, K. Bramham, and S. Hutchings

19.1 Introduction

Contrast-enhanced ultrasound is an approach to clinical imaging involving the injection of microbubbles to delineate perfusion within solid organs such as the liver and kidney. Contrast-enhanced ultrasound has been used to diagnose ischemia, differentiate tumors, characterize complex cysts, identify abscesses, and facilitate invasive procedures [1]. However, it is the ability of contrast-enhanced ultrasound to highlight the small blood vessels of the microcirculation that has led to increasing interest in this technique among critical care specialists as a means of assessing tissue perfusion.

The concept of differential perfusion between the large blood vessels of the macrocirculation and those of the microcirculation is well described in a variety of shock states [2]. An important example of this hemodynamic incoherence is found in septic acute kidney injury (AKI), where serial studies have demonstrated that renal function is reduced despite preserved or even increased systemic blood flow [3]. Until recently, the lack of an imaging modality to assess parenchymal renal blood flow at the bedside has been a limiting factor in both our understanding of and ability to accurately diagnose and treat the causes of sepsis-associated AKI. Contrast-enhanced ultrasound is an emerging technique with the potential to significantly increase our understanding in this area.

J. Watchorn · S. Hutchings (✉)
Department of Inflammation Biology, School of Microbial Sciences, Faculty of Life Sciences and Medicine, King's College London, London, UK

Department of Critical Care, King's College Hospital, London, UK
e-mail: sam.hutchings@nhs.net

K. Bramham
Department of Women and Children's Health, School of Life Course Sciences, Faculty of Life Sciences and Medicine, King's College London, London, UK

J.-L. Vincent (ed.), *Annual Update in Intensive Care and Emergency Medicine 2022*, Annual Update in Intensive Care and Emergency Medicine,
https://doi.org/10.1007/978-3-030-93433-0_19

In this chapter, we provide an overview of the development of contrast-enhanced ultrasound followed by a discussion of the technical aspects of imaging and analysis, its strengths and limitations, and an overview of studies that have used contrast-enhanced ultrasound to evaluate renal perfusion in shock states.

19.2 Principles of Contrast Ultrasonography

Contrast-enhanced ultrasound relies on the physical characteristics of microbubbles, which possess the rheological properties of erythrocytes rendering them a reliable tracer for blood flow and blood pool imaging. However, unlike red blood cells, gas-filled microbubbles are deformed by ultrasound energy, readily resonate, and emit a reflecting sound wave; the properties of the resulting signal are exploited by dedicated ultrasound equipment.

19.2.1 Microbubble Characteristics

Microbubble lifespan is a key characteristic of contrast agents. Microbubbles must have sufficient longevity to remain in the circulation during the timeframe of the examination but also be degradable, permitting the elimination of inert gas and shell components. Initial approaches to increasing bubble lifespan used thick albumin shells to enclose air but these rigid shells deformed insufficiently when insonated and produced little backscatter [4]. The second approach was based on a theory that diffusion from the bubble would be reduced if they were filled with poorly-soluble gas, such as sodium hexafluoride or perfluorocarbons [5]. This is the basis of contemporary microbubble contrast agents, which have either lipid or albumin shells. Common, commercially available contrast agents are presented in Table 19.1.

Elimination of microbubbles from the circulation is caused by the loss of gas from the bubble over time, causing contraction. Eventually, the external compression overcomes the internal pressure maintaining the bubble integrity and it collapses, the free gas within the blood is exhaled, and the shell is metabolized.

A schematic of a typical microbubble used in SonoVue contrast (Bracco, Milan, Italy) is shown in Fig. 19.1.

19.2.2 Microbubble–Ultrasound Interactions

Microbubble destruction occurs continually though both dissolution and cavitation from ultrasound energy. The proportion of bubbles destroyed by ultrasound is subject to the acoustic energy imparted in them; once this energy reaches a sufficient threshold, bubble integrity is lost causing mass fragmentation. Although seemingly detrimental, this allows the life of a microbubble to be controlled and bubble fragmentation can be used for the assessment of tissue perfusion.

Table 19.1 Details of commonly available ultrasound contrast agents

Agent	Shell	Gas core	Manufacturer	Standard bolus dose (ml)	Elimination half-life (min)	Notes
SonoVue	Lipid	Sodium hexafluoride (SF_6)	Bracco, Milan, Italy	1.2–2.4	12	Marketed as Lumason in the USA
Optison	Albumin	Perflutren (C_3F_8)	GE Healthcare, Milwaukee, WI, USA	0.5	1.3	
Luminity	Lipid	Perflutren (C_3F_8)	Lantheus Medical Imaging, N. Billerica, MA, USA	0.2–0.3	1.3	Marketed as Definity in the USA
Sonazoid	Egg phosphatidyl serine	Perflurobutane (C_4F_{10})	GE Healthcare, Milwaukee, WI, USA	0.5–1.0	30–45	Currently only available in Asia

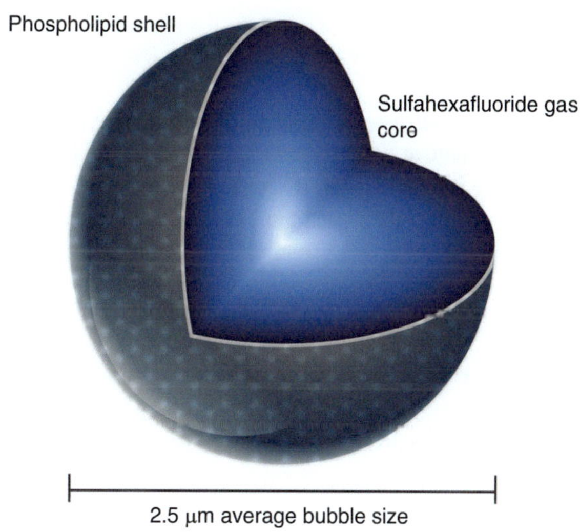

Fig. 19.1 Stylized SonoVue microbubble, comprising a phospholipid (dipalmitoylphosphatidylglycerol) shell, approximately 2 nm thickness and a sulfahexafluoride (SF6) gas core. Average bubble size 2.5 μm (90% <6 μm, 99% <11 μm) [4]. One milliliter SonoVue contains 4×10^7 microbubbles and 1.5 μl of SF6

Standard B-mode ultrasound has several drawbacks when imaging contrast agents: the wave power may cause bubble destruction and tissues are highly echogenic, making the differentiation of contrast difficult. The acoustic properties of bubbles have enabled equipment manufacturers to selectively identify bubbles in preference to tissue [6]. These techniques provide a specific contrast mode, which at baseline has little background noise but displays signal from bubble insonation on

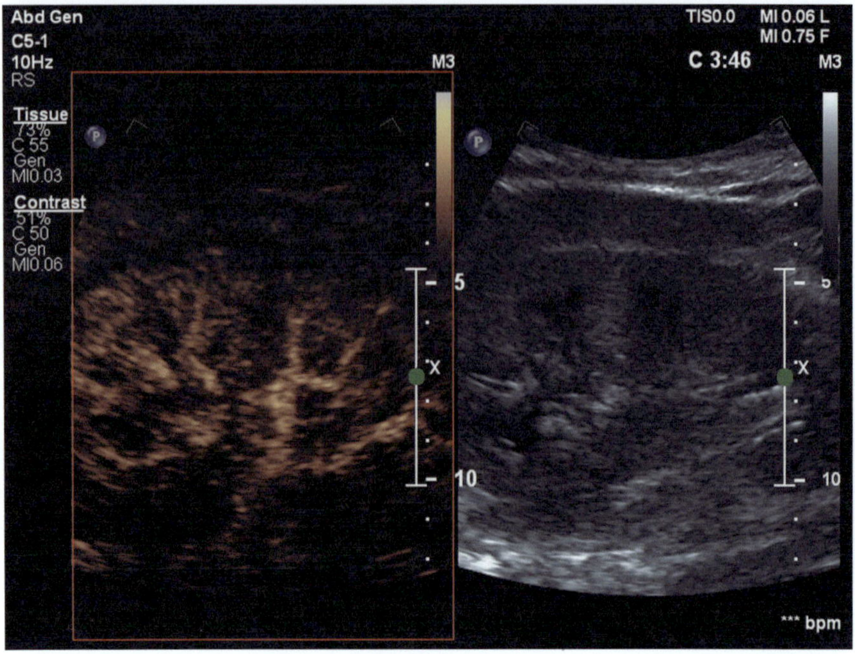

Fig. 19.2 Ultrasound dual-mode mode image of a kidney. Contrast mode is displayed on the left with microbubble specific signal preferentially filtered and B-mode is displayed on the right

delivery of contrast. The filtered image can be presented alongside the non-filtered B-mode image at powers less than the threshold for bubble destruction, as presented in Fig. 19.2. Oscillatory frequencies and bubble destruction thresholds are agent specific and therefore mechanical indices may vary slightly.

19.2.3 Method of Contrast Administration: Bolus vs. Continuous

Ultrasound contrast medium can be administered in a single bolus or via continuous infusion, termed dynamic contrast-enhanced ultrasound (DCE-US). The former method is typically used in oncological imaging with the perfusion of different regions being compared in the same study. Both methods provide tissue perfusion data through the creation of time intensity curves. We believe the latter method has more utility in the quantification of perfusion in critical illness where variables will be compared between patients and alterations in cardiac output may have more influence on the shape of a bolus-method time intensity curve.

When given by infusion, typically 1 ml/min of neat contrast is infused although contrast agents may be diluted and tailored to the specific examination [7]. A wash-in phase occurs until steady-state is achieved. The field of view is then pulsed with high mechanical index ultrasound which causes mass fragmentation and the field of view darkens until it is re-perfused, from which time intensity curves for specific regions of interest are created. Typical kinetics are shown in Fig. 19.3.

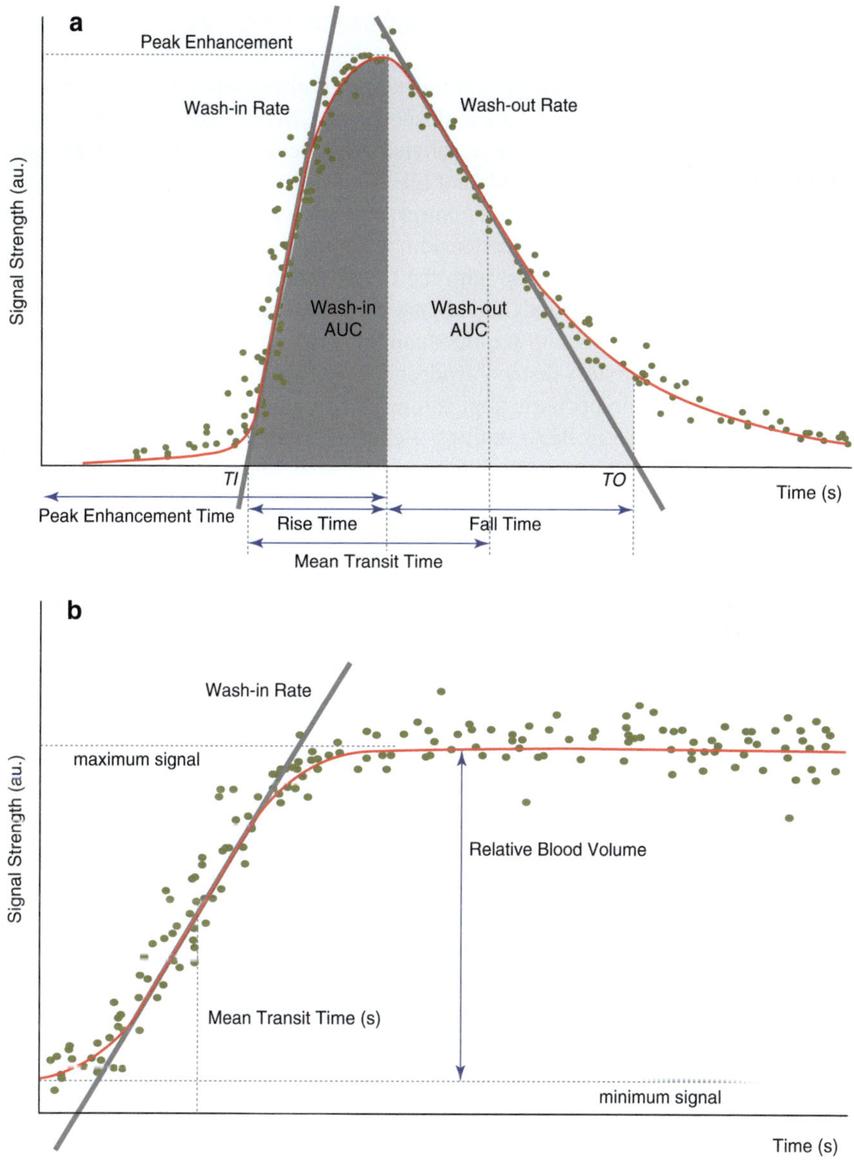

Fig. 19.3 Diagrams of typical time intensity curves. (**a**) bolus-transit kinetics. Assessed values: (1) maximum wash-in rate (WiR) and (2) maximum wash-out rate (WiR) are measured using the maximal slope and the gradients and x-axis intercepts are used to quantify bolus transit kinetics. TI = time in, defined as maximum wash-in rate x-axis intercept; TO = time out, defined as maximum wash-out rate x-axis intercept. (3) Mean transit time (mTT) = wash-in rate x-axis intercept to mid-point wash-out rate. (4) Wash-in area under the curve (WiAUC) = AUC (TI: peak enhancement time). (5) Wash-out AUC (WoAUC) = AUC (peak enhancement time: TO). (6) Rise time = peak enhancement time – TI. (7) Fall time = TO – peak enhancement time. (8) Wash-in perfusion index = WiAUC/Rise Time. (**b**) Destruction-replenishment kinetics. Assessed values: (1) relative blood volume (rBV) = maximum signal - minimum signal. (2) Wash-in rate (WiR) = gradient of maximum slope. (3) Mean transit time (mTT) = time to half maximum signal. (4) Perfusion index (PI) = rBV/mTT

19.3 Safety Profile of Ultrasound Contrast Agents

Reported adverse events following administration of ultrasound contrast agents are rare (<1%), with headache and nausea most common. Serious adverse events occur at a rate of 0.03% and the rate of anaphylactoid reactions is between 0.004 and 0.009% [8]. Such events are typically not IgE mediated and therefore no prior exposure is required. Product labelling for contrast agents continues to warn against their administration in pulmonary hypertension; however several prospective studies have examined this in conjunction with the US Federal Drugs Administration. All have demonstrated stable hemodynamics and no safety concerns [9, 10]. As a result, investigators continue to administer ultrasound contrast agents in pulmonary hypertension and acute respiratory distress syndrome (ARDS). Ultrasound contrast agents have seen limited use in pediatric populations and pregnancy and therefore have an uncertain safety profile in these settings. Being of similar dimensions to erythrocytes, bubble contrast agents are not filtered across the glomerulus, have no renal interactions and are not nephrotoxic; a distinct advantage over contrast agents used in other imaging modalities [1].

19.4 Acquisition and Analysis of Renal Contrast-Enhanced Ultrasound Images

Off-line processing of contrast-enhanced ultrasound imagery is performed using dedicated software. A number of proprietary platforms are available as are bespoke research software [11]. We will focus on VueBox™ (Bracco, Geneva, Switzerland), a commonly used analysis system for quantification. An overall region of delimitation is selected and motion compensation applied. Motion in a clip can occur due to respiratory artefact, a frequent issue in renal imaging, or probe movements.

Cortical signal is uniform although may be attenuated towards the poles and nearer the pelvis as signal is scattered by other bubbles [12]. Provided regions of interest (ROIs) are within well-visualized parenchymal tissue, the exact shape or location of the ROI makes little difference to the reproducibility of the results [13]. Signals from the medullary region are more heterogeneous, calyces produce no signal as contrast agents are not filtered, and vascular regions have high signal. Medullary parenchymal tissue receives approximately one tenth of cortical blood flow and enhances more slowly. The anisotropic nature of medullary perfusion, the complex arrangement of the transiting vasculature, and the avascular calyces extending into the region makes clinical quantification of medullary perfusion challenging.

Pulsed high mechanical intensity ultrasound is used to produce destruction-replenishment kinetics. These time intensity curves have several key components as shown in Fig. 19.3b. The plateau of peak intensity minus the background signal is termed the relative blood volume and is reflective of the total volume of the vascular space within the ROI. However, as 2D ultrasound cannot accurately assess volumetric parameters, the relative blood volume is expressed in arbitrary units. Peak signal intensity is also affected by a number of other factors, such as habitus, distance from the probe, probe position and the mechanical index [14]. The maximal gradient of the wash-in slope is termed the wash-in rate, and the time taken to reach half-maximum signal intensity the mean transit time (mTT). These variables are related to blood velocity and flow: wash-in rate is dependent on signal intensity and time, whereas mTT is a discrete time-based variable. Perfusion index is a composite variable produced by dividing relative blood volume by the mTT and provides a single number representing tissue perfusion [15].

19.5 Validation and Reproducibility of Renal Contrast-Enhanced Ultrasound

19.5.1 Validation Against Standard Measures of Renal Blood Flow

Experimental studies have compared contrast-enhanced ultrasound-derived variables with direct arterial flow measurements, showing good correlation in dogs [16] and rats [17]. In humans, the gold standard for measuring renal blood flow, para-aminohippuric-acid (PAH), is only reliable with stable renal function and does not lend itself to evaluations in AKI in critically ill patients. A study in healthy volunteers attempted pharmacological manipulation of renal blood flow, comparing renal blood flow to cortical perfusion by contrast-enhanced ultrasound analysis, and demonstrating only a moderate degree of correlation [18]. However, renal blood flow provides a measure of blood flow at the organ level and contrast-enhanced ultrasound provides detail of the microcirculation; due to the complex vascular arrangement and regulation of renal perfusion only a limited correlation would be expected [19]. These findings, of a moderate correlation between renal blood flow and cortical perfusion, were echoed in a healthy volunteer study, comparing radionucleotide measurements and PAH measurements with contrast-enhanced ultrasound [20]. Improvements in velocity (time) based variables have been demonstrated with dopamine infusion [21], valsartan administration [22], and a high protein meal [23], and two of these studies used concurrent assessment with PAH to show a significant correlation; however, all three studies demonstrated no significant change in intensity-based variables.

19.5.2 Reproducibility of Contrast-Enhanced Ultrasound Measurements

The reproducibility of contrast-enhanced ultrasound data is a potential issue with both bolus and infusion methods, particularly in the quantification of signal intensity [24]. Potential sources of error have been well described in previous reviews and may be broadly subdivided into issues with microbubbles, ultrasound scanner settings, and patient characteristics [25].

Hudson and colleagues demonstrated an *in vitro* coefficient of variation of 13% using the same ultrasound machine [26]. A North American Quantitative Imaging Biomarkers Alliance (QIBA) Contrast-Enhanced Ultrasound Committee supported a body of work in 2020 promoting standardization across machines and analysis platforms. They demonstrated similar *in vivo* reproducibility to the study by Hudson et al. [26], particularly for time-dependent variables, but found that intensity-dependent variables could not be compared between different systems without standardization [27]. Intensity parameters vary even when imaged and analyzed using the same platform, as they can be altered by signal saturation from dynamic range settings, microbubble concentration, depth and acoustic shadowing from both microbubbles and native structures [24].

19.6 Selected Experimental and Clinical Studies That Have Used Renal Contrast-Enhanced Ultrasound

An experimental study compared a variety of macro- and micro-hemodynamic parameters in pigs with induced septic shock, demonstrating that renal cortical blood flow reduced during shock and, unlike systemic hemodynamic parameters such as cardiac output, did not recover during resuscitation [28].

Harrois et al. [29] used contrast-enhanced ultrasound to study 20 critically ill septic patients and dichotomized the cohort based on the development of KDIGO AKI stage 2 or 3 within the first 72 h of admission. Increased mTT, but not intensity-based parameters predicted the development of AKI and there was no difference in systemic hemodynamic variables, such as cardiac index, between the groups. A notable feature was the widely heterogeneous nature of the contrast-enhanced ultrasound-derived perfusion variables in patients with sepsis. This finding is in keeping with the results of other studies using different modalities, such as sublingual videomicroscopy, which have consistently demonstrated that flow heterogeneity within the microcirculation is almost pathognomonic of septic shock [30].

Yoon and colleagues conducted an observational study of 48 patients with AKI presenting to a nephrology department [31]. Time-based contrast-enhanced ultrasound parameters (wash-in rate, rise time, and mTT), but not those based on signal intensity (such as relative blood volume) predicted the development of KDIGO stage 3 AKI, initiation of renal replacement therapy (RRT) and recovery from AKI. Systemic hemodynamic parameters were not recorded during this study making it difficult to comment on the relative contributions of the macro- and microcirculations to the observed perfusion deficits.

Our research group has recently concluded an observational study, MICROSHOCK-RENAL, investigating renal perfusion in critically ill patients with septic shock [32]. To our knowledge, this is the first study to date that has used contrast-enhanced ultrasound alongside a comprehensive hemodynamic assessment using echocardiography and renal artery Doppler flow analysis. The findings of a substudy of MICROSHOCK-RENAL, investigating critically ill patients with coronavirus disease 2019 (COVID-19) with KDIGO stage 3 AKI, showed very impaired renal cortical perfusion, despite preserved cardiac output [33] .

Several investigators have used contrast-enhanced ultrasound as a tool to assess the effect of therapy on renal perfusion. In a small case series, Schneider and colleagues demonstrated an improvement in cortical perfusion following terlipressin administration in patients with hepatorenal syndrome [34]. The same group also manipulated renal cortical perfusion in critically ill patients using norepinephrine. A targeted mean arterial pressure (MAP) of 60 mmHg was compared with 80 mmHg in a mixed group of 12 patients, within 48 h of ICU admission. The authors noted wide inter-individual variation in response to therapy and, again, this is in keeping with similar studies that have assessed the microcirculatory response to vasoactive drug therapy using different monitoring modalities [35, 36].

19.7 Future Avenues for Renal Contrast-Enhanced Ultrasound Research

19.7.1 Understanding the Pathogenesis of Perfusion Abnormalities in Septic AKI

Although there is an increasing evidence base that renal cortical perfusion is impaired in septic AKI, there is uncertainty about the relative contributions of systemic effects (e.g., venous congestion, right sided heart failure, etc.), flow at the level of the renal vessels, and intrinsic microcirculatory perfusion anomalies. This information is crucial when deciding on therapeutic interventions and further clinical studies that use contrast-enhanced ultrasound alongside monitors of systemic hemodynamic parameters are required.

19.7.2 Prognostication in AKI

If AKI in critically ill patients, especially those with sepsis, is linked to renal perfusion then longitudinal assessment of perfusion may enable new insights about the natural history of the condition. Contrast-enhanced ultrasound-derived variables could be used to study not only the onset of AKI but also the need for, and timing of, RRT. Recovery of renal function may be presaged by recovery in contrast-enhanced ultrasound variables, opening up the potential to use the technique for longer term outcome prediction or prognosis.

19.7.3 Goal-Directed Therapy to Prevent or Ameliorate AKI

There have been many attempts to prevent AKI in vulnerable patients through the use of goal-directed hemodynamic therapy [37, 38]. To date, these interventions have been limited in two respects: first they have targeted macro-hemodynamic variables, which are often not impaired, particularly in septic AKI; second, interventions are not targeted at individual patients but rather toward a "one-size-fits-all" approach to management. The use of contrast-enhanced ultrasound addresses these issues, allowing direct assessment of perfusion in patients undergoing targeted interventions, such as changes in dose or type of vasopressor therapy. Further research could enable the phenotyping of individual patients based on contrast-enhanced ultrasound parameters. These phenotypes could then be identified by clinical or biomarker based parameters and therapies adjusted accordingly.

19.8 Conclusion

Renal contrast-enhanced ultrasound is a technique that is both feasible and safe in critically ill patients and has the potential to produce insight into the pathogenesis of septic AKI. There is a degree of variability in the derived variables that would benefit from a standardized approach to imaging and allowing more effective comparison between studies. In the near future, renal contrast-enhanced ultrasound may enable the development of individualized therapy to mitigate the development of AKI in critically ill patients.

References

1. Selby NM, Williams JP, Phillips BE. Application of dynamic contrast enhanced ultrasound in the assessment of kidney diseases. Curr Opin Nephrol Hypertens. 2021;30:138–43.
2. Ince C, Boerma EC, Cecconi M, et al. Second consensus on the assessment of sublingual microcirculation in critically ill patients: results from a task force of the European Society of Intensive Care Medicine. Intensive Care Med. 2018;44:281–99.
3. Langenberg C, Bellomo R, May C, Wan L, Egi M, Morgera S. Renal blood flow in sepsis. Crit Care. 2005;9:R363.
4. Klibanov AL. Ultrasound contrast: gas microbubbles in the vasculature. Investig Radiol. 2021;56:50–61.
5. Mattrey RF, Wrigley R, Steinbach GC, Schutt EG, Evitts DP. Gas emulsions as ultrasound contrast agents preliminary results in rabbits and dogs. Investig Radiol. 1994;29:S139–41.
6. Dietrich C, Averkiou M, Nielsen M, et al. How to perform contrast-enhanced ultrasound (CEUS). Ultrasound Int Open. 2018;4:E2–15.
7. Chan A, Barrett EJ, Anderson SM, Kovatchev BP, Breton MD. Muscle microvascular recruitment predicts insulin sensitivity in middle-aged patients with type 1 diabetes mellitus. Diabetologia. 2012;55:729–36.
8. Muskula PR, Main ML. Safety with echocardiographic contrast agents. Circ Cardiovasc Imaging. 2018;10:e005459.
9. Wever-Pinzon O, Suma V, Ahuja A, et al. Safety of echocardiographic contrast in hospitalized patients with pulmonary hypertension: a multi-center study. Eur Heart J Cardiovasc Imaging. 2012;13:857–62.
10. Abdelmoneim SS, Bernier M, Scott CG, et al. Safety of contrast agent use during stress echocardiography in patients with elevated right ventricular systolic pressure. Circ Cardiovasc Imaging. 2010;3:240–8.
11. Prada F, Gennari AG, Linville IM, et al. Quantitative analysis of in-vivo microbubble distribution in the human brain. Sci Rep. 2021;11:11797.

12. Sidhu P, Cantisani V, Dietrich C, et al. The EFSUMB guidelines and recommendations for the clinical practice of contrast-enhanced ultrasound (CEUS) in non-hepatic applications: update 2017 (long version). Ultraschall Der Medizin. 2018;39:e2–44.
13. Macrì F, Pietro SD, Liotta L, Piccionello AP, Pugliese M, Majo MD. Effects of size and location of regions of interest examined by use of contrast-enhanced ultrasonography on renal perfusion variables of dogs. Am J Vet Res. 2016;77:869–76.
14. Gauthier M, Leguerney I, Thalmensi J, et al. Estimation of intra-operator variability in perfusion parameter measurements using DCE-US. World J Radiol. 2011;3:70–81.
15. Dietrich C, Averkiou M, Correas J-M, Lassau N, Leen E, Piscaglia F. An EFSUMB introduction into dynamic contrast-enhanced ultrasound (DCE-US) for quantification of tumour perfusion. Ultraschall Med. 2012;33:344–51.
16. Wei K, Le E, Bin JP, Coggins M, Thorpe J, Kaul S. Quantification of renal blood flow with contrast-enhanced ultrasound. J Am Coll Cardiol. 2001;37:1135–40.
17. Kogan P, Johnson KA, Feingold S, et al. Validation of dynamic contrast-enhanced ultrasound in rodent kidneys as an absolute quantitative method for measuring blood perfusion. Ultrasound Med Biol. 2011;37:900–8.
18. Muskiet MHA, Emanuel AL, Smits MM, et al. Assessment of real-time and quantitative changes in renal hemodynamics in healthy overweight males: contrast-enhanced ultrasonography vs para-aminohippuric acid clearance. Microcirculation. 2019;26(7):e12580.
19. Schneider AG, Goodwin MD, Bellomo R. Measurement of kidney perfusion in critically ill patients. Crit Care. 2013;17:220.
20. Hosotani Y, Takahashi N, Kiyomoto H, et al. A new method for evaluation of split renal cortical blood flow with contrast echography. Hypertens Res. 2002;25:77–83.
21. Kishimoto N, Mori Y, Nishiue T, et al. Renal blood flow measurement with contrast-enhanced harmonic ultrasonography: evaluation of dopamine-induced changes in renal cortical perfusion in humans. Clin Nephrol. 2003;59:423–8.
22. Kishimoto N, Mori Y, Nishiue T, et al. Ultrasound evaluation of valsartan therapy for renal cortical perfusion. Hypertens Res. 2004;27:345–9.
23. Kalantarinia K, Belcik JT, Patrie JT, Wei K. Real-time measurement of renal blood flow in healthy subjects using contrast-enhanced ultrasound. Am J Physiol Renal Physiol. 2009;297:F1129–34.
24. Ignee A, Jedrejczyk M, Schuessler G, Jakubowski W, Dietrich CF. Quantitative contrast enhanced ultrasound of the liver for time intensity curves—reliability and potential sources of errors. Eur J Radiol. 2010;73:153–8.
25. Tang M-X, Mulvana H, Gauthier T, et al. Quantitative contrast-enhanced ultrasound imaging: a review of sources of variability. Interface Focus. 2011;1:520–39.
26. Hudson JM, Karshafian R, Burns PN. Quantification of flow using ultrasound and microbubbles: a disruption replenishment model based on physical principles. Ultrasound Med Biol. 2009;35:2007–20.
27. Averkiou MA, Juang EK, Gallagher MK, et al. Evaluation of the reproducibility of bolus transit quantification with contrast-enhanced ultrasound across multiple scanners and analysis software packages—a quantitative imaging biomarker alliance study. Investig Radiol. 2020;55:643–56.
28. Lima A, van Rooij T, Ergin B, et al. Dynamic contrast-enhanced ultrasound identifies microcirculatory alterations in sepsis-induced acute kidney injury. Crit Care Med. 2018;46:1284–92.
29. Harrois A, Grillot N, Figueiredo S, Duranteau J. Acute kidney injury is associated with a decrease in cortical renal perfusion during septic shock. Crit Care. 2018;22:161.
30. De Backer D, Creteur J, Preiser JC, Dubois MJ, Vincent JL. Microvascular blood flow is altered in patients with sepsis. Am J Respir Crit Care. 2002;166:98–104.
31. Yoon HE, Kim DW, Kim D, Kim Y, Shin SJ, Shin YR. A pilot trial to evaluate the clinical usefulness of contrast-enhanced ultrasound in predicting renal outcomes in patients with acute kidney injury. PLoS One. 2020;15:e0235130.
32. Watchorn J, Huang D, Hopkins P, Bramham K, Hutchings S. Prospective longitudinal observational study of the macro and micro haemodynamic responses to septic shock in the renal

and systemic circulations: a protocol for the MICROSHOCK – RENAL study. BMJ Open. 2019;9:e028364.

33. Watchorn J, Huang DY, Joslin J, Bramham K, Hutchings SD. Critically ILL COVID-19 patients with acute kidney injury have reduced renal blood flow and perfusion despite preserved cardiac function; a case-control study using contrast enhanced ultrasound. Shock. 2021;55:479–87.
34. Schneider AG, Schelleman A, Goodwin MD, Bailey M, Eastwood GM, Bellomo R. Contrast-enhanced ultrasound evaluation of the renal microcirculation response to terlipressin in hepatorenal syndrome: a preliminary report. Ren Fail. 2014;37:175–9.
35. Schneider AG, Goodwin MD, Schelleman A, Bailey M, Johnson L, Bellomo R. Contrast-enhanced ultrasonography to evaluate changes in renal cortical microcirculation induced by noradrenaline: a pilot study. Crit Care. 2014;18:653.
36. Redfors B, Bragadottir G, Sellgren J, Swärd K, Ricksten SE. Effects of norepinephrine on renal perfusion, filtration and oxygenation in vasodilatory shock and acute kidney injury. Intensive Care Med. 2011;37:60–7.
37. Asfar P, Meziani F, Hamel JF, et al. High versus low blood-pressure target in patients with septic shock. N Engl J Med. 2014;370:1583–93.
38. Lamontagne F, Richards-Belle A, Thomas K, et al. Effect of reduced exposure to vasopressors on 90-day mortality in older critically ill patients with vasodilatory hypotension. JAMA. 2020;323:938–49.

Focused Clinical Hemodynamic Assessment in Septic Shock

20

E. Kattan, G. Hernández, and J. Bakker

20.1 Introduction

Septic shock is a highly prevalent and lethal condition [1]. From a hemodynamic point of view, several pathogenic mechanisms determine the progression of circulatory dysfunction and tissue hypoperfusion, eventually leading to multiorgan failure and death if not promptly treated [2]. These factors typically change over time. While loss of vascular tone and relative hypovolemia predominate in early phases, more complex mechanisms such as endothelial and microcirculatory dysfunction, distributive abnormalities, vasoplegia, capillary leak, and varying degrees of myocardial dysfunction may be involved in progressive phases of septic shock [2]. In the end, however, these highly dissimilar mechanisms may lead to a common clinical profile of hypotension and hypoperfusion, of which it is not easy to determine the predominant mechanism during the initial evaluation at intensive care unit (ICU) admission.

E. Kattan · G. Hernández
Departamento de Medicina Intensiva, Facultad de Medicina, Pontificia Universidad Católica de Chile, Santiago, Chile

J. Bakker (✉)
Departamento de Medicina Intensiva, Facultad de Medicina, Pontificia Universidad Católica de Chile, Santiago, Chile

Department of Intensive Care Adults, Erasmus MC University Medical Center, Rotterdam, The Netherlands

Department of Pulmonary and Critical Care, New York University School of Medicine, New York, NY, USA

Division of Pulmonary, Allergy, and Critical Care Medicine, Columbia University College of Physicians and Surgeons, New York, NY, USA
e-mail: jb3387@cumc.columbia.edu

J.-L. Vincent (ed.), *Annual Update in Intensive Care and Emergency Medicine 2022*, Annual Update in Intensive Care and Emergency Medicine,
https://doi.org/10.1007/978-3-030-93433-0_20

It is likely that evolution into different profiles of sepsis-related circulatory dysfunction is influenced by the relative preponderance at the individual level of any of the above cited mechanisms. The search for tools to identify hemodynamic phenotypes to individualize therapies has been highlighted as a priority in a septic shock research agenda [3, 4]. A few recent studies have reported on the heterogeneity of hemodynamic and perfusion profiles. Using transesophageal echocardiography, Geri et al. identified five hemodynamic clusters in a cohort of septic shock patients [5]. The clusters incorporated characteristics that marked hypovolemia and left ventricular dysfunction despite similar mean arterial pressure (MAP) levels. In addition, Hernandez et al. proposed that capillary refill time (CRT) at baseline may determine different septic shock phenotypes [6]. Finally, Hilty et al. characterized different clinical types of circulatory dysfunction on the basis of sublingual microcirculatory parameters [7].

Low MAP is the hallmark of sepsis-related acute circulatory dysfunction. As the duration of hypotension is related to morbidity and mortality [8], current guidelines recommend timely correction of the MAP to levels greater than 65 mmHg using fluids and vasopressors [9]. This 'MAP-driven strategy' has probably led to an unwanted adverse effect, a reductionist approach to clinical hemodynamic monitoring in which, among numerous variables provided by the blood pressure signal, only MAP is considered for decision-making. Moreover, this standardized or 'one size fits all' resuscitation strategy is debatable since septic shock patients are highly heterogeneous. For example, a recent study showed that 30% of septic shock patients were fluid unresponsive at ICU admission [10]. Others have suggested a very early administration of norepinephrine instead of fluids could be associated with better outcomes in predominantly vasoplegic patients [11], as was also shown in an experimental model of septic shock [12] and a single center randomized trial [13].

So, the prominent clinical question is: can we do better?

20.2 Insights into Current Hemodynamic Monitoring

In the past 30 years, a myriad of monitoring techniques has been developed, tested, and successfully introduced to clinical practice [14]. Current guidelines recommend advanced hemodynamic monitoring only in selected cases [15, 16]. Bedside monitoring using echocardiography [17] has become a standard of care for patients with septic shock [18]. However, in many healthcare systems, especially in low- and-middle income countries [19], bedside echocardiography is not readily available 24/7, and not all ICU physicians are trained in its use, hindering its immediate applicability.

This technological boom in monitoring techniques has produced a 'shift' in clinicians' agendas, since they have to incorporate overwhelming new information on the functioning, troubleshooting, interpretation, and limitations of each device into daily clinical practice [20]. As an unintended consequence, valuable information derived from standard bedside monitoring tools may get overlooked, with the inherent risk of losing key elements for clinical decision making.

Standard monitoring in the ICU includes placement of a central venous catheter and an arterial line [16]. A paramount question then arises when advanced monitors or echocardiography are not readily available: is it possible to determine hemodynamic phenotypes using classical clinical monitoring tools? An initial approach with already available signals could aid physicians to decide on early resuscitation interventions. The physiological background of the key components of a focused clinical hemodynamic assessment (FCHA) is presented below.

20.2.1 Arterial Line

Arterial lines have been recommended as standard monitoring devices in critically ill patients, since they allow clinicians to obtain accurate and beat-to-beat measurements of MAP, the initial macrocirculatory target to ensure organ perfusion pressure [9]. Moreover, the analysis and interpretation of MAP can deliver valuable information about cardiac function, heart-lung interactions, arterial system, and valvular diseases [21]. In this sense, focusing on MAP alone could be an oversimplification of the instrument, since patients with similar MAP values may have considerable differences in underlying pathophysiological conditions (Fig. 20.1).

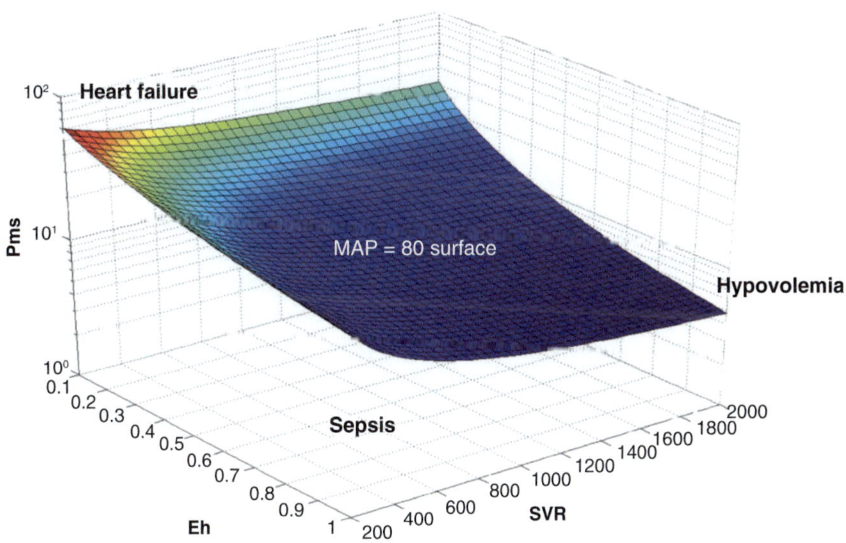

Fig. 20.1 The plot of a surface area for a 70 kg patient, where the mean arterial pressure (MAP) is similar in different clinical syndromes of circulatory failure: heart failure, hypovolemia and sepsis. *Pms* mean systemic filling pressure, *Eh* index of cardiac efficiency, *SVR* systemic vascular resistance. (Provided by M.R. Pinsky, Pittsburgh, USA)

20.2.2 Pulse Pressure as a Surrogate for Stroke Volume

Since the early 1900s, various researchers have tried to study the correlation between arterial pulse pressure and stroke volume [22]. Pulse pressure is an interesting variable as it is easy to obtain and provides a readily accessible monitoring window into the function of the heart and its interaction with the vascular system. According to a 3-compartment Windkessel model, characteristics of the arterial system (one of the main determinants of pulse pressure together with stroke volume) are determined by peripheral resistance, total arterial compliance, and aortic characteristic impedance [23]. Mathematical derivations of this model provided the basis for cardiac output monitors based on pulse-contour analysis [24]. Moreover, multiple studies have shown, both in simulated conditions [25] and patients [26] in different clinical scenarios [27] that pulse pressure can adequately track stroke volume.

The main objective of a fluid challenge is to increase stroke volume and thus cardiac output to restore tissue perfusion [28]. The use of the pulse pressure variation (PPV) [29], when performed in compliance with the test's validity criteria [29], allows clinicians to rapidly assess fluid responsiveness at the bedside, tailor fluid therapy, and avoid unnecessary fluid loading [10]. Other tests, such as end-expiratory occlusion test, could be performed when there are limitations to simple PPV assessment [30].

20.2.3 Diastolic Blood Pressure as a Proxy for Arterial Vascular Tone

According to the previously mentioned model, diastolic blood pressure is determined by a function of total arterial compliance, peripheral resistance, and heart rate [23]. Despite its relevance to organ perfusion, such as coronary flow, diastolic arterial pressure (DAP) has not been traditionally considered in decision-making processes during septic shock resuscitation, even though it provides valuable information to the clinician. Thus, in patients with diastolic 'hypotension' and tachycardia, it could be concluded that vasoplegia could be the main pathological determinant of this hypotension and hypoperfusion [31]. Recently, Ospina-Tascón et al. described the diastolic shock index (DSI), a novel and simple approach to assess severity and clinical patterns of patients with septic shock [32]. In brief, the DSI can be calculated as the heart rate divided by the DAP. A DSI >2.2 was associated with higher mortality, and has been advocated to evaluate an early start of vasopressors [11].

20.2.4 Arterial Waveform Analysis as Qualitative Hemodynamic Fine-Tuning

Arterial waveform analysis provides insight into classic components of cardiovascular semiology, such as *parvus et tardus* arterial tracing in aortic stenosis [33]. Moreover, in the context of circulatory dysfunction, a critical analysis of the arterial trace can provide a valuable aid for interpretation of the clinical scenario:

- In patients with hypovolemic shock, the arterial waveform will be spiked and narrow with a relatively high diastolic pressure. In those with left ventricular dysfunction, the ascending slope during systole will be less steep. Meanwhile, in distributive states, such as septic shock, arterial curves will be wider and present lower diastolic pressures, consistent with vasoplegia [34].
- Another critical component of the arterial tracing, the morphology and position of the dicrotic notch in the waveform, can also deliver relevant clinical information [35]. For example, patients with low cardiac output and high peripheral resistance develop dicrotic waves; and vasodilation and low vascular resistance are associated with more delayed and lower dicrotic notches in the trace [34].
- Even though waveform and arterial notch analysis is more qualitative in nature, and can require certain training, it can be useful as a complementary assessment of the cardiovascular status and enable hemodynamic patterns to be identified.

20.2.5 Central Venous Pressure

Since the description of dynamic predictors of fluid responsiveness, the central venous pressure (CVP) has been inadequately disregarded as a useful hemodynamic parameter, probably due to an oversimplification of its meaning and interpretation [36]. Even though its ability to predict fluid responsiveness is scant [28], the CVP is a rich variable delivering valuable information on cardiac and circulatory functions. As the CVP is the consequence of venous return and myocardial function [37], in its most simple assessment a high CVP thus translates into a state where the right ventricle is limited to accommodate the venous return, hence working at higher filling pressures [38]. In the same thread, CVP is the upstream pressure for venous return, meaning that high values, or relevant changes before and after a fluid challenge, can be used as a safety limit for fluid loading [39]. In addition, systemic perfusion pressure has been calculated from the difference between MAP and CVP, although physiologically the pre- and post-capillary pressure would be a more meaningful parameter of perfusion pressure [40]. Furthermore, the CVP trace curves also deliver valuable information of pathological conditions, as for example 'tall c and v waves' reflect the presence of tricuspid regurgitation [33].

20.2.6 Peripheral Perfusion

The main objective of using hemodynamic parameters during circulatory dysfunction in septic shock is to restore and improve tissue perfusion. Thus, it is relevant to include perfusion markers in a structured clinical approach. Laboratory markers, such as lactate, are not always readily available and can present extended processing times in some clinical scenarios, potentially delaying therapies. Since the original report by Joly and Weil [41], derangements in peripheral perfusion have been identified as a prognostic marker in critically ill patients [42, 43]. Two standardized approaches, CRT and the Mottling Score have been described and associated with mortality [44, 45]. During septic shock resuscitation, peripheral perfusion indices have faster resolution kinetics than lactate [46]. In addition, the use of CRT as a target of resuscitation [47] has been associated with better outcomes than when using lactate levels [48, 49]. Peripheral perfusion can aid to stratify disease severity, allowing for clinical phenotyping [6]. In this sense, peripheral perfusion emerges as a cornerstone tool in clinical practice, enabling perfusion status to be assessed dynamically at the bedside. Eventually, the response of CRT to flow-increasing maneuvers may disclose the status of the hemodynamic coherence between the macro- and microcirculations [50]. This topic is currently being studied in patients with septic shock (ClinicalTrials.gov Identifier: NCT04693923).

20.3 Applicability and Future Directions

Through a sequential analysis of FCHA components, clinicians may rapidly integrate these signals into clinically relevant hemodynamic phenotypes and disclose the relationship between macro- and microcirculatory derangements, which may assist subsequent therapeutic interventions (Fig. 20.2). The simplicity of the FCHA approach makes it a clinical tool that may have broad applicability in a wide variety of settings [51]. This should, however, not result in the avoidance of laboratory measurements, advanced hemodynamic monitoring, or echocardiography, neither lead to nihilism in their use. We believe these are valuable tools, which have both a clinical and educational role, and can help bedside decision making in different scenarios. Moreover, FCHA may provide a systematic cardiovascular assessment when these measurements are not immediately available, allowing the clinician to grasp an initial orientation of the hemodynamic condition of the patient. This

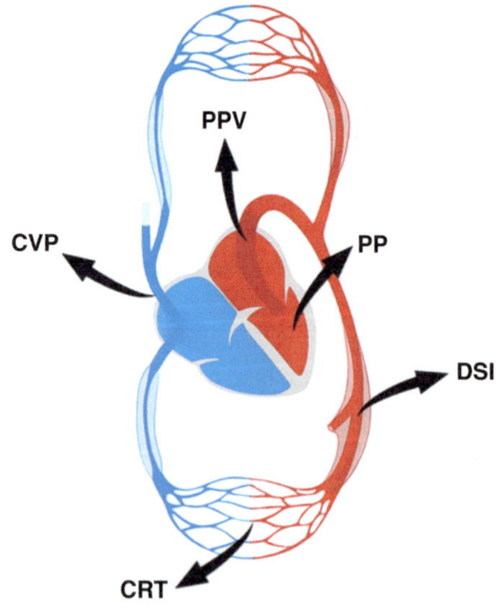

Fig. 20.2 Conceptual integration of focused clinical hemodynamic assessment (FCHA) variables. *CRT* capillary refill time, *PPV* pulse pressure variation, *CVP* central venous pressure, *DSI* diastolic shock index

resuscitation strategy will be tested in the future ANDROMEDA-SHOCK-2 trial (ClinicalTrials.gov Identifier: NCT05057611).

20.4 Conclusion

FCHA may constitute a standardized hemodynamic assessment, easily applicable when advanced monitoring is not readily available. It may provide the clinician at the bedside with valuable information about different key aspects of the cardiovascular system, thus enabling potential clinical phenotypes to be identified and targeted individualized treatment. Future research should validate this approach.

Acknowledgments This manuscript was supported in part by grant FONDECYT-ANID No. 1200246 (GH). We would like to acknowledge Ricardo Castro, Magdalena Vera, Pablo Born, Patricio Vásquez, Leyla Alegria, Sebastián Merino, Gustavo Ospina-Tascón, Adrian Wong, and Jean-Louis Teboul for significant contributions to the conception of this manuscript. We would also like to thank Michael Pinsky for the production of Fig. 20.1.

References

1. Rudd KE, Johnson SC, Agesa KM, et al. Global, regional, and national sepsis incidence and mortality, 1990–2017: analysis for the global burden of disease study. Lancet. 2020;395:200–11.
2. Cecconi M, Evans L, Levy M, Rhodes A. Sepsis and septic shock. Lancet. 2018;392:75–87.
3. Saugel B, Trepte CJ, Heckel K, Wagner JY, Reuter DA. Hemodynamic management of septic shock: is it time for "'individualized goal-directed hemodynamic therapy"' and for specifically targeting the microcirculation? Shock. 2015;43:522–9.
4. Taccone FS, Bond O, Cavicchi FZ, Hites M. Individualized antibiotic strategies. Curr Opin Anesthesiol. 2016;29:166–71.
5. Geri G, Vignon P, Aubry A, et al. Cardiovascular clusters in septic shock combining clinical and echocardiographic parameters: a post hoc analysis. Intensive Care Med. 2019;45: 657–67.
6. Hernández G, Kattan E, Tascón GO, Bakker J, Castro R. Capillary refill time status could identify different clinical phenotypes among septic shock patients fulfilling sepsis-3 criteria: a post hoc analysis of ANDROMEDA-SHOCK trial. Intensive Care Med. 2020;46:816–8.
7. Hilty MP, Akin S, Boerma C, et al. Automated algorithm analysis of sublingual microcirculation in an international multicentral database identifies alterations associated with disease and mechanism of resuscitation. Crit Care Med. 2020;48:E864–75.
8. Maheshwari K, Nathanson BH, Munson SH, et al. The relationship between ICU hypotension and in-hospital mortality and morbidity in septic patients. Intensive Care Med. 2018;44: 857–67.
9. Rhodes A, Evans LE, Alhazzani W, et al. Surviving sepsis campaign: international guidelines for management of sepsis and septic shock: 2016. Intensive Care Med. 2017;43:304–77.
10. Kattan E, Ospina-Tascón GA, Teboul JL, et al. Systematic assessment of fluid responsiveness during early septic shock resuscitation: secondary analysis of the ANDROMEDA-SHOCK trial. Crit Care. 2020;24:23.
11. Ospina-Tascón GA, Hernandez G, Alvarez I, et al. Effects of very early start of norepinephrine in patients with septic shock: a propensity score-based analysis. Crit Care. 2020;24:52.
12. Byrne L, Obonyo NG, Diab SD, et al. Unintended consequences: fluid resuscitation worsens shock in an ovine model of endotoxemia. Am J Respir Crit Care Med. 2018;198:1043–54.

13. Permpikul C, Tongyoo S, Viarasilpa T, Trainarongsakul T, Chakorn T, Udompanturak S. Early use of norepinephrine in septic shock resuscitation (CENSER) a randomized trial. Am J Respir Crit Care Med. 2019;199:1097–105.
14. Funcke S, Sander M, Goepfert MS, et al. Practice of hemodynamic monitoring and management in German, Austrian, and Swiss intensive care units: the multicenter cross-sectional ICU-CardioMan Study. Ann Intensive Care. 2016;6:49.
15. Teboul JL, Saugel B, Cecconi M, et al. Less invasive hemodynamic monitoring in critically ill patients. Intensive Care Med. 2016;42:1350–9.
16. Cecconi M, De Backer D, Antonelli M, et al. Consensus on circulatory shock and hemodynamic monitoring. Task force of the European Society of Intensive Care Medicine. Intensive Care Med. 2014;40:1795–815.
17. Mercado P, Maizel J, Beyls C, et al. Transthoracic echocardiography: an accurate and precise method for estimating cardiac output in the critically ill patient. Crit Care. 2017;21:1–8.
18. Yang Y, Royse C, Royse A, Williams K, Canty D. Survey of the training and use of echocardiography and lung ultrasound in Australasian intensive care units. Crit Care. 2016;20:9–10.
19. Haniffa R, Pubudu De Silva A, et al. Improving ICU services in resource-limited settings: perceptions of ICU workers from low-middle-, and high-income countries. J Crit Care. 2018;44:352–6.
20. Saugel B, Vincent J. Cardiac output monitoring: how to choose the optimal method for the individual patient. Curr Opin Crit Care. 2018;24:165–72.
21. Esper SA, Pinsky MR. Arterial waveform analysis. Best Pract Res Clin Anaesthesiol. 2014;28:363–80.
22. Rosen I, White H. The relation of pulse pressure to stroke volume. Am J Phys. 1926;78:168–84.
23. Westerhof N, Lankhaar JW, Westerhof BE. The arterial windkessel. Med Biol Eng Comput. 2009;47:131–41.
24. Wesseling KH, Jansen JRC, Settels JJ, Schreuder JJ. Computation of aortic flow from pressure in humans using a nonlinear, three-element model. J Appl Physiol. 1993;74:2566–73.
25. Bighamian R, Hahn J. Relationship between stroke volume and pulse pressure during blood volume perturbation: a mathematical analysis. Biomed Res Int. 2014;2014:459269.
26. Marquez J, McCurry K, Severyn DA, Pinsky MR. Ability of pulse power, esophageal Doppler, and arterial pulse pressure to estimate rapid changes in stroke volume in humans. Crit Care Med. 2008;36:3001–7.
27. Convertino VA, Cooke WH, Holcomb JB. Arterial pulse pressure and its association with reduced stroke volume during progressive central hypovolemia. J Trauma. 2006;61:629–34.
28. Michard F, Teboul J-L. Predicting fluid responsiveness in ICU patients. Chest. 2002;121:2000–8.
29. Teboul JL, Monnet X, Chemla D, Michard F. Arterial pulse pressure variation with mechanical ventilation. Am J Respir Crit Care Med. 2019;199:22–31.
30. Monnet X, Teboul JL. Assessment of fluid responsiveness: recent advances. Curr Opin Crit Care. 2018;24:190–5.
31. Ospina-Tascón GA, Hernandez G, Bakker J. Should we start vasopressors very early in septic shock? J Thorac Dis. 2020;12:3893–6.
32. Ospina-Tascón GA, Teboul JL, Hernandez G, et al. Diastolic shock index and clinical outcomes in patients with septic shock. Ann Intensive Care. 2020;10:41.
33. Miller RR. Miller's anesthesia. 8th ed. Philadelphia, PA: Elsevier; 2015.
34. Klein LW, Shahrrava A. The incisura. Cardiol Rev. 2019;27:274–8.
35. Ewy GA, Rios JC, Marcus FI. The dicrotic arterial pulse. Circulation. 1969;39:655–61.
36. Cecconi M, Hofer C, Teboul JL, et al. Fluid challenges in intensive care: the FENICE study: a global inception cohort study. Intensive Care Med. 2015;41:1529–37.
37. Patterson S, Starling E. On the mechanical factors which determine the output of the ventricles. J Physiol. 1914;48:357–279.
38. Berlin DA, Bakker J. Starling curves and central venous pressure. Crit Care. 2014;19:55.
39. De Backer D, Vincent JL. Should we measure the central venous pressure to guide fluid management? Ten answers to 10 questions. Crit Care. 2018;22:43.

40. Bayliss W, Starling E. Observations on venous pressures and their relationship to capillary pressures. J Physiol. 1894;16:159–318.
41. Joly H, Weil MH. Temperature of the great toe as an indication of the severity of shock. Circulation. 1969;39:131–8.
42. Kaplan LJ, Mcpartland K, Santora TA, Trooskin SZ. Start with a subjective assessment of skin temperature to identify hypoperfusion in intensive care unit patients. J Trauma. 2001;50:620–7.
43. Lima A, Jansen TC, Van Bommel J, Ince C, Bakker J. The prognostic value of the subjective assessment of peripheral perfusion in critically ill patients. Crit Care Med. 2009;37:934–8.
44. Dubin A, Henriquez E, Hernández G. Monitoring peripheral perfusion and microcirculation. Curr Opin Crit Care. 2018;24:173–80.
45. Hariri G, Joffre J, Leblanc G, et al. Narrative review: clinical assessment of peripheral tissue perfusion in septic shock. Ann Intensive Care. 2019;9:37.
46. Hernandez G, Pedreros C, Veas E, et al. Evolution of peripheral vs metabolic perfusion parameters during septic shock resuscitation. A clinical-physiologic study. J Crit Care. 2012;27:283–8.
47. Castro R, Kattan E, Ferri G, et al. Effects of capillary refill time-vs. lactate-targeted fluid resuscitation on regional, microcirculatory and hypoxia-related perfusion parameters in septic shock: a randomized controlled trial. Ann Intensive Care. 2020;10:150.
48. Zampieri FG, Damiani LP, Bakker J, et al. Effect of a resuscitation strategy targeting peripheral perfusion status vs serum lactate levels on 28-day mortality among patients with septic shock: a Bayesian reanalysis of the ANDROMEDA-SHOCK trial. Am J Respir Crit Care Med. 2020;201:423–9.
49. Kattan E, Hernández G, Tascón GO, Valenzuela ED, Bakker J. A lactate-targeted resuscitation strategy may be associated with higher mortality in patients with septic shock and normal capillary refill time: a post hoc analysis of the ANDROMEDA-SHOCK study. Ann Intensive Care. 2020;10:114.
50. Ince C. Hemodynamic coherence and the rationale for monitoring the microcirculation. Crit Care. 2015;19:S8.
51. Mekontso Dessap A. Frugal innovation for critical care. Intensive Care Med. 2019;45:252–4.

Vasopressor Choice and Timing in Vasodilatory Shock

21

P. M. Wieruszewski and A. K. Khanna

21.1 Introduction

Vasodilatory shock is the most common form of circulatory shock encountered in patients admitted to the intensive care unit (ICU) [1]. Sepsis is the predominant etiology, but other causes of vasodilatory shock include postoperative vasoplegia, anaphylaxis, spinal cord injury (i.e., neurogenic shock), systemic inflammatory response from acute pancreatitis, and direct vascular relaxation from general and neuraxial anesthetics. Vasodilatory shock is a medical emergency that requires prompt diagnosis and treatment. Regardless of etiology, vasodilatory shock is characterized by reduced systemic vascular resistance and arterial hypotension that warrants intravascular fluid resuscitation and pharmacological vasopressors to restore the vascular tone. Left untreated, perfusion pressures suffer, leading to inadequate cellular oxygen utilization, conversion to anaerobic metabolism, multiorgan failure, and death [2, 3]. For over a decade, norepinephrine has been recommended as the first-line vasopressor choice, with vague guidance on secondary agent selection and timing [4], leading to considerable heterogeneity in intensivist practice at the bedside [5]. Herein, we provide a contemporary review of factors that influence vasopressor selection and timing, challenging the classic treatment paradigms of vasodilatory shock.

P. M. Wieruszewski
Departments of Anesthesiology and Pharmacy, Mayo Clinic, Rochester, MN, USA

A. K. Khanna (✉)
Department of Anesthesiology, Section on Critical Care Medicine, Wake Forest School of Medicine, Atrium Health Wake Forest Baptist Medical Center, Winston-Salem, NC, USA

Outcomes Research Consortium, Cleveland, OH, USA
e-mail: akhanna@wakehealth.edu

J.-L. Vincent (ed.), *Annual Update in Intensive Care and Emergency Medicine 2022*, Annual Update in Intensive Care and Emergency Medicine,
https://doi.org/10.1007/978-3-030-93433-0_21

21.2 A Balanced Vasopressor Approach

The classic approach to fluid-refractory vasodilatory shock treatment is to apply catecholamine vasopressors and titrate to achieve a specified mean arterial pressure (MAP). This stepwise approach traditionally involves initiation of norepinephrine, subsequent up-titration of dosage, often to toxic levels, waiting for a relative catecholamine-refractory state, and then moving on to the next vasopressor [4]. This strategy delays attainment of adequate perfusion pressures and ultimately leads to progressive multiorgan failure, and in turn, the chances of death rise with each progressive increase in the number of total organ failures [6]. Refractory vasodilatory shock is the end point of treatment failure and is clinically characterized by a lack of sustainable adequate MAP despite increasing doses of a single or multiple vasopressors [7]. This state is a molecular combination of a complex set of physiological alterations coming together, including but not limited to altered microcirculatory flow, membrane hyperpolarization, cellular relaxation, and vascular reactivity (Fig. 21.1).

This approach leaves intensivists with many uncertainties, including (1) at what point do you consider norepinephrine-treatment failure, (2) when do you apply a secondary vasopressor, and (3) which secondary vasopressor do you select? It is important to understand these challenges and rationalize an early, multimodal balanced vasopressor strategy as an alternative to the classic stepwise approach. Normal blood pressure homeostasis and pathogenesis in shock, as well as the major

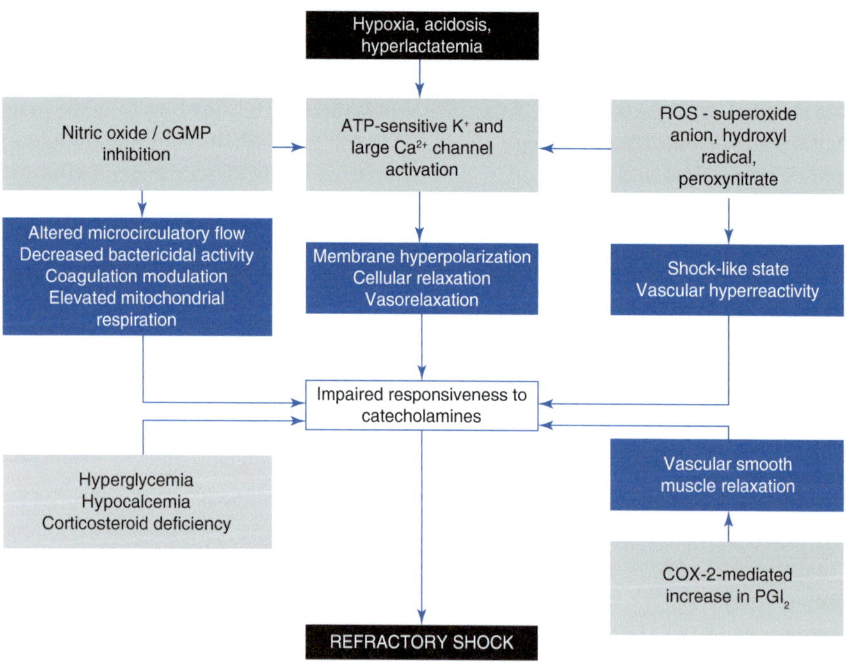

Fig. 21.1 Pathogenic mechanisms leading to refractory vasodilatory shock. *ATP* adenosine triphosphate, *cGMP* cyclic guanosine monophosphate, *COX-2* cyclooxygenase-2, *PGI*$_2$ prostaglandin I_2, *ROS* reactive oxygen species. (From [8] with permission)

determinants of shock outcomes including timing delays in perfusion, hyperlactatemia, and catecholamine burden, particularly as it all relates to the pharmacology of vasopressors, is a critical discussion that deserves mention in this context.

21.3 Blood Pressure Homeostasis and Pathogenesis

Under normal physiological conditions, blood pressure and circulatory function are maintained in homeostasis by a complex counter regulatory interplay of the sympathetic nervous system, vasopressinergic system, and the renin-angiotensin system (Fig. 21.2).

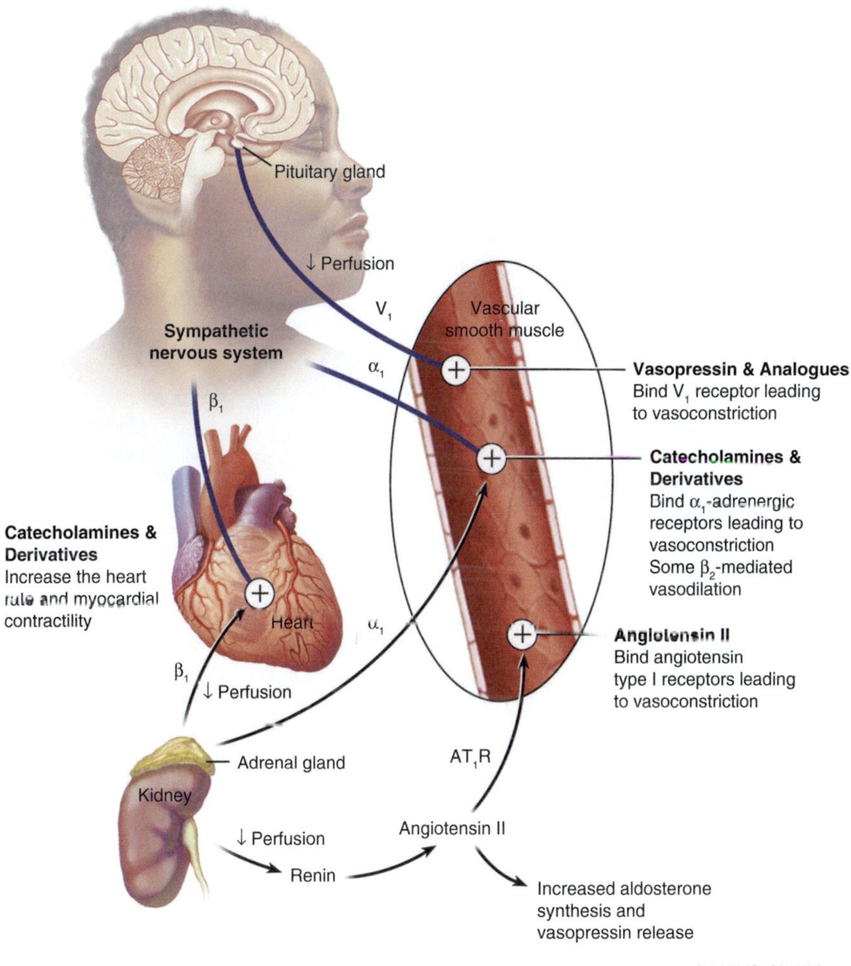

Fig. 21.2 Physiologic concert of the adrenergic, vasopressinergic, and renin-angiotensin systems in blood pressure homeostasis, and select mechanisms of pharmacologic vasopressors. α_1 alpha$_1$-adrenergic receptor, AT_1R angiotensin type 1 receptor, β_1 beta$_1$-adrenergic receptor, β_2 beta$_2$-adrenergic receptor, V_1 vasopressin 1 receptor. (Used with permission of Mayo Foundation for Medical Education and Research, all rights reserved)

When these systems are perturbed by an insult (e.g., sepsis), the homeostatic balance is disrupted. The most obvious objective finding is macrocirculatory dysfunction identified by directly measuring systemic blood pressure, although damage to tissues and the microvasculature regionally occurs in parallel and even preceding global evidence of hypotension [9].

In addition to direct insults from profound systemic inflammatory responses, the very systems responsible for homeostasis are impaired during shock. Although a stress-induced hyperdynamic state often accompanies septic shock, total heart rate variability is reduced suggesting impairment of the sympathetic system [10]. Similarly, in states of hypotension the posterior pituitary is expected to secrete endogenous vasopressin stores, although plasma vasopressin concentrations in vasodilatory septic hypotension have been shown to be inappropriately low (3.1 pg/ml) as compared to other hypotensive states also expected to experience this hormonal response, such as cardiogenic shock (22.7 pg/ml), $p < 0.001$ [11]. Finally, despite activation of the renin-angiotensin system in shock, various angiotensin receptors are downregulated, contributing to vascular hyporeactivity and also impaired endogenous catecholamine secretion [12, 13]. Despite this multifactorial and co-existent hormonal deficiency that is evident during the continuum of vasodilatory shock, the recommended approach remains a step-wise one where catecholamines are started with up-titration, often to toxic levels, and only then a potential introduction of a secondary agent [4].

21.4 Timing

Attainment of a satisfactory perfusion pressure to push arterial blood into capillaries and deliver oxygen to tissues is the ultimate goal of resuscitation in vasodilatory shock. Delays in restoring adequate perfusion are consistently associated with worse organ failures and an increased risk of death in vasodilatory shock [6, 14, 15]. Specifically, after adjustment for severity of illness, delay in vasopressor initiation was associated with an increase in in-hospital death (OR 1.02, 95% CI 1.01–1.03, $p < 0.001$), which was most profound when delays were in excess of 14.1 h (OR 1.34, 95% CI 1.03–1.76, $p = 0.048$) [6]. Similar to the time-dependent mortality risk of delayed antimicrobials in sepsis, the risk of death has been shown to increase by 5.3% for every hour that vasopressor initiation is delayed [16]. In another cohort study, those who received vasopressors within 6 h of shock onset achieved goal MAPs twice as fast (1.5 vs. 3.0 h, $p < 0.01$), spent more time off vasopressors in the first 72 h of shock (34.5 vs. 13.1 h, $p = 0.03$), and were independently nearly 3 times as likely to survive at 30-days (mortality for vasopressors after 6 h; OR 2.9, 95%CI 1.3–7.0, p not reported) [15]. On the other hand, when vasopressor initiation is delayed beyond 4 h, the odds of worsening organ failure increase fourfold (OR 4.34, 95% CI 1.47–12.79, $p = 0.008$), when compared to those receiving vasopressors in <4 h [14]. Indeed, a 2018 update to the Surviving Sepsis Campaign recommends including vasopressor initiation in the crucial 1-h bundle for fluid-resistant hypotension [17], although most recently in 2021, guidance regarding timing of vasopressor initiation is ambiguous [4].

Despite the evidentiary knowledge of worse outcomes with a delay in vasopressor initiation, there has been limited effort to drive protocolized practice in support of such a strategy. The CENSER study was an early pioneer of this concept in which norepinephrine initiation within 1 h of septic shock was evaluated in a prospective, double-blind, randomized setting [18]. Those that were randomized to early norepinephrine had greater likelihood (OR 3.4, 95% CI 2.09–5.53, $p < 0.001$) of shock reversal (MAP >65 mmHg for 2 readings, urine output >0.5 ml/kg/h for 2 h, and 10% reduction in lactate from baseline) at 6 h. There were no differences in hospital or 28-day mortality, although this phase II study was not powered for mortality. It is interesting, however, that early norepinephrine recipients were less likely to experience cardiogenic pulmonary edema (OR 0.70, 95% CI 0.56–0.87, $p = 0.004$) or arrhythmias (OR 0.74, 95% CI 0.56–0.94, $p = 0.03$).

While it is clear that earlier vasopressor initiation is better than later, timing of a secondary agent is less clear. However, recently, a large retrospective cohort study found that when vasopressin was added as a second-line agent to norepinephrine in septic shock, the risk of in-hospital mortality increased by an order of 12–18% with delay in initiation of vasopressin from shock onset (2.1–12.2 h) and increasing lactate concentration [19]. Perhaps these are all signals that more rapid attention to and an earlier opportunity for non-catecholamine vasopressors to act—while the physiological milieu is still favorable, or shock has not progressed to a point of irreversibility—is key to improving outcomes in these patients.

21.5 Hyperlactatemia

In pathologic shock, arterial hypotension reduces oxygen delivery, leading to regional and global tissue hypoxia [20]. Consequently, oxygen utilization at the cellular level is impaired with inadequate mitochondrial oxidation. Concurrently, vasodilatory shock is often accompanied by a hyperdynamic state secondary to stress (e.g., sepsis) leading to aerobic glycolysis further contributing to excess lactate production [20]. The net result is a state of hyperlactatemia that is exacerbated by acidemia impairing hepatic lactate clearance.

Hyperlactatemia has consistently been a hallmark of poor prognosis in vasodilatory shock. In a cohort of severe sepsis and septic shock, initial lactate concentrations were higher (7.3 mmol/l) in those who died within 24 h of presentation compared to those alive after 24 h (3.3 mmol/l) [21]. In a multivariable analysis in this population, this initial lactate concentration (OR 1.19, 95% CI 1.05–1.35, $p = 0.004$) and organ failures as measured by the modified sequential organ failure assessment (mSOFA) score (OR 1.17, 95% CI 1.00–1.36, $p = 0.046$) were independent predictors of early death [21]. Similarly, outside of the immediate presentation period, lactate >4 mmol/l has been independently associated with a threefold greater risk of 28-day death in septic shock (OR 3.0, 95% CI 2.1–4.1, $p < 0.001$), regardless of vasopressor use [22]. Even among patients with shock from sepsis requiring vasopressors, those experiencing at least one lactate concentration greater than 2.5 mmol/l at any time during their shock course, have nearly half the survival

(57.1%) than those without hyperlactatemia (92.3%) at 100 days ($p < 0.0001$) [23]. Interestingly, even when the lactate concentration is within the generally considered 'normal limits', those with relative increases to the higher end of the normal range experience greater likelihood of death [24]. Taken altogether, hyperlactatemia in vasodilatory shock appears to epitomize a serious deficit in adequate organ perfusion. Indeed, the risk of multiorgan failure and death increases with increasing lactate concentration [25].

In addition to prognosis, lactate concentration may provide valuable insight into vasopressor selection and timing considerations, particularly when it comes to non-adrenergic vasopressors added to catecholamines. Although only less than half of patients receiving vasopressin experience a favorable hemodynamic response, response is twice as likely among those with lower lactate concentrations (OR 2.15, 95% CI 1.39–3.32, $p < 0.001$), which in turn, is associated with a greater likelihood of ICU survival [26]. Recently in a cohort study of patients with septic shock, when the addition of vasopressin to first-line norepinephrine was delayed, the odds of in-hospital death increased with an increasing lactate concentration as much as 18% per mmol/l at 12.2 h from the shock onset (95% CI 1.07–1.32) [19]. Similarly, post-marketing experience with synthetic angiotensin II demonstrates a similar hemodynamic and survival response as it relates to lactate concentration. Despite a profound baseline severity illness amongst recipients of synthetic angiotensin II (baseline SOFA of 12 and APACHE II of 30), hemodynamic responders had a lower baseline lactate concentration (6.5 mmol/l) compared to non-responders (9.5 mmol/l), and in a multivariable model the likelihood of hemodynamic response was greater with lower lactate (OR 1.11 per mmol/l, 95% CI 1.05–1.17, $p < 0.001$) and 30-day mortality was lower with lower lactate (OR 0.94 per mmol/l, 95% CI 0.91–0.96, $p < 0.001$) [27].

21.6 Catecholamine Burden

The most obvious consequence to the classic stepwise vasopressor approach is overall catecholamine burden. With its potent vasoconstrictive effects at alpha-adrenergic receptors throughout the vascular periphery, excess stimulation may be detrimental, with distal vessels remaining most susceptible leading to ischemic digits and splanchnic hypoxia and resulting in necrosis and serious morbidity [28, 29]. In addition to the desired vasoconstrictive effects of catecholamines, beta-receptor stimulation at the level of the myocardium (Fig. 21.2) has made these agents particularly intolerable. Arrhythmia is common and occurs in up to one-third of norepinephrine recipients in septic shock, and is associated with increased risk of death [30]. Duration and dosage of norepinephrine have shown value in predicting dysrhythmia, and the risk increases by 6% for every 5 μg/min increase in maximum norepinephrine dosage [30].

Cumulative dosage of norepinephrine exposure has been an easily identifiable objective measure for predicting prognosis in septic shock. Compared to an approximate 90-day mortality of 25% amongst >3000 international patients with septic

Table 21.1 Norepinephrine dose and mortality

Study	Norepinephrine dose	Death type	Death rate (%)
Jenkins et al. 2009 [35]	>100 μg/min	ICU	94
Brown et al. 2013 [32]	≥1 μg/kg/min	90-days	83
Dopp-Zemel et al. 2013 [34]	≥0.9 μg/kg/min	28-days	65
Martin et al. 2015 [29]	>1 μg/kg/min	90-days	90
Auchet et al. 2017 [33]	>1 μg/kg/min	28-days	60
		90-days	66
Brand et al. 2017 [36]	≥90 μg/min	Hospital	90

shock in the PRISM meta-analysis [31], those that required high-dose norepinephrine had mortality rates ranging from 60% to in excess of 90% [29, 32–36] (Table 21.1).

In addition to prognosis, catecholamine dosage is an easy, bedside marker for deciding on vasopressor escalation. In the landmark VASST trial, patients who received vasopressin when the norepinephrine dosage was <15 μg/min experienced lower 28-day (26.5% vs. 35.7%, $p = 0.05$) and 90-day (35.8% vs. 46.1%, $p = 0.04$) mortality [37]. Similarly, in a recent analysis of >1500 septic shock patients, the risk of in-hospital mortality was increased by 20.7% for every 10 μg/min increase in norepinephrine dosage at the time of vasopressin addition as the second-line agent [19]. Most importantly, regardless of response rate and baseline severity of illness, risk of mortality is independently lower if there is a positive hemodynamic response to vasopressin (OR 0.51, 95% CI 0.35–0.76, $p = 0.001$) and angiotensin II (HR 0.50, 95% CI 0.35–0.71, $p < 0.001$) [26, 27]. All these data suggest that hemodynamic restoration and shock reversal is a crucial determinant in survival probability.

21.7 A Path Towards Personalization: Early Multimodal Vasopressor Therapy

To tailor vasopressor therapy in vasodilatory shock, phenotypic prognostication and pharmacologic response need to be characterized. There have been several emerging candidate biomarkers that have demonstrated association with vasopressor response and outcomes in septic shock (Table 21.2). Genetic variations in ARDβ2 encoding the β_2-adrenergic receptor have been found to be associated with a higher norepinephrine requirement, greater renal, hematologic, hepatic, and neurologic dysfunction, and an increased 28-day mortality in septic shock [38]. Similarly, variants in AGTRAP, the angiotensin II receptor type 1 associated protein, have been associated with reduced MAP, lower vascular tone, and an increase in 28-day mortality [39]. Interestingly, defects in LNPEP (leucyl and cystinyl aminopeptidase), also known as vasopressinase, have been associated with increased clearance of plasma vasopressin and increased 28-day mortality [40]. Elevations of plasma angiopoietin-2 concentrations, an endothelial growth factor that promotes vascular leakage, have been associated with renal, hepatic, and coagulation dysfunction, as well as increased 7- and 28-day mortality [41]. While there is a so-called relative

Table 21.2 Potential biomarkers for vasopressor therapy

Biomarker	Pathologic variant/ threshold of harm	Vasopressor	Clinical association
Genetic polymorphisms			
ADRβ2	SNP rs1042717	Norepinephrine, epinephrine	↑organ dysfunction, ↑norepinephrine requirement, ↑septic shock mortality [38]
AGTRAP	SNP rs11121816	Angiotensin II	↓vascular tone, ↑septic shock mortality [39]
LNPEP	SNP rs4869317	Vasopressin and analogues	↑vasopressin clearance, ↑septic shock mortality [40]
Circulating peptides			
Angiopoeitin-2	>5807 pg/ml	Vasopressin and analogues	↑organ failure, ↑septic shock mortality [41]
Renin	>40 pg/ml	Angiotensin II	↓hemodynamic response, ↑shock mortality [42, 43]
Vasopressin	Variable	Vasopressin	Mixed outcomes, variable hemodynamic response [44, 45]

ADRβ2 beta$_2$-adrenergic receptor gene, *AGTRAP* angiotensin II receptor type 1 associated protein gene, *LNPEP* leucyl/cystinyl aminopeptidase gene

vasopressin deficiency in the early stages of septic shock [11], plasma vasopressin concentrations have not been shown to predict positive response to exogenous vasopressin administration, and outcome correlations are mixed [44, 45].

Although lactate has long been a prognosticator in critical illness and shock, serum renin is rapidly emerging as a potentially superior predictor of mortality in various shock states in the ICU. Two separate studies have shown that an absolute renin threshold concentration and a rate of rise of renin were both superior to lactate in associations with ICU and in-hospital mortality in critically ill patients [42, 46]. Importantly, renin appeared to be stable, and concentrations were not influenced appreciably by renal replacement therapy or drugs that alter the renin-angiotensin cascade (i.e., ACE inhibitors and angiotensin receptor blockers) [46]. Administration of exogenous angiotensin II has been shown to favorably benefit survival outcomes in those with high-renin shock [43, 47]. One of the biggest clinical barriers to the use of this biomarker in conjunction with or as an alternative to lactate is the lack of a true point-of-care assay that would allow targeted resuscitation at the bedside in response to concentrations in a timely manner [48, 49].

Our approach speaks to the use of early multimodal vasopressors, also termed 'broad-spectrum vasopressors' by others. This is analogous to the use of broad-spectrum and early antimicrobials in suspected and confirmed sepsis. While there are not currently convincing data, as there are for the analogy with antimicrobials, there is certainly a physiological premise for the use of lower doses of multiple different classes of vasopressors as we initiate therapy in vasodilatory shock. This will need to be combined with the extensive use of biomarkers and de-escalation from multiple to a single agent could occur if one biomarker stands out as a clear signal of harm for a particular patient. For example, a patient with septic shock where vasopressin levels are disproportionately low compared with the increase in lactate and increase in angiotensin II (i.e., low renin), and where initial use of vasopressin has shown clinical benefit and laboratory correction of this anomaly could be slowly transitioned to a vasopressin-heavy approach after an initial broad-spectrum strategy that rapidly achieves perfusion targets. Similarly, an exquisite response to synthetic angiotensin II in the setting of high serum renin, would be an obvious rationale for continuing an angiotensin II predominant vasopressor approach. Indeed, the value of testing angiotensin II responsiveness has been proven in clinical studies and portends an excellent prognosis in appropriately chosen patients [50]. There will also be those with benign shock, where very low dose catecholamines may be all that is necessary and clearly not all patients will necessitate combination vasopressors. Finally, the use of non-vasoconstricting adjuncts (e.g., corticosteroids) targeted at the underlying pathology, as catecholamine-sparing strategies, should not be ignored to provide a balanced approach to the overall resuscitation of vasodilatory shock [7, 51].

21.8 Conclusion

The classic approach to vasodilatory shock management consists of a stepwise escalation of vasopressors which leads to prolonged states of hypoperfusion, hyperlactatemia, excessive catecholamine exposure, and poor outcome. An early, balanced, multimodal vasopressor therapy strategy provides a physiologic-guided approach to the complex, multifactorial pathogenesis of vasodilatory shock. Data are desperately needed in the development and deployment of biomarkers in the individualized approach to vasopressor therapy to improve shock outcomes.

References

1. Vincent JL, De Backer D. Circulatory shock. N Engl J Med. 2013;369:1726–34.
2. Khanna AK, Maheshwari K, Mao G, et al. Association between mean arterial pressure and acute kidney injury and a composite of myocardial injury and mortality in postoperative critically ill patients. Crit Care Med. 2019;47:910–7.
3. Maheshwari K, Nathanson BH, Munson SH, et al. The relationship between ICU hypotension and in-hospital mortality and morbidity in septic patients. Intensive Care Med. 2018;44:857–67.
4. Evans L, Rhodes A, Alhazzani W, et al. Surviving sepsis campaign: international guidelines for management of sepsis and septic shock 2021. Intensive Care Med. 2021;47:1181–247.
5. Scheeren TWL, Bakker J, De Backer D, et al. Current use of vasopressors in septic shock. Ann Intensive Care. 2019;9:20.
6. Beck V, Chateau D, Bryson GL, et al. Timing of vasopressor initiation and mortality in septic shock: a cohort study. Crit Care. 2014;18:R97.
7. Jentzer JC, Vallabhajosyula S, Khanna AK, Chawla LS, Busse LW, Kashani KB. Management of refractory vasodilatory shock. Chest. 2018;154:416–26.
8. Vallabhajosyula S, Jentzer JC, Khanna AK. Vasodilatory shock in the ICU: perils, pitfalls and therapeutic options. In: Vicnent JL, editor. Annual update in intensive care and emergency medicine. Basel: Springer; 2018. p. 99–111.
9. Dünser MW, Takala J, Brunauer A, Bakker J. Re-thinking resuscitation: leaving blood pressure cosmetics behind and moving forward to permissive hypotension and a tissue perfusion-based approach. Crit Care. 2013;17:326.

10. Garrard CS, Kontoyannis DA, Piepoli M. Spectral analysis of heart rate variability in the sepsis syndrome. Clin Auton Res. 1993;3:5–13.
11. Landry DW, Levin HR, Gallant EM, et al. Vasopressin deficiency contributes to the vasodilation of septic shock. Circulation. 1997;95:1122–5.
12. Mederle K, Schweda F, Kattler V, et al. The angiotensin II AT1 receptor-associated protein Arap1 is involved in sepsis-induced hypotension. Crit Care. 2013;17:R130.
13. Bucher M, Hobbhahn J, Kurtz A. Nitric oxide-dependent down-regulation of angiotensin II type 2 receptors during experimental sepsis. Crit Care Med. 2001;29:1750–5.
14. Black LP, Puskarich MA, Smotherman C, Miller T, Fernandez R, Guirgis FW. Time to vasopressor initiation and organ failure progression in early septic shock. J Am Coll Emerg Physicians Open. 2020;1:222–30.
15. Colon Hidalgo D, Patel J, Masic D, Park D, Rech MA. Delayed vasopressor initiation is associated with increased mortality in patients with septic shock. J Crit Care. 2020;55:145–8.
16. Bai X, Yu W, Ji W, et al. Early versus delayed administration of norepinephrine in patients with septic shock. Crit Care. 2014;18:532.
17. Levy MM, Evans LE, Rhodes A. The surviving sepsis campaign bundle: 2018 update. Intensive Care Med. 2018;44:925–8.
18. Permpikul C, Tongyoo S, Viarasilpa T, Trainarongsakul T, Chakorn T, Udompanturak S. Early use of norepinephrine in septic shock resuscitation (CENSER). A randomized trial. Am J Respir Crit Care Med. 2019;199:1097–105.
19. Sacha GL, Lam SW, Wang L, Duggal A, Reddy AJ, Bauer SR. Association of catecholamine dose, lactate, and shock duration at vasopressin initiation with mortality in patients with septic shock. Crit Care Med. 2021; Sep 24. https://doi.org/10.1097/CCM.0000000000005317. Epub ahead of print.
20. Kraut JA, Madias NE. Lactic acidosis. N Engl J Med. 2014;371:2309–19.
21. Javed A, Guirgis FW, Sterling SA, et al. Clinical predictors of early death from sepsis. J Crit Care. 2017;42:30–4.
22. Thomas-Rueddel DO, Poidinger B, Weiss M, et al. Hyperlactatemia is an independent predictor of mortality and denotes distinct subtypes of severe sepsis and septic shock. J Crit Care. 2015;30:e1–6.
23. Hernandez G, Castro R, Romero C, et al. Persistent sepsis-induced hypotension without hyperlactatemia: is it really septic shock? J Crit Care. 2011;26:435.e9–14.
24. Nichol AD, Egi M, Pettila V, et al. Relative hyperlactatemia and hospital mortality in critically ill patients: a retrospective multi-centre study. Crit Care. 2010;14:R25.
25. Jansen TC, van Bommel J, Woodward R, Mulder PGH, Bakker J. Association between blood lactate levels, sequential organ failure assessment subscores, and 28-day mortality during early and late intensive care unit stay: a retrospective observational study. Crit Care Med. 2009;37:2369–74.
26. Sacha GL, Lam SW, Duggal A, et al. Predictors of response to fixed-dose vasopressin in adult patients with septic shock. Ann Intensive Care. 2018;8:35.
27. Wieruszewski PM, Wittwer ED, Kashani KB, et al. Angiotensin II infusion for shock. Chest. 2021;159:596–605.
28. Landry GJ, Mostul CJ, Ahn DS, et al. Causes and outcomes of finger ischemia in hospitalized patients in the intensive care unit. J Vasc Surg. 2018;68:1499–504.
29. Martin C, Medam S, Antonini F, et al. Norepinephrine: not too much, too long. Shock. 2015;44:305–9.
30. Wieruszewski ED, Jones GM, Samarin MJ, Kimmons LA. Predictors of dysrhythmias with norepinephrine use in septic shock. J Crit Care. 2021;61:133–7.
31. Rowan KM, Angus DC, Bailey M, et al. Early, goal-directed therapy for septic shock—a patient-level meta-analysis. N Engl J Med. 2017;376:2223–34.
32. Brown SM, Lanspa MJ, Jones JP, et al. Survival after shock requiring high-dose vasopressor therapy. Chest. 2013;143:664–71.
33. Auchet T, Regnier M-A, Girerd N, Levy B. Outcome of patients with septic shock and high-dose vasopressor therapy. Ann Intensive Care. 2017;7:43.

34. Döpp-Zemel D, Groeneveld AJ. High-dose norepinephrine treatment: determinants of mortality and futility in critically ill patients. Am J Crit Care. 2013;22:22–32.
35. Jenkins CR, Gomersall CD, Leung P, Joynt GM. Outcome of patients receiving high dose vasopressor therapy: a retrospective cohort study. Anaesth Intensive Care. 2009;37:286–9.
36. Brand DA, Patrick PA, Berger JT, et al. Intensity of vasopressor therapy for septic shock and the risk of in-hospital death. J Pain Symptom Manag. 2017;53:938–43.
37. Russell JA, Walley KR, Singer J, et al. Vasopressin versus norepinephrine infusion in patients with septic shock. N Engl J Med. 2008;358:877–87.
38. Nakada T, Russell JA, Boyd JH, et al. β2-adrenergic receptor gene polymorphism is associated with mortality in septic shock. Am J Respir Crit Care Med. 2010;181:143–9.
39. Nakada T, Russell JA, Boyd JH, et al. Association of angiotensin II type 1 receptor-associated protein gene polymorphism with increased mortality in septic shock. Crit Care Med. 2011;39:1641–8.
40. Nakada T, Russell JA, Wellman H, et al. Leucyl/cystinyl aminopeptidase gene variants in septic shock. Chest. 2011;139:1042–9.
41. Fisher J, Douglas JJ, Linder A, Boyd JH, Walley KR, Russell JA. Elevated plasma angiopoietin-2 levels are associated with fluid overload, organ dysfunction, and mortality in human septic shock. Crit Care Med. 2016;44:2018–27.
42. Jeyaraju M, McCurdy MT, Levine AR, et al. Renin kinetics are superior to lactate kinetics for predicting in-hospital mortality in hypotensive critically ill patients. Crit Care Med. 2022;50:50–60.
43. Bellomo R, Forni LG, Busse LW, et al. Renin and survival in patients given angiotensin II for catecholamine-resistant vasodilatory shock. A clinical trial. Am J Respir Crit Care Med. 2020;202:1253–61.
44. Yerke JR, Sacha GL, Scheraga RG, et al. Vasopressin plasma concentrations are not associated with hemodynamic response to exogenous vasopressin for septic shock. Pharmacotherapy. 2020;40:33–9.
45. Russell JA. Bench-to-bedside review: vasopressin in the management of septic shock. Crit Care. 2011;15:226.
46. Gleeson PJ, Crippa IA, Mongkolpun W, et al. Renin as a marker of tissue perfusion and prognosis in critically ill patients. Crit Care Med. 2019;47:152–8.
47. Bellomo R, Wunderink RG, Szerlip H, et al. Angiotensin I and angiotensin II concentrations and their ratio in catecholamine-resistant vasodilatory shock. Crit Care. 2020;24:43.
48. Khanna AK. Tissue perfusion and prognosis in the critically ill-Is renin the new lactate? Crit Care Med. 2019;47:288–90.
49. Khanna AK. Renin kinetics and mortality-same, same but different? Crit Care Med. 2022;50:153–7.
50. Ham KR, Boldt DW, McCurdy MT, et al. Sensitivity to angiotensin II dose in patients with vasodilatory shock: a prespecified analysis of the ATHOS-3 trial. Ann Intensive Care. 2019;9:63.
51. Venkatesh B, Khanna AK, Cohen J. Less is more: catecholamine-sparing strategies in septic shock. Intensive Care Med. 2019;45:1810–2.

Part VII

Cardiac Arrest

Advanced Life Support Update

22

G. D. Perkins and J. P. Nolan

22.1 Introduction

Cardiac arrest remains a significant cause of morbidity and mortality around the world. The International Liaison Committee on Resuscitation (ILCOR) is a collaboration of resuscitation councils from around the world that work together with the shared vision of saving more lives globally through resuscitation [1]. ILCOR has been synthesizing evidence relating to resuscitation to produce consensus on science and treatment recommendations for many years. Recent evidence evaluations have been informed by systematic reviews of the literature and the Grading of Recommendations Assessment, Development and Evaluation (GRADE) method to assess the certainty in evidence and the strength of recommendations [2]. These evidence evaluations are translated into practice by regional resuscitation councils from around the world. In Europe, the European Resuscitation Council (ERC) produces high quality, multi-disciplinary, evidenced-based guidelines for resuscitation [3]. In this chapter, we summarize key practice recommendations drawn from the most recent guideline updates relating to advanced life support (ALS) [4, 5], post-resuscitation care, and prognostication [6].

G. D. Perkins (✉)
Warwick Clinical Trials Unit, Warwick Medical School, University of Warwick, Coventry, UK

Critical Care Unit, Heartlands Hospital, University Hospital Birmingham, Birmingham, UK
e-mail: g.d.perkins@warwick.ac.uk

J. P. Nolan
Warwick Clinical Trials Unit, Warwick Medical School, University of Warwick, Coventry, UK

Critical Care Unit, Royal United Hospital Bath, Bath, UK

J.-L. Vincent (ed.), *Annual Update in Intensive Care and Emergency Medicine 2022*, Annual Update in Intensive Care and Emergency Medicine,
https://doi.org/10.1007/978-3-030-93433-0_22

22.2 Setting the Scene: Epidemiology and Outcomes

Data from the ERC Registries for Cardiac Arrest (EuReCa) studies report that the incidence of resuscitation attempts for out-of-hospital cardiac arrest (OHCA) ranges from 19 to 104 per 100,000 population per year [7, 8]. An international review of registries reported an incidence within these ranges in the USA, Canada, Australia, Asia, and Japan [9]. Most OHCAs in Europe have medical/cardiac causes and present with an initially non-shockable rhythm (80%) [7]. Return of spontaneous circulation (ROSC) is achieved in one third of patients with OHCA (range 8–42%) and the overall rate of survival to discharge is in the region of 8% (range 0–18%) [7]. Those with a witnessed cardiac arrest, with early bystander cardiopulmonary resuscitation (CPR), and with public access defibrillation have the best chances of survival [10].

Fewer data are available on the epidemiology of in-hospital cardiac arrest (IHCA) [11, 12]. The incidence of IHCA in the UK and USA is between 1.6 and 10 cases per 1000 admissions. Like OHCA, the majority of IHCAs are associated with non-shockable rhythms from a combination of respiratory and cardiac causes. A higher proportion of arrests are witnessed, and CPR is started almost simultaneously with the arrival of the ALS team within minutes. The rate of survival to hospital discharge is approximately 25%, 2–3 times higher than for OHCA [11].

Differences in case numbers likely reflect differences in system responses to cardiac arrest, the threshold as to when resuscitation is commenced and continued, as well as differences in risk from the resident population characteristics [11, 12]. Differences in outcomes can often be explained by the proportion of cardiac arrests where resuscitation is attempted and, where relevant, the community response to cardiac arrest (particularly bystander CPR and defibrillation). The time taken for the ALS team to arrive, how health systems approach discontinuation of resuscitation, access to and the quality of post-resuscitation care as well as neuroprognostication and withdrawal of life sustaining treatment practices likely also contribute to variation in outcomes [12].

The importance of functional recovery beyond the blunt categorization of outcomes into favorable or unfavorable neurological outcomes has been emphasized in recent reviews [12, 13]. Many patients classified as surviving with a favorable neurological outcome have significant functional impairments. Common problems reported in survivors of cardiac arrest include fatigue, cognitive problems (slowing or problems with attention or memory), emotional problems (anxiety, depression, post-traumatic stress), and physical impairments. These problems adversely affect health related quality of life and can reduce ability to return to work and social participation. Guidelines highlight the paucity of detailed follow-up for cardiac arrest survivors and lack of a strong evidence base to inform rehabilitation strategies [12].

22.3 Advanced Life Support Treatment Algorithm

The ALS treatment algorithm (Fig. 22.1) provides a framework for the assessment and treatment of cardiac arrest. Agonal breathing (also known as terminal gasping) is relatively common in the early stages after cardiac arrest [14]. Therefore, a

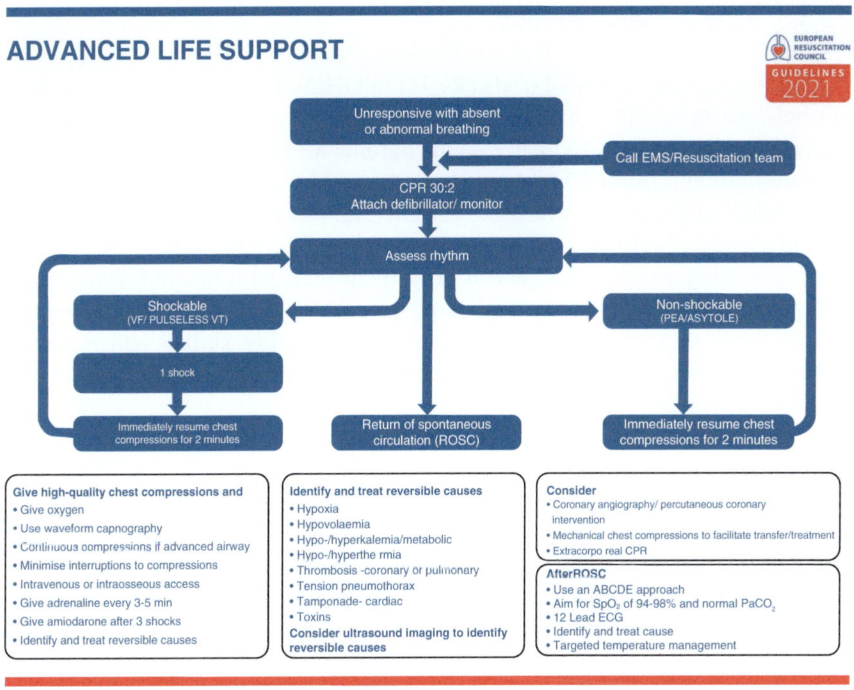

Fig. 22.1 Advanced life support treatment algorithm. (Reproduced with permission from the European Resuscitation Council [5]). *ABCDE* airway, breathing, circulation, disability, exposure, *CPR* cardiopulmonary resuscitation, *ECG* electrocardiogram, *EMS* emergency medical system, *PEA* pulseless electrical activity, $PaCO_2$ arterial partial pressure of carbon dioxide, *ROSC* return of spontaneous circulation, SpO_2 arterial oxygen saturation, *VF* ventricular fibrillation, *VT* ventricular tachycardia

diagnosis of cardiac arrest should be considered in any patient who is unresponsive with absent or abnormal breathing [14]. The use of advanced monitoring (e.g., electrocardiograph [EKG], arterial blood pressure, and capnography) may aid rapid diagnosis [5, 10]. Palpation of a central pulse to confirm cardiac arrest should be undertaken with caution and with an awareness of a high false positive rate (i.e., a pulse is thought to be present but is actually absent) [15]. Resuscitation should be started with chest compressions first, unless the person is attached to a defibrillator at the time of a witnessed cardiac arrest, in which case up to three successive shocks may be delivered. Cough CPR, fist pacing, and precordial thump are generally ineffective and their use should not delay definitive treatment with CPR and defibrillation [16].

The algorithm splits treatments according to whether the initial rhythm is shockable or non-shockable. Whilst the person remains in a shockable rhythm, the priority is high quality CPR and attempted defibrillation. It is important to minimize interruptions in CPR, particularly before and after delivering a shock. For non-shockable rhythms, high quality CPR with minimal interruptions remains a key priority alongside drug therapy and seeking to identify and treat reversible causes.

22.3.1 Airway Management

Large randomized controlled trials (RCTs) in OHCA have failed to show a benefit between the options of bag-mask ventilation, supraglottic airway use, and tracheal intubation [17]. Evidence on the optimal airway device during in-hospital resuscitation is limited, but should be addressed by the upcoming AIRWAYS-3 trial. Based on the current evidence, ILCOR suggests that the decision on which type of airway should be used in cardiac arrest is tailored to reflect the skills of those providing airway management [18]. In systems with low to medium intubation success rates, priority should be given to using supraglottic airways. Where those providing airway management are highly skilled and regularly undertaking tracheal intubation with a high success rate (>95%), tracheal intubation may be considered [5].

22.3.2 Drugs

The PARAMEDIC2 trial, which enrolled 8014 patients with OHCA, showed that epinephrine (1 mg given every 3–5 min) was highly effective at restarting the heart [19]. The effects on long-term survival were less pronounced with a number needed to treat of 112 to improve survival at 30 days. The study did not find evidence of improved survival with a favorable neurological outcome but there was a higher rate of organ donation in those treated with epinephrine [20]. An economic evaluation reported that when the societal benefits of organ donation were included in economic modeling, treatment with epinephrine had a 90% chance of being cost effective with a threshold of 34,500 Euro. A post hoc analysis highlighted that the earlier ALS was initiated, the greater were the chances of survival with a favorable neurological outcome [21]. ILCOR recommends the administration of epinephrine during CPR for both shockable and non-shockable rhythms [18]. The ALS Task Force highlights that neurological injury occurs following several minutes of cardiac arrest and that it is not possible at the time of starting resuscitation to identify those most at risk of neurological injury. Therefore, administering a drug that improves ROSC and survival gives an opportunity to provide high quality post-resuscitation care with the aim of reducing adverse neurological outcomes.

Meta-analyses of high dose epinephrine, vasopressin and the combination of epinephrine and vasopressin compared with standard dose (1 mg) epinephrine found low certainty evidence of improved ROSC for high dose epinephrine only. There was no improvement in long-term survival or favorable neurological outcome for any of these interventions [22]. ILCOR therefore suggests not using vasopressin routinely with or without epinephrine [18]. A trial which assessed the combination of vasopressin and steroids in addition to standard care amongst 512 patients with IHCA was published after the most recent ILCOR treatment recommendations [23]. The trial showed a 9.6% (95% confidence interval [CI] 1.1–18.0%) increase in ROSC but no difference in survival to 30 days or survival with a favorable neurological outcome. While the evidence will be assessed by ILCOR, it seems unlikely, given the absence of benefit on long-term outcomes, that treatment guidelines will change as a consequence.

A systematic review identified 14 randomized trials and 17 observational studies assessing the use of anti-arrhythmic drugs in patients with in- or out-of-hospital cardiac arrest and shock-refractory pulseless ventricular tachycardia/fibrillation (VT/VF) [24]. ILCOR's assessment of the evidence led to a weak recommendation in support of amiodarone or lidocaine based on the pre-defined subgroup analysis of bystander witnessed cardiac arrest observed in the ROC-ALPS study [25, 26]. The certainty of evidence was too low for ILCOR to make a recommendation about the use of bretylium, nifekalant, or sotolol for the treatment of adults in shock-refractory cardiac arrest.

22.3.3 Route of Drug Administration

Given the time critical nature of cardiac arrest, the route of drug administration is an important consideration. Early guidelines described the use of intracardiac epinephrine, but this practice was subsequently abandoned because of the risk of misplacement and complications. Enthusiasm for endobronchial delivery via a tracheal tube also reduced based on experimental studies showing sub-optimal absorption [27]. Drug delivery through a correctly positioned central venous cannula will deliver drugs to the central circulation more rapidly than a peripheral venous cannula. However, the time taken to cite a central venous catheter *de novo* during CPR and the risk of complications likely outweigh the benefits [28].

The peripheral venous route is used most frequently during cardiac arrest treatment, supplemented with a fluid bolus to reduce drug transit time to the central circulation. The intraosseous route provides access to the rich intra-medullary venous network. Experimental studies have shown similar transit times and drug concentrations compared with the intravenous route [27]. Both observational studies and RCTs suggest that the intraosseous access is quicker and has a higher first attempt success rate than venous access. Meta-analyses of observational studies are often limited by resuscitation time bias as it is difficult to separate the effects of time of drug administration from route (intravenous versus intraosseus) [29]. ILCOR has called for further research on the optimal route of drug administration, something which is hoped will be answered through the PARAMEDIC3 trial (ISRCTN: 14223494).

22.3.4 Extracorporeal Cardiopulmonary Resuscitation

Extracorporeal cardiopulmonary resuscitation (eCPR) has been used during IHCA and OHCA when traditional attempts to achieve ROSC have failed. A recent systematic review identified 25 observational studies [30]. Although eCPR was feasible, there was wide heterogeneity in study design and outcomes and inconsistency between results. Studies were assessed as being at critical risk of bias leading to overall very low certainty evidence. Authors of two small RCTs have published their experience of eCPR. In a single-center RCT in Minnesota (USA), 30 patients with OHCA were randomized to eCPR or standard ALS after arrival in the emergency department. Six of 14 (43%) patients in the eCPR arm survived to hospital discharge compared with 1 of 15 (7%) in the standard care arm (risk difference 36.2%, 3.7–59.2; posterior probability of eCPR superiority 0.9861) [31]. A small feasibility trial randomized in a 4:1 ratio adults with OHCA to expedited transport for eCPR or standard care. Among 151 patients assessed, 15 were enrolled of which only 5 were eligible for and treated with eCPR [32]. None of the patients enrolled in the study survived with a good neurological outcome. Both studies were characterized by low enrolment rates compared with the overall population of OHCA, matching clinical experience that only few patients with cardiac arrest may be eligible for eCPR. This raises uncertainty about the equality of access to this treatment. ILCOR's most recent treatment recommendation is to consider eCPR as a rescue therapy for selected patients with cardiac arrest when conventional CPR is failing in settings in which it can be implemented (weak recommendation, very low-certainty evidence) [33].

22.4 Post-resuscitation Care

Most patients who achieve ROSC will be comatose in the hours to days that follow [34]. Although there are factors in the initial history and response to treatment that are associated with adverse outcome (e.g., prolonged cardiac arrest duration, unwitnessed event, absence of bystander CPR, initial non-shockable rhythm), none are able to predict outcome with sufficient precision to guide treatment escalation decisions by themselves [35]. Clinicians are advised to consider the specific circumstances of an individual's cardiac arrest, their response to treatment, associated comorbidities and frailty, alongside the patient's values and preferences (where known) in relation to the range of outcomes that can occur after cardiac arrest (death, severe neurological impairment through to good quality survival). An individualized treatment plan can then be developed for the patient [35].

Guidelines for the initial phase of care following ROSC take the clinician through a systematic assessment of the patient which seeks to normalize physiology and identify and treat the underlying cause of cardiac arrest (Fig. 22.2).

22.4.1 Coronary Angiography and Percutaneous Coronary Intervention

A 12-lead EKG may help identify evidence of an acute coronary syndrome as a potential cause of the cardiac arrest. Those who have ST elevation on their EKG should be considered for urgent coronary angiography and, if indicated, percutaneous coronary intervention (PCI) if this can be achieved within 120 min of diagnosis [4]. Where this is not possible, consideration should be given to providing

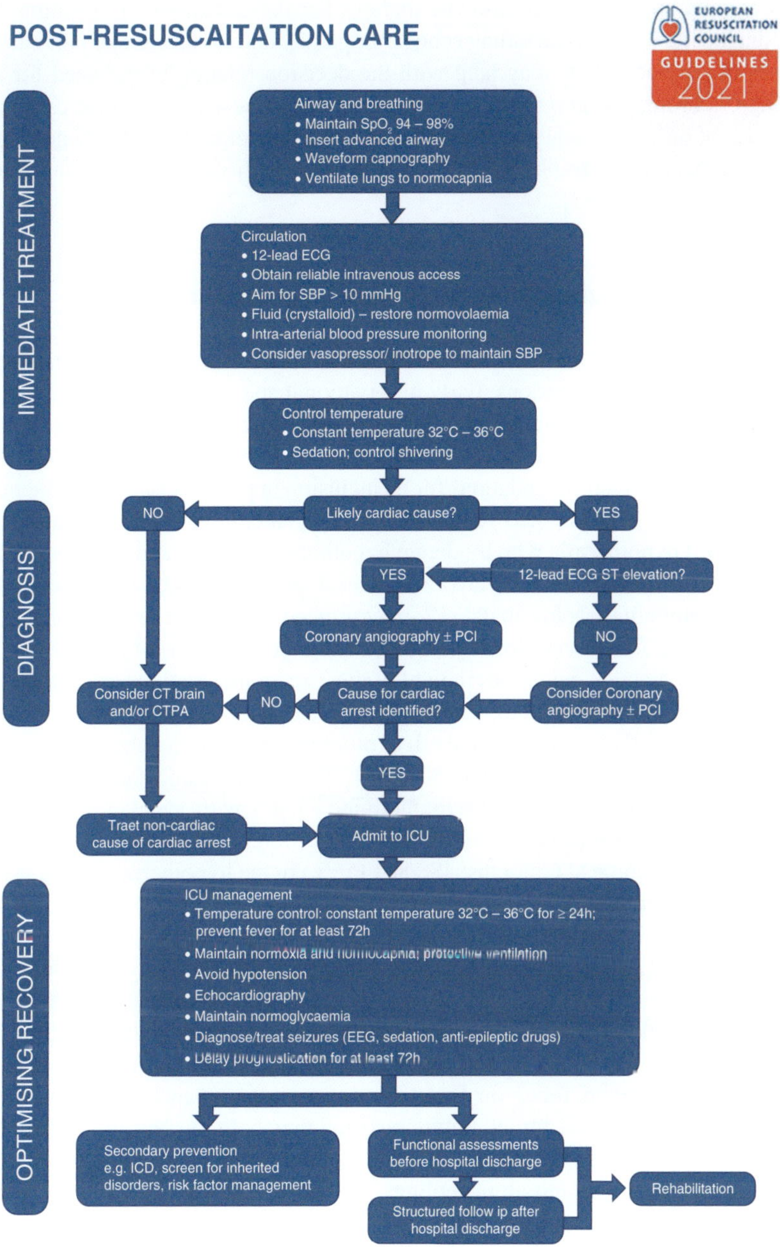

Fig. 22.2 Post resuscitation care algorithm. (Reproduced with permission from the European Resuscitation Council [6]). *SBP* systolic blood pressure, *PCI* percutaneous coronary intervention, *CTPA* computed tomography pulmonary angiogram, *ICU* intensive care unit, *EEG* electroencephalography, *ICD* implanted cardioverter defibrillator

pre-coronary angiography fibrinolytic therapy. For those without ST elevation, further diagnostic work up (including echocardiography and exploration of non-cardiac causes of cardiac arrest) may help with the decision relating to the need for and timing of coronary angiography [4, 36]. Those with a suspected cardiac cause and evidence of on-going ischemia and/or hemodynamic compromise may benefit from early coronary angiography +/- PCI and should be discussed within the multidisciplinary team [4, 33].

22.4.2 Temperature Management After Cardiac Arrest

Temperature management after cardiac arrest has been one of the most studied post-resuscitation care interventions. Early observational and randomized controlled trials suggested that treating those who were comatose after cardiac arrest with controlled hypothermia (circa 32-34 °C) improved survival and neurological outcomes, leading to recommendations for its inclusion in post-resuscitation care treatment guidelines. The Targeted Temperature Management (TTM) 1 study compared mild (36 °C) hypothermia with moderate hypothermia (33 °C) and found no difference in the rate of survival or favorable neurological outcomes between groups, leading to guidelines being updated to recommend a constant temperature in the range of 32-36 °C. Observational studies tracking the outcomes of patients following change to practice guidelines in light of these recommendations have suggested an increase in mortality, although there is some uncertainty in these findings because of likely confounding caused by the effect of temperature on the physiological values used for statistical adjustment [37, 38]. The most recent, large multicenter TTM2 trial compared moderate hypothermia (33 °C) with avoidance of pyrexia (≤37.5 °C) over 28 h [39]. The study found no difference in death or unfavorable neurological outcome at 6 months: 488/881 (55%) in the hypothermia group versus 479/866 (55%) in the normothermia group (relative risk 1.00 [95% CI 0.92–1.09]). The rate of cardiac arrhythmia was higher in the intervention group (25% versus 17%). The TTM2 study prompted ILCOR and others to update a systematic review [40] and undertake a network meta-analysis [41]. The conclusion from these reviews was that the evidence does not support the routine use of induced hypothermia following cardiac arrest. ILCOR recommendations are in the process of being updated (see costr.ilcor.org) to focus on fever prevention rather than routinely inducing hypothermia to a specific target. Future research may help to identify whether specific sub-groups of patients may benefit from active cooling, as well as the optimal timing and methods for initiating cooling.

22.5 Neuroprognostication

Prognostication is an important part of the care pathway for the post-cardiac arrest comatose patient. For people who are predicted to make a good recovery, it can provide hope for the person's family and justification for the continuation of life support. For those predicted to have a poor outcome (death or survival with severe disability or unresponsive wakefulness syndrome), it enables an informed

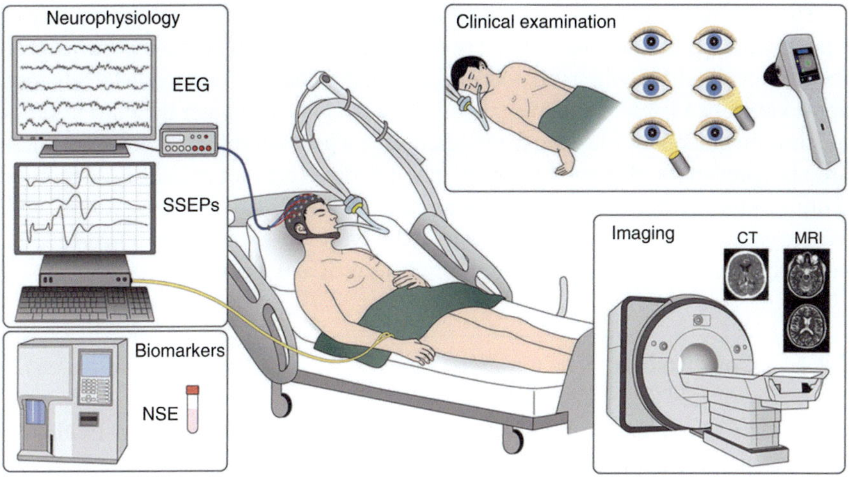

Fig. 22.3 Key testing modalities used for neuroprognostication after cardiac arrest. (Reproduced with permission from the European Resuscitation Council [6]). *EEG* electroencephalography, *NSE* neuron specific enolase, *SSEP* somatosensory evoked potential, *CT* computed tomography

discussion with families about treatment options which might include withdrawal of life sustaining treatment. Given the high stakes of the outcome following prognostication it is important that assessments for an adverse outcome have a very low false positive rate—otherwise there is a risk of premature withdrawal of life sustaining treatment in patients who might otherwise survive.

Most initially comatose patients who will go on to make a good neurological recovery wake up within the first few days of intensive care admission [42, 43]. The ERC and the European Society of Intensive Care Medicine (ESICM) prognostic algorithm recommends that clinicians consider prognostication at least 72 h after intensive care unit (ICU) admission in patients who have a motor response of ≤3 on the Glasgow Coma Scale [6, 44]. Care is advised to avoid major confounders which include analgesia and sedation, neuromuscular blocking drugs, hypothermia, severe hemodynamic instability, or significant metabolic disturbance (e.g., glucose, blood gases, electrolytes). No single predictor is 100% accurate, therefore a multimodal strategy is required to minimize the risk of false positive tests leading to premature withdrawal of life sustaining treatment. Figure 22.3 illustrates the main testing modalities used in neuroprognostication.

Factors associated with a lower false positive rate for an adverse neurological outcome include [6, 43, 44]:

- No pupillary and corneal reflexes at ≥72 h.
- Bilateral absence of N20 somatosensory evoked potential wave.
- Highly malignant electroencephalogram (EEG).
- Neuron specific enolase >60 μg/l at 48 and or 72 h.
- Status myoclonus within the first 72 h.
- Diffuse and extensive anoxic injury on brain computed tomography (CT) or magnetic resonance imaging (MRI).

The presence of at least two of these adverse signs suggests a high probability of a poor neurological outcome. Where none or only one of these tests is positive, then the patient should be observed and reassessed. Among this intermediate category, approximately 14% will achieve a good recovery [45]. Although the current prognostication guidelines focus on the prediction of a poor neurological outcome, there are also predictors of a good neurological outcome (e.g., a benign EEG recorded within 24 h of ROSC [46]) and guidelines on the use of these are being formulated. Where predictors of a good outcome coexist with those of a poor outcome (i.e., conflicting predictors) it may be appropriate to wait and reassess.

22.6 Conclusion

Cardiac arrest remains an important cause of morbidity and mortality. Evidence-based resuscitation treatment guidelines enable clinicians to incorporate best evidence into practice. High quality CPR, rapid defibrillation, and early treatment with epinephrine improve survival. Anti-arrhythmic drugs may be considered in those with shock-refractory cardiac arrest. Post-resuscitation care should focus on identifying and treating reversible causes of cardiac arrest and restoring normal physiology. The evidence highlights that clinicians should prioritize avoidance of pyrexia over any specific hypothermia temperature targets. Careful attention to the timing of prognostication (no earlier than 72 h) and use of multimodal tests to assess prognosis will help inform difficult decisions regarding the continuation or withdrawal of life-sustaining treatments.

Acknowledgement GDP is supported by the National Institute for Health Research (NIHR) Applied Research Collaboration (ARC) West Midlands. The views expressed are those of the author(s) and not necessarily those of the NIHR or the Department of Health and Social Care.

References

1. Perkins GD, Neumar R, Monsieurs KG, et al. The International Liaison Committee on Resuscitation-Review of the last 25 years and vision for the future. Resuscitation. 2017;121:104–16.
2. Morley PT, Atkins DL, Finn JC, et al. Evidence evaluation process and management of potential conflicts of interest. Resuscitation. 2020;156:A23–34.
3. Perkins GD, Graesner JT, Semeraro F, et al. European Resuscitation Council Guidelines 2021: executive summary. Resuscitation. 2021;161:1–60.
4. Lott C, Truhlar A, Alfonzo A, et al. European Resuscitation Council Guidelines 2021: cardiac arrest in special circumstances. Resuscitation. 2021;161:152–219.
5. Soar J, Bottiger BW, Carli P, et al. European Resuscitation Council Guidelines 2021: adult advanced life support. Resuscitation. 2021;161:115–51.
6. Nolan JP, Sandroni C, Bottiger BW, et al. European Resuscitation Council and European Society of Intensive Care Medicine Guidelines 2021: post-resuscitation care. Resuscitation. 2021;161:220–69.
7. Grasner JT, Wnent J, Herlitz J, et al. Survival after out-of-hospital cardiac arrest in Europe—results of the EuReCa TWO study. Resuscitation. 2020;148:218–26.

8. Grasner JT, Lefering R, Koster RW, et al. EuReCa ONE-27 Nations, ONE Europe, ONE Registry: a prospective one month analysis of out-of-hospital cardiac arrest outcomes in 27 countries in Europe. Resuscitation. 2016;105:188–95.
9. Kiguchi T, Okubo M, Nishiyama C, et al. Out-of-hospital cardiac arrest across the world: first report from the International Liaison Committee on Resuscitation (ILCOR). Resuscitation. 2020;152:39–49.
10. Perkins GD, Jacobs IG, Nadkarni VM, et al. Cardiac arrest and cardiopulmonary resuscitation outcome reports: update of the Utstein resuscitation registry templates for out-of-hospital cardiac arrest. Resuscitation. 2015;96:328–40.
11. Andersen LW, Holmberg MJ, Berg KM, Donnino MW, Granfeldt A. In-hospital cardiac arrest: a review. JAMA. 2019;321:1200–10.
12. Grasner JT, Herlitz J, Tjelmeland IBM, et al. European Resuscitation Council Guidelines 2021: epidemiology of cardiac arrest in Europe. Resuscitation. 2021;161:61–79.
13. Haywood K, Whitehead L, Nadkarni VM, et al. COSCA (Core Outcome Set for Cardiac Arrest) in adults: an Advisory Statement From the International Liaison Committee on Resuscitation. Resuscitation. 2018;127:147–63.
14. Olasveengen TM, Semeraro F, Ristagno G, et al. European Resuscitation Council Guidelines 2021: basic life support. Resuscitation. 2021;161:98–114.
15. Cummins RO, Hazinski MF. Guidelines based on fear of type II (false-negative) errors why we dropped the pulse check for lay rescuers. Resuscitation. 2000;46:439–42.
16. Dee R, Smith M, Rajendran K, et al. The effect of alternative methods of cardiopulmonary resuscitation—cough CPR, percussion pacing or precordial thump—on outcomes following cardiac arrest. A systematic review. Resuscitation. 2021;162:73–81.
17. Granfeldt A, Avis SR, Nicholson TC, et al. Advanced airway management during adult cardiac arrest: a systematic review. Resuscitation. 2019;139:133–43.
18. Soar J, Berg KM, Andersen LW, et al. Adult advanced life support: 2020 international consensus on cardiopulmonary resuscitation and emergency cardiovascular care science with treatment recommendations. Resuscitation. 2020;156:A80–A119.
19. Perkins GD, Ji C, Deakin CD, et al. A randomized trial of epinephrine in out-of-hospital cardiac arrest. N Engl J Med. 2018;379:711–21.
20. Achana F, Petrou S, Madan J, et al. Cost-effectiveness of adrenaline for out-of-hospital cardiac arrest. Crit Care. 2020;24:579.
21. Perkins GD, Kenna C, Ji C, et al. The influence of time to adrenaline administration in the paramedic 2 randomised controlled trial. Intensive Care Med. 2020;46:426–36.
22. Finn J, Jacobs I, Williams TA, Gates S, Perkins GD. Adrenaline and vasopressin for cardiac arrest. Cochrane Database Syst Rev. 2019;1:CD003179.
23. Andersen LW, Isbye D, Kjaergaard J, et al. Effect of vasopressin and methylprednisolone vs placebo on return of spontaneous circulation in patients with in-hospital cardiac arrest: a randomized clinical trial. JAMA. 2021;326:1586–94.
24. Ali MU, Fitzpatrick-Lewis D, Kenny M, et al. Effectiveness of antiarrhythmic drugs for shockable cardiac arrest: a systematic review. Resuscitation. 2018;132:63–72.
25. Soar J, Donnino MW, Maconochie I, et al. 2018 international consensus on cardiopulmonary resuscitation and emergency cardiovascular care science with treatment recommendations summary. Resuscitation. 2018;133:194–206.
26. Kudenchuk PJ, Brown SP, Daya M, et al. Amiodarone, lidocaine, or placebo in out-of-hospital cardiac arrest. N Engl J Med. 2016;374:1711–22.
27. Burgert JM, Johnson AD, O'Sullivan JC, et al. Pharmacokinetic effects of endotracheal, intraosseous, and intravenous epinephrine in a swine model of traumatic cardiac arrest. Am J Emerg Med. 2019;37:2043–50.
28. Lee PM, Lee C, Rattner P, Wu X, Gershengorn H, Acquah S. Intraosseous versus central venous catheter utilization and performance during inpatient medical emergencies. Crit Care Med. 2015;43:1233–8.

29. Hsieh YL, Wu MC, Wolfshohl J, et al. Intraosseous versus intravenous vascular access during cardiopulmonary resuscitation for out-of-hospital cardiac arrest: a systematic review and meta-analysis of observational studies. Scand J Trauma Resusc Emerg Med. 2021;29:44.
30. Holmberg MJ, Geri G, Wiberg S, et al. Extracorporeal cardiopulmonary resuscitation for cardiac arrest: a systematic review. Resuscitation. 2018;131:91–100.
31. Yannopoulos D, Bartos J, Raveendran G, et al. Advanced reperfusion strategies for patients with out-of-hospital cardiac arrest and refractory ventricular fibrillation (ARREST): a phase 2, single centre, open-label, randomised controlled trial. Lancet. 2020;396:1807–16.
32. Hsu CH, Meurer WJ, Domeier R, et al. Extracorporeal cardiopulmonary resuscitation for refractory out-of-hospital cardiac arrest (EROCA): results of a randomized feasibility trial of expedited out-of-hospital transport. Ann Emerg Med. 2021;78:92–101.
33. Wyckoff M, Singletary EM, Soar J, et al. 2021 international consensus on cardiopulmonary resuscitation and emergency cardiovascular care science with treatment recommendations summary from the basic life support; advanced life support; neonatal life support; education, implementation, and teams; first aid task forces; and the COVID-19 working group. Resuscitation. 2021;169:229–311.
34. Perkins GD, Callaway CW, Haywood K, et al. Brain injury after cardiac arrest. Lancet. 2021;398:1269–78.
35. Mentzelopoulos SD, Couper K, Voorde PV, et al. European Resuscitation Council Guidelines 2021: ethics of resuscitation and end of life decisions. Resuscitation. 2021;161:408–32.
36. Nikolaou NI, Netherton S, Welsford M, et al. A systematic review and meta-analysis of the effect of routine early angiography in patients with return of spontaneous circulation after out-of-hospital cardiac arrest. Resuscitation. 2021;163:28–48.
37. Nolan JP, Orzechowska I, Harrison DA, Soar J, Perkins GD, Shankar-Hari M. Changes in temperature management and outcome after out-of-hospital cardiac arrest in United Kingdom intensive care units following publication of the targeted temperature management trial. Resuscitation. 2021;162:304–11.
38. Salter R, Bailey M, Bellomo R, et al. Changes in temperature management of cardiac arrest patients following publication of the target temperature management trial. Crit Care Med. 2018;46:1722–30.
39. Dankiewicz J, Cronberg T, Lilja G, et al. Hypothermia versus normothermia after out-of-hospital cardiac arrest. N Engl J Med. 2021;384:2283–94.
40. Granfeldt A, Holmberg MJ, Nolan JP, et al. Targeted temperature management in adult cardiac arrest: systematic review and meta-analysis. Resuscitation. 2021;167:160–72.
41. Fernando SM, Di Santo P, Sadeghirad B, et al. Targeted temperature management following out-of-hospital cardiac arrest: a systematic review and network meta-analysis of temperature targets. Intensive Care Med. 2021;47:1078–88.
42. Lybeck A, Cronberg T, Aneman A, et al. Time to awakening after cardiac arrest and the association with target temperature management. Resuscitation. 2018;126:166–71.
43. Lee DH, Cho YS, Lee BK, et al. Late awakening is common in settings without withdrawal of life-sustaining therapy in out-of-hospital cardiac arrest survivors who undergo targeted temperature management. Crit Care Med. 2021; Sep 15. https://doi.org/10.1097/CCM.0000000000005274. Epub ahead of print.
44. Nolan JP, Sandroni C, Bottiger BW, et al. European Resuscitation Council and European Society of Intensive Care Medicine guidelines 2021: post-resuscitation care. Intensive Care Med. 2021;47:369–421.
45. Moseby-Knappe M, Westhall E, Backman S, et al. Performance of a guideline-recommended algorithm for prognostication of poor neurological outcome after cardiac arrest. Intensive Care Med. 2020;46:1852–62.
46. Rossetti AO, Tovar Quiroga DF, Juan E, et al. Electroencephalography predicts poor and good outcomes after cardiac arrest: a two-center study. Crit Care Med. 2017;45:e674–82.

Brain Injury Biomarkers for Predicting Outcome After Cardiac Arrest

23

J. Humaloja, N. J. Ashton, and M. B. Skrifvars

23.1 Introduction

Accurate prognostication is a key aspect of the management of unconscious patients after cardiac arrest [1]. The focal points include not only avoiding fruitless and expensive treatment in the intensive care unit (ICU) but also needing to continue care for patients who have a realistic chance of survival but whose awakening and neurological recovery takes longer than usual. It is, of course, paramount not to withdraw care too early in patients who have a reasonable chance of full recovery. Current post-cardiac arrest care guidelines recommend a multimodal approach using a combination of clinical examination, neurophysiological investigations, such as electroencephalogram (EEG) and somatosensory evoked potentials (SSEP), radiological imaging with computed tomography (CT) or magnetic resonance imaging (MRI) of the brain, and brain injury biomarkers [1]. The strategy in unconscious patients is to use several investigative means, and if two or more investigations point toward a high risk of severe brain injury, to initiate family discussion and consider withdrawal of intensive care. Conversely, if the findings are contradictory, continuing care is recommended unless there are other reasons (e.g., comorbid conditions) for the withdrawal of care. Biomarkers have been an important part of many cardiac arrest prognostication algorithms for almost 20 years [2, 3]. The fundamental concept is that all biomarkers derived from neuronal tissue measure the severity of brain injury. However, as many patients do not survive due to multiorgan failure,

J. Humaloja · M. B. Skrifvars (✉)
Department of Emergency Care and Services, Helsinki University Hospital, University of Helsinki, Helsinki, Finland
e-mail: markus.skrifvars@hus.fi

N. J. Ashton
Department of Psychiatry and Neurochemistry, Institute of Neuroscience and Physiology, The Sahlgrenska Academy at the University of Gothenburg, Mölndal, Sweden

J.-L. Vincent (ed.), *Annual Update in Intensive Care and Emergency Medicine 2022*, Annual Update in Intensive Care and Emergency Medicine,
https://doi.org/10.1007/978-3-030-93433-0_23

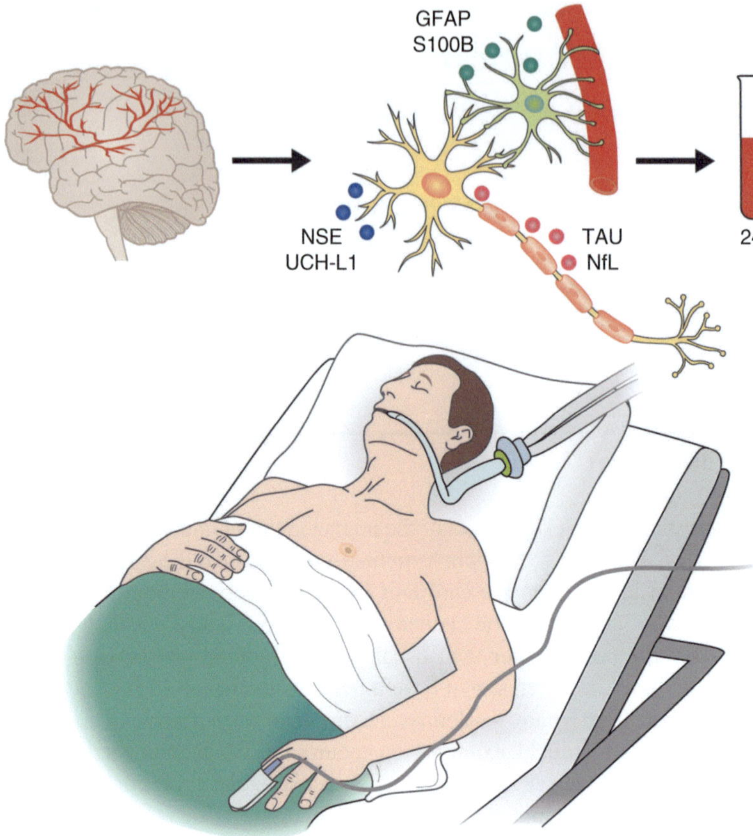

Fig. 23.1 Central nervous system histological origin of six brain injury biomarkers studied in patients after cardiac arrest. Green dots represent biomarkers released after glial cell injury, blue dots represent biomarkers derived from injured neurons, and pink dots represent biomarkers of axonal injury. *GFAP* glial fibrillary acidic protein, *NSE* neuron-specific enolase, *NfL* neurofilament light, *UCH-L1* ubiquitin C-terminal hydrolase-L1, *S100B* S100 calcium-binding protein B

severe circulatory shock, and comorbid conditions, a biomarker predicting brain injury is of limited utility in these conditions.

In recent years, many novel brain injury biomarkers originating from slightly different parts of the brain have been introduced (Fig. 23.1). A deeper understanding of these will aid clinicians' use of brain injury biomarkers together with other means of prognostication. Compared to other investigations, biomarkers have certain advantages, as their results are, for example, not affected by sedative or pain medication or muscle relaxants. Biomarkers are easily obtained if standardized methods for determination are available. However, interpretation can be difficult, since confident and conclusive thresholds may vary, even for neuron-specific enolase (NSE), a biomarker studied in cardiac arrest for over 20 years [1]. The ideal brain injury biomarker should only be expressed in the central nervous tissue to avoid elevated levels due to other situations. For instance, several studies have shown the influence of blood sample hemolysis on NSE concentrations, which is the main disadvantage of NSE.

Several promising novel biomarkers have been proposed and preliminary evidence has emerged: neurofilament light (NfL), ubiquitin carboxy-terminal hydrolase L1 (UHC-L1), glial fibrillary acidic protein (GFAP), and tau protein (tau) (Fig. 23.1). Two studies using NfL showed an excellent ability to predict the outcome after cardiac arrest, and NfL may even replace NSE in the future [4–6]. The latest joint guidelines of the European Resuscitation Council (ERC) and the European Society of Intensive Care Medicine (ESICM) recommend against the use of S100 calcium-binding protein B (S100B) and the novel biomarkers NfL, GFAP, and tau for prognostication, given the lack of conclusive evidence [1].

In this chapter, we discuss six biomarkers—two familiar ones (NSE, S100B) and four more recently studied in relation to cardiac arrest (NfL, UCH-1, TAU, and GFAP)—focusing on their use for neurological outcome prediction in patients at risk of hypoxic brain injury after cardiac arrest. Table 23.1 presents a selection of recent studies on the performance of these biomarkers to predict neurological outcome after cardiac arrest. These biomarkers appear to originate histologically from slightly different parts of brain tissue, and a deeper understanding may aid the clinician in using biomarkers for determining the magnitude of brain injury in clinical practice.

23.2 Neuron-Specific Enolase

NSE is a neuronal glycolytic enzyme that is abundant in the neurons of brain gray matter and involved in axonal transport [7]. NSE has a half-life of between 24 and 30 h, and its production is upregulated during ischemia and axon injuries. Extracerebrally, NSE is present in red blood cells (RBCs) and in thrombocytes; hence, assessing the degree of hemolysis in the blood sample is always essential, but especially when NSE is used in patients undergoing treatments that may result in hemolysis (extracorporeal membrane oxygenation [ECMO], renal replacement therapy [RRT], or use of an intra-arterial balloon pump [IABP]) [8, 9]. Additionally, neuroendocrine cells and small cell carcinomas express NSE; thus, malignant tumors or hematologic malignancy can affect the concentration [7]. Importantly, variations in NSE levels differ between laboratories, which can influence thresholds between studies and concentrations measured in the clinical setting [10].

Studies suggest that NSE levels peak at 48–72 h after cardiac arrest, and the prognostic accuracy is also highest at 48 h [7]. The ERC/ESISCM 2021 guidelines for post-resuscitation care specify a threshold for poor prognosis of >60 μg/l at 48 or 72 h [1]. However, there is no international consensus on the threshold [11]. Previously, a NSE concentration >33 ng/ml at 48 h after cardiac arrest was considered to indicate poor neurological prognosis, but this was mainly based on one study by Zandbergen et al. [12], which was published in 2006 before the widespread introduction of standardized post-cardiac arrest care and targeted temperature

Table 23.1 Selected studies on the prognostic ability of six brain injury biomarkers after cardiac arrest (CA)

Biomarker	Study	N	CA location	24-h threshold	48-h threshold	72-h threshold
NSE ng/ml	*Zandbergen, 2006* [12]	231	NS	31.7	23.8	32.3
	AUROC			NA	NA	NA
	Sensitivity (%)			NA	NA	NA
	Lee, 2013 [14]	224	NS	80.8	52.7	NA
	AUROC			0.80	0.90	
	Sensitivity (%)			27	60	
	Larsson, 2014 [15]	125	OHCA/IHCA	49	40	22
	AUROC			0.73	0.79	0.85
	Sensitivity (%)			27	37	50
	Stammet, 2015 [16]	686	OHCA	107	120	50
	AUROC			0.75	0.85	0.86
	Sensitivity (%)			9	27	52
	Helwig, 2017 [17]	100	OHCA	NA	34	NA
	AUROC				0.63	
	Sensitivity (%)				44	
	Streitberger, 2017 [9]	828	OHCA	NA	NA	85.5
	AUROC					0.90
	sensitivity (%)					49
	Streitberger, 2017 [9]	225	IHCA	NA	NA	1227
	AUROC					0.79
	Sensitivity (%)					0
	Nakstad, 2020 [19]	237	OHCA	172	87	79
	AUROC			NA	NA	NA
	Sensitivity (%)			8	36	39
S100B ng/ml	*Larsson, 2014* [15]	125	OHCA + IHCA	1.3	0.61	0.38
	AUROC			0.78	0.75	0.83
	Sensitivity (%)			23	21	30
	Stammet, 2017 [24]	687	OHCA	2.59	3.67	1.83
	AUROC			0.80	NA	NA
	Sensitivity (%)			10	5	5
	Duez, 2018 [23]	115	OHCA	1.05	0.95	0.72
	AUROC			0.81	0.81	0.74
	Sensitivity (%)			23	17	11
	Jang, 2019 [22]	97	OHCA	0.19	0.16	0.20
	AUROC			0.93	0.92	0.86
	Sensitivity (%)			78	78	61
NfL pg/ml	*Rana, 2013* [26]	61	OHCA	321	405	309
	AUROC			0.93	0.85	0.92
	Sensitivity (%)			79	57	75
	Moseby-Knappe, 2019 [5]	717	OHCA	1232	1539	1756
	AUROC			0.94	0.94	0.94
	Sensitivity (%)			53	65	64
	Wihersaari, 2021 [4]	112	OHCA	150	359	390
	AUROC			0.98	0.99	0.98
	Sensitivity (%)			78	83	85

Table 23.1 (continued)

Biomarker	Study	N	CA location	24-h threshold	48-h threshold	72-h threshold
UCH-L1 pg/ml	*Ebner, 2020* [36]	717	OHCA	12,175	7945	9170
	AUROC			0.85	0.87	0.86
	Sensitivity (%)			4	9	1
GFAP pg/ml	*Larsson, 2014* [15]	125	OHCA + IHCA	1090	300	530
	AUROC			0.59	0.63	0.67
	Sensitivity (%)			16	23	14
	Helwig, 2017 [17]	100	OHCA	NA	80	NA
	AUROC				0.65	
	Sensitivity (%)				21	
	Ebner, 2020 [36]	717	OHCA	3425	2952	3581
	AUROC			0.88	0.88	0.89
	Sensitivity (%)			17	19	12
Tau pg/ml	*Mattsson, 2017* [48]	689	OHCA	874.5	148.8	72.7
	AUROC			0.81	0.90	0.91
	Sensitivity (%)			4	33	42

AUROC area under the receiver operating characteristic curve, *CA* cardiac arrest, *NA* not applicable, *NS* not specified, *OHCA* out-of-hospital cardiac arrest, *IHCA* in-hospital cardiac arrest, *Nfl* neurofilament light protein, *S100B* S100 calcium-binding protein B, *GFAP* glial fibrillary acidic protein, *UCH-L1* ubiquitin C-terminal hydrolase L1

management (TTM), which may have influenced the threshold specified in the prognostication guidelines used at that time [12, 13]. Since that study, high serum NSE levels have been demonstrated to have moderate accuracy in predicting neurological outcomes at 48–72 h after cardiac arrest with area under the receiver operating characteristic (AUROC) curves of between 0.63 and 0.90 (Table 23.1) [14–17]. Most studies considered in this review have been conducted on out-of-hospital cardiac arrest (OHCA) patients, but a few studies included in-hospital cardiac arrest (IHCA) patients [9, 15]. Only Streitberger et al. presented the predictive accuracy separately for both cohorts, and NSE predicted outcome more accurately after OHCA than after IHCA (AUROC 0.90 vs. 0.79) in their study [9]. As most studies do not differentiate between the causes of death, this may partly explain the discrepancy, (e.g., hypoxic brain injury may not be the most likely cause of death after IHCA [18]).

NSE has confounding sources, and it is not unusual to see high outlier values in patients who recover with good neurological outcome, which can increase the determined threshold value of poor prognosis with a 0% false positive rate to impractically high levels, also compromising the test's sensitivity [16, 19]. In a study by Stammet et al., the threshold of poor prognosis for a 0% false positive rate at 48 h was as high as 120 ng/ml [16]. In turn, the threshold values with a 1–5% false positive rate were between 68 and 42 ng/ml, retaining moderate sensitivity (47–61%) [16]. Correspondingly, in the study by Streitberger et al., the threshold for poor prognosis at 72 h with a 0% false positive rate was 85.5 ng/ml, but with a 5% false positive rate the threshold decreased to 59.2 ng/ml, simultaneously increasing the test sensitivity from 49% to 60% [20]. As NSE's prognostic accuracy is adequate only when used as part of a multimodal approach, it is acceptable to allow a small number of false positives to achieve at least moderate sensitivity. The smallest threshold (34 ng/ml) for poor prognosis at 48 h with a 0% false positive rate was reported in the study by Helwig et al.; thus, in that study, the prognostic accuracy of NSE was rather low (AUROC 0.63) [17]. Furthermore, ascending concentration in serial measurements has been found to improve prognostic accuracy; however, the optimal sample timing is still uncertain [7, 16].

23.3 S100 Calcium-Binding Protein B

S100B is abundant in glial cells and specifically expressed in specific astrocytes surrounding the blood vessels in the brain [7, 21]. Extra-cerebrally, S100B is present in Schwann cells of the peripheral nervous system. Healthy adults express very low levels of S100B, and S100B does not move freely over an intact blood–brain barrier [21]. Of non-neuronal sources, muscle cells, adipocytes, and chondrocytes are found to express S100B, which may create a confounding source of S100B in CA patients receiving chest compressions [7, 21]. However, the half-life of S100B is only about 30 min, and compression-originated S100B possibly soon vanishes from blood [7]. S100B is considered an early biomarker after cardiac arrest, as the level usually peaks at 24 h. Four studies in the last decade examined S100B after cardiac arrest (Table 23.1) [15, 22–24]. In three studies, the best prognostic accuracy appeared 24 h after cardiac arrest (AUROC of between 0.78 and 0.93). In the study by Larsson et al., the best accuracy was, interestingly, found at 72 h (AUROC 0.83) [15]. The thresholds to predict poor neurological outcome with a 0% false positive rate at 24 h had great variability (0.19–2.59 ng/ml). The highest threshold was reported in the largest study included in this review, that was conducted by Stammet et al. with the TTM After Cardiac Arrest trial cohort [24]. Other studies reported low sensitivities (<24%), but Jang et al. reported a sensitivity of 78% [22]. In the study by Jang et al., the primary endpoint was 3-month neurological outcome, while in all the other studies, the outcome was assessed after a 6-month follow-up [15, 22–24]. Two of the included studies reported prognostic accuracy for both S100B and NSE, or the prognostic accuracy of NSE for the same patient cohort was reported in another manuscript: in both cases, S100B predicted the outcome better at 24 h, but, at later time points, NSE was more accurate than S100B [15, 16, 24].

23.4 Neurofilament Light

Neurofilaments (light [NfL], medium [NfM], heavy [NfH], and β-internexin), are approximately 10 nm in size, and are abundant structural scaffolding proteins exclusively expressed in neurons, predominantly within large, myelinated axons within the cerebral white matter [25]. Their function is largely unknown but hypothesized to be essential for radial growth and enabling rapid nerve conduction. Pathological processes that cause axonal damage release neurofilaments into the extracellular fluids, cerebrospinal fluid (CSF), and peripheral blood. However, even under normal circumstances, NfL is continuously released from axons in an age-dependent manner, with typical NfL reference ranges in the CSF increasing by twofold between ages 20 and 50 years and further doubling by the age of 70. A similar age-dependent increase is also seen in blood.

NfL has been extensively studied as a biomarker of neural injury in neurodegenerative disorders, with mild increases in Alzheimer's disease but more dynamic changes in disorders with a greater intensity of neurodegeneration (e.g., frontotemporal dementia or amyotrophic lateral sclerosis [25]). However, the large increases in NfL in blood following hypoxic brain injury suggest that NfL may better serve as a prognostic biomarker for acute neurological injury than for chronic neurodegeneration. Studies using conventional enzyme-linked immunosorbent assay (EILSA) technology have demonstrated the large increases and predictive power of plasma neurofilaments in cardiac arrest [26, 27]. Now, semi-automated ultra-sensitive immunoassays (e.g., single molecular array [Simoa]) can quantify plasma NfL at low levels, even in healthy individuals [25].

In the Carbon dioxide, Oxygen and Mean arterial pressure After Cardiac Arrest and REsuscitation (COMACARE) trial using the Simoa platform, individuals with a poor outcome (Cerebral Performance Category [CPC] scale ≥3) had a median plasma NfL level >2300 pg/ml [4]. In contrast, those with a good outcome had levels <20 pg/ml. Consequently, NfL predicted the outcome of OHCA patients with an AUROC of 0.98 (95% CI 0.97–1.00) as early as 24 h after the event (Table 23.1) [4]. While admission levels of plasma NfL were elevated in individuals with subsequent poor outcomes compared to good outcomes, the considerable overlap means that NfL is unlikely to be useful at this early stage (AUROC 0.65). This study by Wihersaari et al. [4] corroborates earlier findings in a larger sample size by Moseby-Knappe et al., who also demonstrated a vastly superior prognostic performance of serum NfL in comparison to other plasma biomarkers (e.g., tau, NSE, and S100b) and clinical data in the TTM After Cardiac Arrest trial [5]. Despite these encouraging results, it has been reported that one-third of individuals with a good outcome had high levels of plasma NfL; thus, NfL has only modest specificity [28]. This leads to the conclusion that plasma NfL thresholds for normal ranges for continuing care should be applied rather than thresholds for poor outcome and terminating care.

NfL has several key advantages as a plasma biomarker. First, there is a consensus on the assay of choice (Simoa), which clinical laboratories in Sweden, the Netherlands, and France have validated for broad use in clinical laboratory practice. This gives a greater chance of thresholds being transferrable between research cohorts and, eventually, clinical routines. Furthermore, NfL in plasma is very stable, largely unaffected by preanalytical variabilities or hemolysis, and the sample can remain at room temperature >48 h without compromising measurement quality or accuracy. In addition, an accurate measurement of NfL does not require immediate centrifugation and can even be extracted as a whole blood dry spot for longer term storage/transportation for remote setting assessment [29]. Plasma or serum NfL is also not susceptible to freeze-thaw cycling, which is useful for research settings or external laboratory testing [30]. Plasma NfL is predominately derived from the central nervous system but, however, is elevated in peripheral neuropathies [31]. However, based on the reported high levels in cardiac arrest patients with poor outcomes, this mild magnitude of change in peripheral neuropathies is unlikely to be a confounder.

23.5 Ubiquitin C-Terminal Hydrolase L1

Ubiquitin C-terminal hydrolase L1 (UCH-L1) is a 26 kDa neuronal deubiquitinase primarily expressed in neurons and neuroendocrine cells [32]. UCH-L1 is important not only for neuroaxonal stability but also for repair after brain injury [33]. Specifically, it is involved in the process of ubiquitination of proteins destined for degradation via the proteasomal pathway. Therefore, it has an essential role in the removal of oxidized or misfolded proteins in both normal and pathological conditions [34]. UCH-L1 is more commonly evaluated in traumatic brain injury (TBI), where it has been permitted for use by the U.S. Food and Drug Administration (FDA) for indicators of good outcome to avoid unnecessary CT scans following concussion [35].

Use of UCH-L1 in cardiac arrest patients has been evaluated in only two studies that were both conducted with the same patient cohort (the patient cohort from the TTM trial) [28, 36]. UCH-L1 was shown to predict poor outcome after cardiac arrest with good accuracy (AUROC of between 0.85 and 0.87), was significantly better than NSE at 24 and 48 h, and the prognostic accuracy was further improved by the addition of GFAP (AUROC of between 0.90 and 0.91) [36]. At 72 h, both UCH-L1 and NSE performed to the same degree. This is in line with the reported short half-life of UCH-L1 (<12 h) in comparison to NSE [36, 37]. Moseby-Knappe et al. demonstrated that UCH-L1 levels were within normal ranges in 63.8% of patients with good outcome at 24 h, however this increased to 88.1% at 72 h [28]. By contrast, predicting poor outcome diminished overtime with elevated UCH-L1 above normal levels in 85.3% of poor outcome patients at 24 h but 70.3% at 72 h. Ability to predict poor outcome was inferior to NfL, Tau, and GFAP [4, 5] but ranked highly in specificity, suggesting UCH-L1 may have a role in the diagnostic challenge of cardiac arrest. The successful FDA approval of serum UCH-L1 paves the way for UCH-L1 to be used for purposes other than TBI particularly as multiple plex assays with NfL, Tau, and GFAP are available. However, further independent studies defining normal reference ranges and their added value over and above other putative biomarkers for cardiac arrest are still lacking. Lastly, given the limited number of studies available, the impact of high expression of UCH-L1 from the pancreas and kidney, as a potential confounder, has largely been unexplored.

23.6 Glial Fibrillary Acidic Protein

GFAP is a structural component of intermediate filaments in the astrocyte cytoskeleton that is considered a highly brain-specific marker [38]. GFAP production is upregulated following ischemia, which is believed to be a neuroprotective mechanism, but can also lead to glial scarring [38]. As a structural protein, GFAP is released from damaged astrocytes and elevated levels are not in general detected in healthy individuals [7]. Serum GFAP has been found to predict neurological outcome after head trauma, and elevated blood levels have been measured after cardiac arrest, intracerebral hemorrhage, and ischemic stroke [15, 38].

To the best of our knowledge, GFAP has been investigated after cardiac arrest in six studies [15, 17, 36, 39–41]. Three studies [39–41] were conducted before the introduction of a highly sensitive method (immunoassay) to measure serum GFAP [42], and we did not include their results in this review. The accuracy of GFAP to predict neurological outcome seems to be better at 48 and 72 h after cardiac arrest compared to earlier time points, with AUROC values of between 0.65 and 0.89; see Table 23.1 [15, 17, 36]. The largest study included in this review, which was conducted in the TTM trial cohort by Ebner et al., reported a threshold of 2952 pg/ml with a 0% false positive rate for poor prognosis 48 h after cardiac arrest, but again the sensitivity remained low (Table 23.1) [36]. The corresponding thresholds determined in the two other included studies were much lower (300 and 80 pg/ml), but these studies have methodological differences compared to the study by Ebner et al. Helwig et al. [17] determined the neurological outcome with a modified Glasgow Outcome Scale at 4 weeks, and a study by Larsson et al. [15] included both IHCA and OHCA patients. All the GFAP studies included in this review compared the predictive accuracy of GFAP to other biomarkers [15, 17, 36]. In the study by Larsson et al., NSE and S100B were more accurate in predicting poor neurological outcomes, and they were more sensitive compared to GFAP, with AUROC values at 48 h for NSE, S100B, and GFAP of 0.79, 0.75 and 0.63, respectively [15]. In the study by Helwig et al., both NSE and GFAP showed rather modest accuracy in predicting the outcome at 48 h, and NSE was more sensitive than GFAP [17]. In turn, in the study conducted by Ebner et al., GFAP predicted the outcome more accurately at every determined time point after the arrest (at 24, 48, and 72 h) compared to NSE, but, as stated above, GFAP presented low sensitivity [36].

23.7 Tau Protein

Tau is a protein molecule that stabilizes the structures of microtubules in neuroaxonal processes and is mainly located in the white matter of the central nervous system [43, 44]. Ischemia causes hyperphosphorylation of tau molecules, detaching them from microtubules [45]. Detached tau molecules aggregate to insoluble masses, interrupting axonal signaling. Elevated serum tau concentrations have been reported after ischemic stroke and cardiac arrest [46–49]. Among patients with neurodegenerative disease (e.g., Alzheimer's disease or Creutzfeldt-Jacob disease), elevated tau levels are present in CSF [50], but this is not reflected in blood as mild elevations are confounded by peripheral expression. Determination of accurate serum tau concentrations requires a highly sensitive immunoassay method, which is only available at specialized laboratories [42]. So far, only one large study has examined tau after cardiac arrest [48], and two other studies were small pilot studies [46, 47]. Mattsson et al. studied tau in the TTM trial cohort, and the predictive power of tau was better in the later samples (the AUROC at 24, 48, and 72 h was 0.81, 0.90, and 0.91, respectively [48]). Further, tau predicted poor neurological outcome between 24 and 72 h after cardiac arrest more accurately than NSE [48]. The thresholds for poor prognosis with a 0% false positive rate seemed high (at 48 h 148.8 pg/ml and at 72 h 72.7 pg/ml), and sensitivity remained low, but already allowing a false positive rate of 2%, the sensitivity increased above 60% and the thresholds decreased to 18.9 pg/ml at 48 h and 11.2 pg/ml at 72 h [5]. Bimodal tau release (early and late) was reported in the two pilot studies of tau and cardiac arrest; the delayed peak was absent or significantly lower in patients with good outcomes [46, 47]. Tau has a half-life of about 10 h, and late elevations in tau concentrations likely reflect ongoing neuronal injury [5].

23.8 Conclusion

Biomarkers will undoubtedly continue to be an important part of outcome prediction in patients with hypoxic brain injury after cardiac arrest. Further research will improve accuracy and may propose new strategies for the way biomarkers are used. The traditional approach of using high threshold levels to identify patients with no chance of a good functional outcome may well be complemented with a strategy of using low biomarker levels to predict a good outcome [27]. As these different biomarkers originate from different areas of the brain, it could be an option to use some of them together (e.g., one biomarker reflecting injury to gray matter, one reflecting axonal injury, and one reflecting injury to the glia). A study by Ebner et al. showed that combining GFAP and UHC-L1 predicted neurological outcomes more accurately than NSE alone [36]. Additionally, unpublished evidence suggests that high levels of tau as a marker of axonal injury identify different poor-outcome patients than those identified with GFAP, a marker of glial injury (Humaloja, personal communication October 14, 2021). It seems logical to combine several hypoxic brain injury biomarkers for improved accuracy. Whether this concept is cost-effective and accurate and whether it has a role as part of a multimodal prognostication approach should be assessed in future large-scale studies.

References

1. Nolan JP, Sandroni C, Böttiger BW, et al. European Resuscitation Council and European Society of Intensive Care Medicine Guidelines 2021: post-resuscitation care. Resuscitation. 2021;161:220–69.
2. Oksanen T, Tiainen M, Skrifvars MB, Varpula T, Kuitunen A, Castrén M, Pettilä V. Predictive power of serum NSE and OHCA score regarding 6-month neurologic outcome after out-of-hospital ventricular fibrillation and therapeutic hypothermia. Resuscitation. 2009;80:165–70.

3. Tiainen M, Roine RO, Pettilä V, Takkunen O. Serum neuron-specific enolase and S-100B protein in cardiac arrest patients treated with hypothermia. Stroke. 2003;34:2881–6.
4. Wihersaari L, Ashton NJ, Reinikainen M, et al. Neurofilament light as an outcome predictor after cardiac arrest: a post hoc analysis of the COMACARE trial. Intensive Care Med. 2021;47:39–48.
5. Moseby-Knappe M, Mattsson N, Nielsen N, et al. Serum neurofilament light chain for prognosis of outcome after cardiac arrest. JAMA Neurol. 2019;76:64–71.
6. Leithner C. Neuron specific enolase after cardiac arrest: from 33 to 60 to 100 to NFL? Resuscitation. 2021;168:234–6.
7. Gul SS, Huesgen KW, Wang KK, Mark K, Tyndall JA. Prognostic utility of neuroinjury biomarkers in post out-of-hospital cardiac arrest (OHCA) patient management. Med Hypotheses. 2017;105:34–47.
8. Ramont L, Thoannes H, Volondat A, Chastang F, Millet M-C, Maquart FX. Effects of hemolysis and storage condition on neuron-specific enolase (NSE) in cerebrospinal fluid and serum: implications in clinical practice. Clin Chem Lab Med. 2005;43:1215–7.
9. Streitberger KJ, Leithner C, Wattenberg M, et al. Neuron-specific enolase predicts poor outcome after cardiac arrest and targeted temperature management: a multicenter study on 1,053 patients. Crit Care Med. 2017;45:1145–51.
10. Mlynash M, Buckwalter MS, Okada A, et al. Serum neuron-specific enolase levels from the same patients differ between laboratories: assessment of a prospective post-cardiac arrest cohort. Neurocrit Care. 2013;10:161–6.
11. Berg KM, Soar J, Andersen LW, et al. Adult advanced life support: 2020 international consensus on cardiopulmonary resuscitation and emergency cardiovascular care science with treatment recommendations. Circulation. 2020;142:S92–S139.
12. Zandbergen EGJ, Hijdra A, Koelman JHTM, Hart AAM, Vos PE, Verbeek MM, de Haan RJ. Prediction of poor outcome within the first 3 days of postanoxic coma. Neurology. 2006;66:62–8.
13. Wijdicks EFM, Hijdra A, Young GB, Bassetti CL, Wiebe S. Practice parameter: prediction of outcome in comatose survivors after cardiopulmonary resuscitation (an evidence-based review). Neurology. 2006;67:203–10.
14. Lee BK, Jeung KW, Lee HY, Jung YH, Lee DH. Combining brain computed tomography and serum neuron specific enolase improves the prognostic performance compared to either alone in comatose cardiac arrest survivors treated with therapeutic hypothermia. Resuscitation. 2013;84:1387–92.
15. Larsson IM, Wallin E, Kristofferzon ML, Niessner M, Zetterberg H, Rubertsson S. Post-cardiac arrest serum levels of glial fibrillary acidic protein for predicting neurological outcome. Resuscitation. 2014;85:1654–61.
16. Stammet P, Collignon O, Hassager C, et al. Neuron-specific enolase as a predictor of death or poor neurological outcome after out-of-hospital cardiac arrest and targeted temperature management at 33°C and 36°C. J Am Coll Cardiol. 2015;65:2104–14.
17. Helwig K, Seeger F, Hölschermann H, Lischke V, Gerriets T, Niessner M, Foerch C. Elevated serum glial fibrillary acidic protein (GFAP) is associated with poor functional outcome after cardiopulmonary resuscitation. Neurocrit Care. 2017;27:68–74.
18. Witten L, Gardner R, Holmberg M, et al. Reasons for death in patients successfully resuscitated from out-of-hospital and in-hospital cardiac arrest. Resuscitation. 2019;136:93.
19. Nakstad ER, Stær-Jensen H, Wimmer H, et al. Late awakening, prognostic factors and long-term outcome in out-of-hospital cardiac arrest—results of the prospective Norwegian Cardio-Respiratory Arrest Study (NORCAST). Resuscitation. 2020;149:170–9.
20. Streitberger KJ, Endisch C, Ploner CJ, et al. Timing of brain computed tomography and accuracy of outcome prediction after cardiac arrest. Resuscitation. 2019;145:8–14.
21. Sen J, Belli A. S100B in neuropathologic states: the CRP of the brain? J Neurosci Res. 2007;85:1373–80.
22. Jang JH, Park WB, Lim YS, et al. Combination of S100B and procalcitonin improves prognostic performance compared to either alone in patients with cardiac arrest: a prospective observational study. Medicine (Baltimore). 2019;98:e14496.

23. Duez CHV, Grejs AM, Jeppesen AN, Schrøder AD, Søreide E, Nielsen JF, Kirkegaard H. Neuron-specific enolase and S-100b in prolonged targeted temperature management after cardiac arrest: a randomised study. Resuscitation. 2018;122:79–86.
24. Stammet P, Dankiewicz J, Nielsen N, et al. Protein S100 as outcome predictor after out-of-hospital cardiac arrest and targeted temperature management at 33 °C and 36 °C. Crit Care. 2017;21:1–10.
25. Ashton NJ, Janelidze S, al Khleifat A, et al. A multicentre validation study of the diagnostic value of plasma neurofilament light. Nat Commun. 2021;12:1–12.
26. Rana OR, Schröder JW, Baukloh JK, et al. Neurofilament light chain as an early and sensitive predictor of long-term neurological outcome in patients after cardiac arrest. Int J Cardiol. 2013;168:1322–7.
27. Rundgren M, Friberg H, Cronberg T, Romner B, Petzold A. Serial soluble neurofilament heavy chain in plasma as a marker of brain injury after cardiac arrest. Crit Care. 2012;16:R45.
28. Moseby-Knappe M, Mattsson-Carlgren N, Stammet P, et al. Serum markers of brain injury can predict good neurological outcome after out-of-hospital cardiac arrest. Intensive Care Med. 2021;47:984–94.
29. Simrén J, Ashton NJ, Blennow K, Zetterberg H. Blood neurofilament light in remote settings: alternative protocols to support sample collection in challenging pre-analytical conditions. Alzheimers Dement (Amst). 2021;13:e12145.
30. Ashton NJ, Suárez-Calvet M, Karikari TK, et al. Effects of pre-analytical procedures on blood biomarkers for Alzheimer's pathophysiology, glial activation, and neurodegeneration. Alzheimers Dement (Amst). 2021;13:e12168.
31. Sandelius Å, Zetterberg H, Blennow K, et al. Plasma neurofilament light chain concentration in the inherited peripheral neuropathies. Neurology. 2018;90:e518–24.
32. Thelin EP, Zeiler FA, Ercole A, et al. Serial sampling of serum protein biomarkers for monitoring human traumatic brain injury dynamics: a systematic review. Front Neurol. 2017;8:300.
33. Bishop P, Rocca D, Henley JM. Ubiquitin C-terminal hydrolase L1 (UCH-L1): structure, distribution and roles in brain function and dysfunction. Biochem J. 2016;473:2453–62.
34. Gong B, Leznik E. The role of ubiquitin C-terminal hydrolase L1 in neurodegenerative disorders. Drug News Perspect. 2007;20:365–70.
35. Anderson TN, Hwang J, Munar M, Papa L, Hinson HE, Vaughan A, Rowell SE. Blood-based biomarkers for prediction of intracranial hemorrhage and outcome in patients with moderate or severe traumatic brain injury. J Trauma Acute Care Surg. 2020;89:80–6.
36. Ebner F, Moseby-Knappe M, Mattsson-Carlgren N, et al. Serum GFAP and UCH-L1 for the prediction of neurological outcome in comatose cardiac arrest patients. Resuscitation. 2020;154:61–8.
37. Diaz-Arrastia R, Wang KKW, Papa L, et al. Acute biomarkers of traumatic brain injury: relationship between plasma levels of ubiquitin C-terminal hydrolase-l1 and glial fibrillary acidic protein. J Neurotrauma. 2014;31:19.
38. Hol EM, Pekny M. Glial fibrillary acidic protein (GFAP) and the astrocyte intermediate filament system in diseases of the central nervous system. Curr Opin Cell Biol. 2015;32:121–30.
39. Kaneko T, Kasaoka S, Miyauchi T, Fujita M, Oda Y, Tsuruta R, Maekawa T. Serum glial fibrillary acidic protein as a predictive biomarker of neurological outcome after cardiac arrest. Resuscitation. 2009;80:790–4.
40. Mörtberg E, Zetterberg H, Nordmark J, Blennow K, Rosengren L, Rubertsson S. S-100B is superior to NSE, BDNF and GFAP in predicting outcome of resuscitation from cardiac arrest with hypothermia treatment. Resuscitation. 2011;82:26–31.
41. Hayashida H, Kaneko T, Kasaoka S, et al. Comparison of the predictability of neurological outcome by serum procalcitonin and glial fibrillary acidic protein in postcardiac-arrest patients. Neurocrit Care. 2009;12:252–7.
42. Rissin DM, Fournier DR, Piech T, et al. Simultaneous detection of single molecules and singulated ensembles of molecules enables immunoassays with broad dynamic range. Anal Chem. 2011;83:2279–85.

43. Weingarten MD, Lockwood AH, Hwo SY, Kirschner MW. A protein factor essential for microtubule assembly. Proc Natl Acad Sci U S A. 1975;72:1858–62.
44. Williams DR. Tauopathies: classification and clinical update on neurodegenerative diseases associated with microtubule-associated protein tau. Intern Med J. 2006;36:652–60.
45. Pluta R, Ułamek-Kozioł M, Januszewski S, Czuczwar SJ. Tau protein dysfunction after brain ischemia. J Alzheimers Dis. 2018;66:429–33.
46. Randall J, Mörtberg E, Provuncher GK, et al. Tau proteins in serum predict neurological outcome after hypoxic brain injury from cardiac arrest: results of a pilot study. Resuscitation. 2013;84:351–6.
47. Mörtberg E, Zetterberg H, Nordmark J, et al. Plasma tau protein in comatose patients after cardiac arrest treated with therapeutic hypothermia. Acta Anaesthesiol Scand. 2011;55:1132–8.
48. Mattsson N, Zetterberg H, Nielsen N, et al. Serum tau and neurological outcome in cardiac arrest. Ann Neurol. 2017;82:665–75.
49. Wunderlich MT, Lins H, Skalej M, Wallesch CW, Goertler M. Neuron-specific enolase and tau protein as neurobiochemical markers of neuronal damage are related to early clinical course and long-term outcome in acute ischemic stroke. Clin Neurol Neurosurg. 2006;108:558–63.
50. Blennow K, Hampel H, Weiner M, Zetterberg H. Cerebrospinal fluid and plasma biomarkers in Alzheimer disease. Nat Rev Neurol. 2010;6:131–44.

Part VIII

Neurocritical Care and Neuromonitoring

The Emerging Role of the Microbiota in Neurocritical Care

24

D. Battaglini, P. Pelosi, and C. Robba

24.1 Introduction

The intestinal microbiota plays a critical role in human physiology and pathology, participating in food digestion, production of vitamins, absorption of energy, modulation of intestinal homeostasis, and regulation of immune functions [1]. The microbiota reflects the 'diversity' of our microbial community and is composed of commensal, symbiotic and pathogenic microorganisms, whereas the microbiome represents the genetic material of the microbiota; both these systems are frequently unbalanced during critical illness [2]. Critically ill patients are highly susceptible to microbiome imbalance due to antibiotic use, multiple drug administration, mechanical ventilation, nutritional therapy, and increased metabolism with consequent hyperinflammation [2]. The dysregulated microbial diversity has been strongly associated with worse outcomes in critical illness [3]. Despite progress in translational medicine, little is known about the microbiota in neurocritically ill patients. Evolution in the management and treatment of acute neurologic injury has not been primarily focused on microbiota modulation and its effect on outcome [3]. Microbial dysbiosis in experimental models of acute brain pathology has been associated with alterations of the blood–brain barrier (BBB), altered permeability, and microglial

D. Battaglini (✉)
Anesthesia and Critical Care, San Martino Policlinico Hospital, IRCCS for Oncology and Neuroscience, Genoa, Italy

Department of Medicine, University of Barcelona, Barcelona, Spain
e-mail: denise.battaglini@hsanmartino.it

P. Pelosi · C. Robba
Anesthesia and Critical Care, San Martino Policlinico Hospital, IRCCS for Oncology and Neuroscience, Genoa, Italy

Department of Surgical Science and Integrated Diagnostics, University of Genoa, Genoa, Italy

J.-L. Vincent (ed.), *Annual Update in Intensive Care and Emergency Medicine 2022*, Annual Update in Intensive Care and Emergency Medicine,
https://doi.org/10.1007/978-3-030-93433-0_24

activation but evidence is lacking in the critically ill setting; the study of microbiota in chronic neurological disorders has made much more progress [1, 3]. Therefore, dysbiosis in neurocritical care remains a very poorly studied but fascinating theme that deserves further investigation [3]. The aim of this chapter is to provide an overview about the progress made in translational biology concerning the study of the microbiota and microbial dysbiosis in the most common pathologies in the neurocritical care setting.

24.2 Mechanisms of Dysbiosis

The human microbiota is a complex system composed of trillions of microbes (around 1000 species in the digestive tract), which, under physiological conditions, can regulate maturation and function of the host's immune system, while under pathological conditions it can cause microbial dysbiosis with systemic complications [4]. Evidence suggests that the gut microbiome can alter neuronal development, cognitive assessment, brain function, and behavior. This mechanism is mediated by bidirectional communication pathways between the gut-lung-heart and the brain through several neural, immune, and endocrine-metabolic pathways in which microbiota composition plays a central role [5]. The typical composition of a healthy and pathological microbiota in critically ill and neurocritically ill patients is summarized in Table 24.1.

24.2.1 Local and Systemic Responses to Acute Brain Injury

The local and systemic responses to acute brain injury involve the activation of the immune innate and adaptive systems, which become susceptible to injury because of the breakdown of protective barriers [4]. The innate immune system immediately activates physical, chemical, and cellular (i.e., lymphoid cells, granulocytes, and phagocytes) defenses against pathogens at the central nervous system (CNS) level (i.e., microglia and astrocytes). Following cell damage, damage-associated molecular patterns (DAMPs) and pathogen-associated molecular patterns (PAMPs) are activated, interacting with pattern recognition receptors (PRRs) on phagocytes (i.e., dendritic cells, macrophages, chemokines, cytokines, and complement), which can recruit other immune cells and amplify the immune response to a systemic level with the liberation of prostaglandins, leukotrienes, platelet activating factor, histamine, serotonin, complement fragments, proteases, and chemokines [4].

After brain injury, damaged cells secrete inflammatory chemokines and cytokines that activate adaptive immunity. The adaptive immunity concurrently starts by recognizing antigens through antigen-presenting cells (APC), which interact with T or B lymphocytes. B lymphocytes exert a fundamental role in homeostasis through the secretion of immunoglobulin-A (IgA) [1]. After proliferating, effector T cells (Th1, Th2, Th17) and regulatory T cells (Treg) can produce cytokines and chemokines to protect the host from pathogens [4]. Usually, Th1 secretes interleukin

Table 24.1 Characteristics of microbiota composition in critically ill patients and in key neurocritical conditions

Population	Microbiota composition
Critically ill patient	↓*Bacteroidetes*, ↓*Firmicutes*
	↑*Proteobacteria*, ↑*Firmicutes* (↑*Streptococcus*, ↑*Veilonella*), ↑*Bacterioidetes*, ↑*Verrucomicrobia*
Traumatic brain injury	↓*Bacteroidetes*, ↓*Fusobacteria*, ↓*Verrucomicrobia*
	↑*Clostridiales*, ↑*Firmicutes* (↑*Enterococcus*), ↑*Proteobacteria* (↑*Escherichia coli*, ↑*Klebsiella pneumoniae*, ↑*Proteus mirabilis*, ↑*Enterobacter cloacae*, ↑*Pseudomonas aeruginosa*), ↑*Acinetobacteria* (↑*Acinetobacter baumanii*)
Ischemic stroke	↓*Bacteroidetes* (↓*Prevotella*), ↓*Firmicutes* (↓*Lactobacillus sakei*, ↓*Faecalibacterium*)
	↑*Proteobacteria* (↑*Escherichia*, ↑*Klebsiella*, ↑*Shigella*, ↑*Proteus*, ↑*Haemophilus*, ↑*Enterobacter*, ↑*Desulfovibrio*), ↑*Firmicutes* (↑*Eubacterium*, ↑*Enterococcus*, ↑*Oscillibacter megasphaera*, ↑*Ruminococcaceae*, ↑*Christensenellaceae*, ↑*Lactobacillus ruminis*), ↑*Acinetobacteria* (↑*Colinsella*), ↑*Bacterioidetes* (↑*Alistipes*), *Verrucomicrobia* (↑*Akkermansia*), ↑*Lentisphaerae* (↑*Victivallis*), ↑*Actinobacteria* (↑*Atopobium*)
Intracerebral hemorrhage	Few data in humans
Subarachnoid hemorrhage	↓*Firmicutes* (↓*Hungatella hathewayi*)
	↑*Bacterioidetes* (↑*B. thetaiotaomicron*, ↑*B. massiliensis*, ↑*B. nordii*, ↑*B. intestinalis*, ↑*B. cellulosilyticus*), ↑*Firmicutes* (↑*Clostridium bartelettii*, ↑*C. nexile*, ↑*C. boltae*)
Spinal cord injury	↓*Firmicutes* (↓*Pseudobutyrivibrio*, ↓*Dialister*, ↓*Megamonas*, ↓*Marvinbryantia*, ↓*Roseburia*, ↓*Subdoligranium*, ↓*Faecalibacteria*, ↓*Laachnoclostridium*, ↓*Phascolarctobacterium*), ↓*Bacteroidetes* (↓*Prevotella*)
	↑*Proteobacteria* (↑*Escheria*, ↑*Shigella*), ↑*Verrucomicrobia*, ↑*Bacteroidetes* (↑*Bacteroides*, ↑*Probacteroides*)

↑ Increased or ↓ decreased phylum of bacteria

(IL)-2, IL-12, tumor necrosis factor-α (TNF-α), and interferon-γ (IFNγ), Th2 secretes IL-4, IL-5 and IL-13, Th17 with the release of IL-17 which activates a pro-inflammatory response, while Treg act by reducing and regulating the inflammatory response via IL-10 and transforming growth factor-β (TGF-β), also inhibiting the secretion of IL-17 from Th17 in the gut [4]. Some experimental and clinical evidence has demonstrated that Treg cells are essential for neuronal survival and play a neuroprotectant role, whereas patients with a higher neutrophil/lymphocyte ratio are more predisposed to death [4]. These together suggest that the role of adaptive immunity is mainly related to the progression of neurological injury and prognosis.

24.2.2 Bidirectional Communication

24.2.2.1 Gut–Brain Axis

The gut microbiota plays a crucial role in regulation of the intestinal barrier. The disturbance in gut bacterial composition may determine neurological derangements and *vice versa* [1]. Dysfunction of the intestinal barrier may lead to enhanced innate-immune response and hyper-inflammation, thus promoting systemic inflammation and poor functional outcome [4]. At the intestinal level, the epithelial intestinal cells express Toll-like receptors (TLRs, among PRRs) which recognize commensal microbes and regulate the innate immune response [4]. Several TLRs control the homeostasis of the intestinal tract thus increasing the burden of commensals (e.g., TLR-5 and nucleotide-binding oligomerization domain-containing protein [NOD-2]) [1]. NOD-like receptors (NLR) may create a multiprotein complex named the inflammasome, which, when activated, increases the liberation of cytokines and chemokines [1].

The gut microbiota may influence the physiologic function of the CNS and of the endocrine nervous system through dedicated pathways, thus modulating brain function [1]. The main pathways between the gut and the brain involve the autonomic nervous system, the hypothalamic-pituitary-adrenal axis (HPA), and the immune-inflammatory system that continuously communicate through peripheral and central connections (via top-down and bottom-up signaling) and through the release of mediators like serotonin, catecholamines, cholecystokinin, gamma-amino butyric acid (GABA), glucagon-like peptide-1, neuropeptide Y, endocrine hormones, microbial compounds, and metabolites [1]. The autonomic nervous system is deputized to the modulation of intestinal homeostasis, gut motility, permeability, bile secretion, mucus, and bicarbonate production [1]. Figure 24.1 summarizes the main pathways involved in the gut-brain axis.

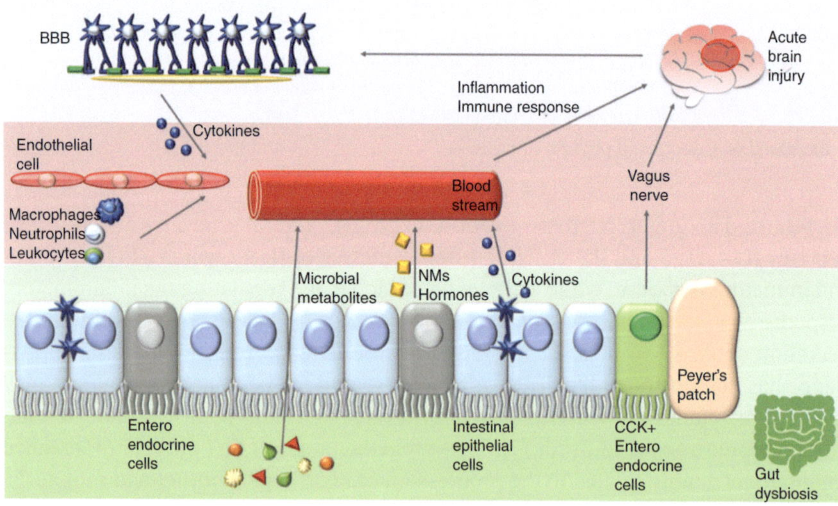

Fig. 24.1 Microbiota brain–gut axis. Brain damage induces local inflammatory response followed by the activation of systemic inflammatory immune response. The intestinal barrier is disrupted, compromising the ability of the microbiota to defend against intestinal pathogens. Microbial metabolites, neurotransmitters (NMs), and cytokines are released into the blood stream. These molecules therefore activate the adaptive and innate immune systems and enhance the systemic inflammatory response. Vagal afferents activate the neuroendocrine system to release peptides, and the inflammatory response to release pro-inflammatory cytokines. Neutrophils, macrophages, and leukocytes are the main actors in this phase. Additionally, T lymphocytes can migrate from Peyer's patch in the small intestine to the brain. *CCK* cholecystokinin, *DC* dendritic cells, *NMs* neurotransmitters, *BBB* blood–brain barrier

24.2.2.2 Heart–Brain Axis

Neurocritically ill patients are at high risk of cardiovascular complications and the existence of a bidirectional interaction between the brain and the heart has been widely discussed [5]. Sympathetic hyperactivity, HPA, immune and inflammatory responses, and gut dysbiosis are the main pathways involved in brain–heart axis dysregulation [5]. According to recent evidence, the occurrence of cardiovascular and cerebrovascular complications in brain injured patients might be associated with dysbiosis [1]. Some clinical studies have identified trimethylamine-N-oxide (TMAO) as the principal marker and predictor of cardiovascular events [5]. Other toxins and metabolites, frequently associated with microbiota imbalance, have been identified as potential factors for the development of cardiovascular and cerebrovascular disease, including lipopolysaccharide [6]. The mechanisms of brain–gut–heart interactions are reported in Fig. 24.2.

24.2.2.3 Lung–Brain Axis

The brain–lung axis represents an integrated physiological ensemble. Neurocritically ill patients often present with pulmonary disorders like acute lung injury, acute respiratory distress syndrome (ARDS), and pulmonary edema, and the mechanical

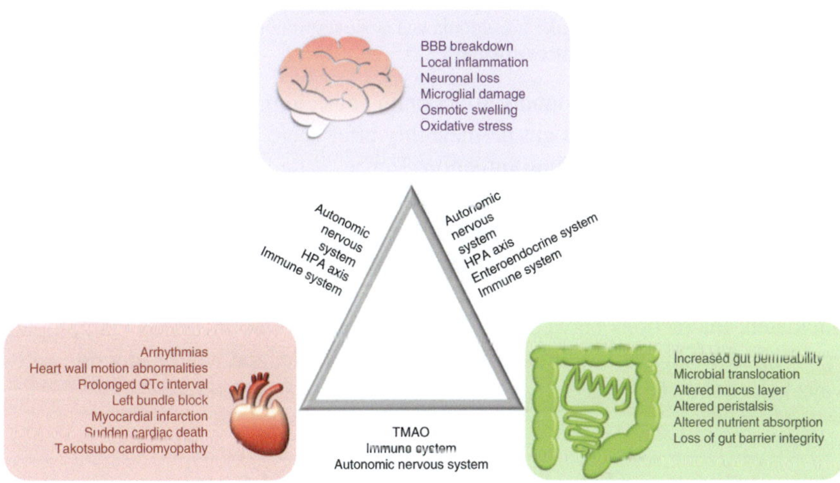

Fig. 24.2 Microbiota gut–brain–heart axis. The main mechanisms involved in the microbiota gut–brain–heart axis include the hypothalamic–pituitary–adrenal axis (HPA), the immune and inflammatory responses, and gut dysbiosis. After brain injury, the blood–brain barrier (BBB) is altered with local inflammation, neuronal loss, microglial damage, with possible osmotic swelling and activation of oxidative processes. The local inflammatory response thus extends to a systemic level via liberation of pro-inflammatory mediators and activation of the innate and adaptive immune responses. Additionally, the autonomic nervous system and the vagus nerve, which commonly control the heart's activity, are altered with possible cardiac complications. At the same time, microbial dysbiosis of the intestinal tract is activated by immune systemic mediators with increased gut permeability and loss of barrier integrity that favors microbial translocation, altered mucus layer, dysregulated peristalsis, which all contribute to the maintenance of systemic inflammation thus sustaining brain injury and consequent cardiac dysfunction. *TMAO* trimethylamine-N-oxide

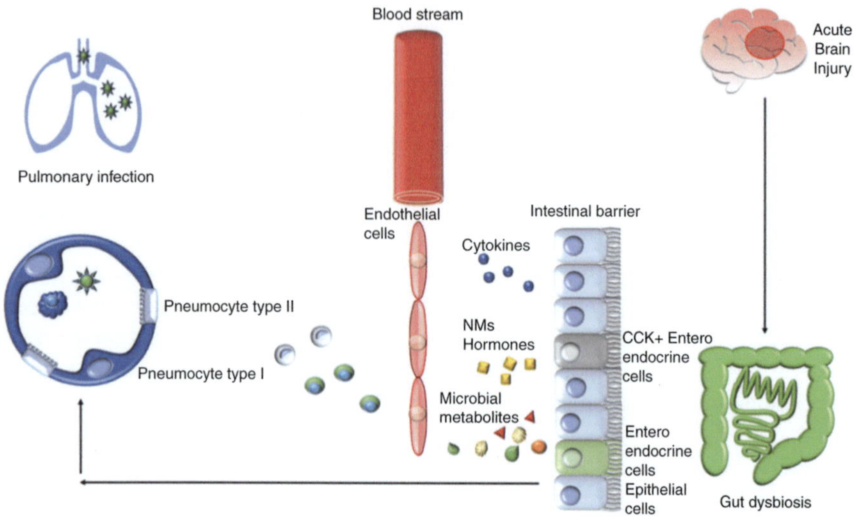

Fig. 24.3 The gut and lung microbiota in neurocritical illness. In the neurocritically ill patient, brain derangements cause dysbiosis of the intestinal microbiota and lungs (via translocation of pathogens through the intestinal barrier–blood stream–pulmonary circulation–lung epithelium), which can contribute to diseases like pneumonia and acute respiratory distress syndrome (ARDS). *NMs* neurotransmitters, *CCK* cholecystokinin

ventilation settings can profoundly affect brain physiology [7]. Experiments in mice demonstrated that increased gut permeability after acute brain injury can result in bacterial translocation and lung infection. Hence, patients with acute brain injury are more susceptible to pneumonia and pulmonary infections, as demonstrated by the high rate of stroke-associated pneumonia and ventilator-associated pneumonia (VAP) in this patient population, and this can also influence patient outcomes [8, 9]. However, this complex connection and potential therapeutic strategies are still being elucidated. Interactions between the brain and the lung are mediated via complex signaling involving neural, inflammatory, immunologic, and neuroendocrine pathways [7], as shown in Fig. 24.3.

24.3 Influence of Dysbiosis on Neurological Outcome

The following sections discuss preclinical and clinical evidence about microbiota dysbiosis in the main neurological pathologies encountered in the intensive care unit (ICU) and the association of microbiome imbalance with outcome in neurocritical care patients.

24.3.1 Traumatic Brain Injury

Traumatic brain injury (TBI) is one of the leading causes of disability and death globally, affecting millions of people each year. Despite a growing body of guidelines and advances in treatment, a large number of TBI survivors still have long-term physical, mental, and cognitive disabilities [10]. The pathophysiology of TBI is complex and includes an immediate injury resulting from external factors (few minutes), followed by secondary brain damage resulting from the primary events as a cascade of biochemical and molecular events that can last for months/years [10]. Particularly at a cellular level, TBI pathophysiology is characterized by inadequate perfusion, oxidative stress, excitotoxicity, cerebral edema, and release of pro-inflammatory mediators that can further damage the brain tissue [10]. Long term manifestations of secondary brain injury include memory deficits, altered attention, reduced executive function, and dysexecutive syndrome with associated anxiety and depression [11]. Recent advances in translational biology suggest that TBI complications might be partially modulated by the maintenance of a homeostatic microbiota. At the gut level, sequelae of TBI include mucosal damage with altered permeability and passage of electrolytes and metabolites [12]. This is followed by reactive gliosis for mucosal repair and barrier function, and, additionally, by the release of local inflammatory mediators, which recall immune cells and amplify the systemic response [12]. Early effects of brain injury on the gut include gastroparesis and altered intestinal function with changes in microbial composition and intestinal epithelial barrier integrity, until a state of dysautonomia is reached [12]. Evidence from animal models has revealed that the intestinal microbiota becomes dysfunctional after 72 h from TBI, changing the normal composition in favor of pathogens like *Pseudomonas aeruginosa* and *Escherichia coli*, increasing intestinal inflammation, reducing antimicrobial peptides, and damaging the mucosal barrier. This pro-inflammatory status has been associated with multiple organ dysfunction, life-threatening systemic complications, and possible death [4]. Microbiota dysbiosis caused by antibiotic administration has been associated with reduced hippocampal neurogenesis and memory retention, increased neuronal loss, with altered microglia and peripheral immune response in a mouse TBI model [13]. Recent reports suggest the role of homocystcine accumulation in dysfunction of the BBB, microvascular disorders, visual dysfunction, and oxidative stress in TBI [11]. Other experimental evidence from a mouse TBI model includes that the presence of *Clostridium butyricum* and *Lactobacillus acidophilus* in the gut microbiota can improve neurological status, BBB function, and neurodegeneration [14], and the use of multiple antibiotics showed anti-inflammatory and neuroprotective effects in mice with TBI [4]. Stimulation of the vagus nerve in a TBI model resulted in neuroprotective effects, reducing cerebral edema and the concentration of pro-inflammatory cytokines. Moreover, vagal stimulation inhibits oxidative stress and apoptosis via nuclear factor-kappa B (NF-κB)/NLRP3 signaling [15]. In the clinical setting, a clear connection between microbiota dysregulation and TBI is still far from being clarified. Characteristics of microbiome composition in TBI patients are reported in Table 24.1, but correlation with outcome and neurological function are still lacking.

24.3.2 Ischemic Stroke

Acute ischemic stroke represents the second leading cause of death worldwide [1]. After acute ischemic stroke, altered intestinal permeability with disruption of the gut-blood barrier and dysregulation of the microbiota may occur, thus leading to an imbalance of gut pathogens compared to commensals [1]. Gut pathogens contribute to enhance the inflammatory response also by increasing the production of TMAO. TMAO may contribute to platelet hyperactivity, foam cell formation, altered steroid and bile metabolism, and to activate macrophages, platelets and dendritic cells [1]. Moreover, in a preclinical model, an important trigger receptor expressed on myeloid cells (TREM-1), which synergically interacts with PRRs, was found to be involved in the enhancement of pro-inflammatory response of intestinal myeloid cells, while its modulation reduced the inflammatory response in acute ischemic stroke [1]. Another animal model demonstrated that Treg can reduce cerebral infarction and improve neurological outcome, acting through the suppression of inflammation [16]. In the clinical setting, changes in the gut microbiota composition were found in patients with acute ischemic stroke with an increase in opportunistic pathogens over commensals [17]. Characteristics and gut microbiota composition in acute ischemic stroke are reported in Table 24.1. A score, the stroke dysbiosis index, was developed to quantify gut dysbiosis in patients with acute ischemic stroke, and was positively associated with unfavorable outcome [18]. A meta-analysis including 87 studies of stroke-associated pneumonia found an incidence rate of around 30% and an association with mortality [19]. In 2017, a meta-analysis confirmed that TMAO increases cardiovascular risk and mortality in patients with acute ischemic stroke [20]. Additionally, psychological studies have demonstrated that 1 year after acute ischemic stroke, 34% of patients have cognitive impairment and that this is associated with TMAO levels [21]. Cognitive decline and dementia are common in acute ischemic stroke survivors, with an incidence rate of 20–53% from 6-months to 2-years after acute ischemic stroke [6]. Several factors are associated with a higher risk of developing cognitive impairment in acute ischemic stroke, including diabetes, hypertension, cerebral deposition of amyloid, and mixed vascular and non-vascular triggers [6]. Patients with acute ischemic stroke who develop cognitive impairment frequently exhibit a deficiency in short-chain fatty acids and microbiota metabolites, with a prevalence of *Fusobacterium* [22].

24.3.3 Intracerebral Hemorrhage

Intracerebral hemorrhage is often included in the broad definition of hemorrhagic stroke, accounting for approximately 20% of strokes. Regardless of the exact location of bleeding, intracerebral hemorrhage has a poor prognosis, with long-term disability and high mortality [23]. Surgical evacuation is a possible therapeutic strategy for operable hemorrhage in order to reduce a mass effect and related complications. However, this method often fails to improve long-term neurological outcome [23] and new strategies are required. The pathological mechanism of intracerebral hemorrhage is characterized by hematoma growth and secondary brain damage with neuroinflammation. As with the brain–gut axis interaction, intracerebral hemorrhage brain injury can determine dysbiosis of the gut microbiota, with gastrointestinal paralysis and altered intestinal barrier integrity in a mouse model [24]. This effect is mediated by T cells at a central level, which can increase vascular permeability, release inflammatory cytokines, and promote microglial polarization into an M1 pro-inflammatory phenotype, thus enhancing a systemic inflammatory response [24]. Microglial polarization is probably mediated by the NLRP3 inflammasome after intracerebral hemorrhage, which, when inhibited, reduces the production of pro-inflammatory cytokines [25].

Experimental studies suggest that bacteria able to produce TMAO and butyrate play a key role in the progression of stroke, also acting on functional outcomes [26]. In contrast, short-chain fatty acids, which are products of dietary fiber fermentation by the gut microbiota, can cross the BBB and induce maturation of microglial cells of the brain. This has been associated also with improved outcome after stroke, attenuating brain inflammation and improving neurogenesis [27]. Few clinical studies on microbiota modulation in intracerebral hemorrhage are currently available. One study investigated clinical functional outcomes at 3-months in patients with intracerebral hemorrhage with altered microbiota, detecting early neurological deterioration, hematoma enlargement, and poor outcome in 19%, 18%, and 45% of cases, respectively. There was a linear correlation between TMAO levels and poor outcome at 3-months, suggesting the regulating role of TMAO in prognosis and outcome after intracerebral hemorrhage [28]. A recent case-controlled study in patients with ischemic and hemorrhagic stroke concluded that after stroke the intestinal communities are highly subverted compared to controls. Moreover, the authors observed an enrichment in bacteria implicated in TMAO production and a reduction in butyrate-producing bacteria, that was also an independent predictor of post-stroke infection [26].

24.3.4 Subarachnoid Hemorrhage

The pathogenetic mechanisms of aneurysm rupture responsible for the majority of cases of subarachnoid hemorrhage (SAH) have still to be elucidated, but it seems that a genetic predisposition as well as environmental factors might play a crucial role [29]. Dysbiosis of gut microbiota has been associated with the occurrence of cerebrovascular and cardiovascular disease and with cognitive impairment in patients with brain injury. Hence, the suspicion that microbiota imbalance could be involved in aneurysm rupture and development of SAH is high [29]. An experimental study in mice, in which intracranial aneurysms and microbiota dysbiosis were induced, demonstrated that dysbiosis can be associated with aneurysm formation and modulation of inflammation [30]. Other factors related to dysbiosis can act in the pathogenesis of aneurysm formation, including lymphocytes [31], and TNF-α liberation [32], typical phases of the pro-inflammatory response that appear after microbiota imbalance. In patients with unruptured cerebral aneurysm, the gut microbiota was altered with an abundance of *Hungatella hathewayi*, which is responsible for modulating taurine levels in the serum. Taurine supplementation in these patients reversed the progression of intracranial aneurysms [29]. The composition of the microbiota in patients with SAH is summarized in Table 24.1. A recent systematic review including studies in preclinical and clinical settings concluded that IL-6 plays a crucial role in the pathogenesis of post-SAH complications like delayed cerebral ischemia and cerebral vasospasm. Indeed, IL-6 is a well-known marker of intracranial inflammation, but its release can also be associated with microbial dysbiosis [33].

24.3.5 Spinal Cord Injury

Spinal cord injury is a disabling condition usually caused by polytrauma, which frequently requires ICU admission and comprehensive critical care, and may culminate in paraplegia or tetraplegia [34]. Unfortunately, neuronal regeneration, tissue repair, and plasticity are limited, due to the loss of regulatory function in the brain and upper spinal cord, with possible evolution to multiple organ dysfunction [34]. The pathogenetic mechanism of dysbiosis in spinal cord injury is even more pronounced than in central nervous system diseases, because the autonomic nervous system is often destroyed and axonal descending fibers below the injury level cannot innervate motor neurons, while ascending fibers cannot transmit information to the brain [34]. This means the brain is unable to control the intestinal system, thus causing an imbalance of sympathetic and parasympathetic pathways with gastrointestinal dysfunction, altered intestinal motility, imbalanced mucosal secretion, dysregulated vascular tone, and altered immune function [35]. The composition of the microbiota of patients with spinal cord injury is summarized in Table 24.1. Experimental studies in rat models demonstrated that an abnormal gut microbial community is involved in the pathogenesis of spinal cord injury [36]. In spinal cord injury, intestinal permeability with bacterial translocation and immune activation in the gut-associated lymphoid tissue (GALT) increases, causing significant changes in microbiota that persist for at least 1 month, predicting the potential locomotor impairment. An experimental study in naïve mice showed that induction of gut dysbiosis before spinal cord injury was associated with neurological impairment, whereas feeding spinal cord injury mice with commercial probiotics produced a protective immune response in GALT, conferring neuroprotection and locomotor recovery [37]. In these animal models, the gut microbiota was altered with an increase in *Clostridaiceae* and *Bifidobacterium* species and an increased production of IL-1ß, IL-12 and macrophage inflammatory protein (MIP)-2 [38]. Another experimental study demonstrated that the endotoxin-responsive, cAMP-specific, Pde4 subfamily-b enzyme (PDE4B) plays a role in inducing neuro-inflammation and white matter loss; genetic ablation of the PDE4B prevented the changes in microbiota with improved functional recovery via inflammatory modulation [39]. Clinical evidence concerning microbiota imbalance in spinal cord injury is still limited. A clinical study concluded that the production of butyrate was reduced in patients with spinal cord injury in comparison to healthy subjects [40]. Another study demonstrated that the composition of the gut microbiota of patients with spinal cord injury was different between those with cervical and with thoracolumbar injury. However, no correlation with the recovery of motor function was found [41]. A study in patients with spinal cord injury showed a significantly different intestinal microbiota compared to a healthy control group, confirming the role of microbiota disorders in spinal cord injury pathogenesis and clinical symptoms [42]. However, there is still no study that reports the potential role of microbiota on motor function improvement [38].

24.4 Modulation of the Human Microbiota

Several factors can influence the gut microbiota composition and its alteration in critically ill patients. Mechanical ventilation, enteral or parenteral feeding, antibiotics, vasopressors, proton pump inhibitors, opioids may alter the health of microbiome. Additionally, invasive procedures like endotracheal intubation, intravascular catheterization, and surgical interventions can facilitate the access of microbes and proliferation [43]. Control and modulation of the administered medications and nutritional goals can improve microbiota imbalance in critical illnesses. The following sections summarize the actions that can be taken to restore microbiota deregulation in neurocritically ill patients.

24.4.1 Nutritional Therapy

Nutritional therapy is a main determinant of microbiota homeostasis, which can be easily modulated or altered during the ICU stay by adjusting the timing and the composition of the diet [43]. Current guidelines on nutritional therapy in the ICU state that enteral nutrition should be started as soon as possible or at least within 48 h from admission. However, in critical care patients this is not always possible, with the consequence that the gastrointestinal tract is not activated, the mucosa is not stimulated, and cellular activities are impaired with possible microbiota dysregulation [43]. Enteral and parenteral nutrition affect the microbiota in different ways. It seems that parenteral nutrition enriches the microbiota of *Proteobacteria* with loss of bacterial diversity and alteration of the barrier function with potential increase in pathogenic bacteria over commensals [43]. On the other hand, enteral nutrition is enriched with synthetic dietary emulsifiers and preservatives, including carboxymethyl cellulose, soy lecithin, arabic gum, soy polysaccharide, and glycerol derivatives, which have been associated with gut dysbiosis [43]. In addition, enteral nutrition, by activating the luminal tract, reduces the release of pro-inflammatory cytokines and exerts a protective effect on dysbiosis [44]. Gastrointestinal motility disturbances are very common in patients with acute brain or spinal cord injuries, affecting with various degrees the esophagus, stomach, small bowel, and colon. Moreover, because the tone of the lower esophageal sphincter is reduced, brain injured patients may manifest increased rates of aspiration. Indeed, the gastric emptying time is prolonged in around 80% of patients with TBI [45]. The main reason for failure of early enteral feeding in brain injured patients is the activation of a fasting motor pattern during feeding with an inhibitory feedback to the proximal small bowel, thus delaying gastric emptying [45]. Some nutritional therapies, such as a high-fat diet and a ketogenic diet, have been proposed in brain injured patients because of the increase in TMAO concentration, whereas use of high-protein diets has given conflicting results although amino acids are fundamental for the synthesis of new neurotransmitters. Finally, short-chain fatty acids, such as propionate, butyrate, and acetate, seem to improve brain recovery [1].

24.4.2 Probiotics and Prebiotics

Probiotics are nutritional supplements that act through acid lactic fermentation in the colon in order to maintain the balance between commensals and pathogens. In the ICU, the use of probiotics did not seem to reduce mortality, but reduced the rate of infection, while exerting contrasting results on length of stay; their effects in brain injured patients are still controversial [1, 11]. Prebiotics are defined as food additives that stimulate the growth and activity of specific gut bacteria. Prebiotics are selectively fermented by probiotics to produce short-chain fatty acids in order to downregulate inflammation, modulate oxidative stress, enhance gut barrier function, and prevent adhesion of pathogens that try to attach to the epithelial lining [46]. The use of prebiotics and probiotics in patients with brain or spinal cord injury is still controversial, although preclinical studies showed promising results.

24.4.3 Fecal Microbiota Transplantation

Fecal microbiota transplantation is an innovative and emerging technique that uses the fecal microbiota of a healthy donor to transplant in to sick people. In clinical settings, fecal microbiota transplantation is approved for the treatment of antibiotic-associated diarrhea and intestinal bowel diseases with proved efficacy in reducing dysbiosis, but in a few cases, bacteremia with *E. coli* developed, thus raising doubts about the safety of fecal microbiota transplantation [1]. In the neurocritical setting, fecal microbiota transplantation has been applied in hepatic encephalopathy; duodenal mucosal diversity, reduced dysbiosis, and antimicrobial-peptide expression were observed [47]. In primarily brain injured subjects, fecal microbiota transplantation mitigated CNS damage in animals with TBI, spinal cord injury, and acute ischemic stroke [48]. Other preclinical studies reported a reduced brain lesion size and improvement of outcome with fecal microbiota transplantation in brain damaged subjects, while in ischemic stroke fecal microbiota transplantation restored microglial function [11]. A meta-analysis of clinical and preclinical models concluded that fecal microbiota transplantation may be a promising treatment option for several neurological disorders, despite the limited number of clinical models [49].

24.5 Conclusion

Microbial dysbiosis is common in critically ill and neurocritically ill patients. Modulation of the microbiome has given promising results on neurological outcomes and complications. To date, nutritional therapy, probiotics, prebiotics, and control of medication administration are the most feasible strategies to modulate the microbiota, while fecal microbiota transplantation represents the most promising therapeutic strategy, although its application in the clinical setting is still very limited.

References

1. Battaglini D, Pimentel-Coelho PM, Robba C, et al. Gut microbiota in acute ischemic stroke: from pathophysiology to therapeutic implications. Front Neurol. 2020;11:598.
2. Martin-Loeches I, Dickson R, Torres A, et al. The importance of airway and lung microbiome in the critically ill. Crit Care. 2020;24:537.
3. Xu R, Tan C, Zhu J, et al. Dysbiosis of the intestinal microbiota in neurocritically ill patients and the risk for death. Crit Care. 2019;23:195.
4. Zhang Y, Wang Z, Peng J, Gerner ST, Yin S, Jiang Y. Gut microbiota-brain interaction: an emerging immunotherapy for traumatic brain injury. Exp Neurol. 2021;337:113585.
5. Battaglini D, Robba C, Lopes da Silva A, et al. Brain–heart interaction after acute ischemic stroke. Crit Care. 2020;24:163.
6. Koszewicz M, Jaroch J, Brzecka A, et al. Dysbiosis is one of the risk factor for stroke and cognitive impairment and potential target for treatment. Pharmacol Res. 2021;164:105277.
7. Stevens RD, Puybasset L. The brain–lung–brain axis. Intensive Care Med. 2011;37:1054–6.
8. Vermeij FH, Scholte op Reimer WJM, de Man P, et al. Stroke-associated infection is an independent risk factor for poor outcome after acute ischemic stroke: data from the Netherlands Stroke Survey. Cerebrovasc Dis. 2009;27:465–71.
9. Robba C, Rebora P, Banzato E, et al. Incidence, risk factors, and effects on outcome of ventilator-associated pneumonia in patients with traumatic brain injury. Chest. 2020;158:2292–303.
10. Battaglini D, Siwicka-Gieroba D, Rocco PR, et al. Novel synthetic and natural therapies for traumatic brain injury. Curr Neuropharmacol. 2021;19:1661–87.
11. George AK, Behera J, Homme RP, Tyagi N, Tyagi SC, Singh M. Rebuilding microbiome for mitigating traumatic brain injury: importance of restructuring the gut-microbiome-brain axis. Mol Neurobiol. 2021;58:3614–27.
12. Hanscom M, Loane DJ, Shea-Donohue T. Brain-gut axis dysfunction in the pathogenesis of traumatic brain injury. J Clin Invest. 2021;131:e143777.
13. Celorrio M, Abellanas MA, Rhodes J, et al. Gut microbial dysbiosis after traumatic brain injury modulates the immune response and impairs neurogenesis. Acta Neuropathol Commun. 2021;9:40.
14. Li H, Sun J, Du J, et al. Clostridium butyricum exerts a neuroprotective effect in a mouse model of traumatic brain injury via the gut-brain axis. Neurogastroenterol Motil. 2018;30:e13260.
15. Tang Y, Dong X, Chen G, et al. Vagus nerve stimulation attenuates early traumatic brain injury by regulating the NF-κB/NLRP3 signaling pathway. Neurorehabil Neural Repair. 2020;34:831–43.
16. Li S, Huang Y, Liu Y, et al. Change and predictive ability of circulating immunoregulatory lymphocytes in long-term outcomes of acute ischemic stroke. J Cereb Blood Flow Metab. 2021;41:2280–94.
17. Yin J, Liao S, He Y, et al. Dysbiosis of gut microbiota with reduced trimethylamine-N-oxide level in patients with large-artery atherosclerotic stroke or transient ischemic attack. J Am Heart Assoc. 2015;4:e002699.

18. Xia GH, You C, Gao XX, et al. Stroke Dysbiosis Index (SDI) in gut microbiome are associated with brain injury and prognosis of stroke. Front Neurol. 2019;10:397.
19. Westendorp WF, Nederkoorn PJ, Vermeij JD, Dijkgraaf MG, van de Beek D. Post-stroke infection: a systematic review and meta-analysis. BMC Neurol. 2011;11:110.
20. Schiattarella GG, Sannino A, Toscano E, et al. Gut microbe-generated metabolite trimethylamine-N-oxide as cardiovascular risk biomarker: a systematic review and dose-response meta-analysis. Eur Heart J. 2017;38:2948–56.
21. Zhu C, Li G, Lv Z, et al. Association of plasma trimethylamine-N-oxide levels with post-stroke cognitive impairment: a 1-year longitudinal study. Neurol Sci. 2020;41:57–63.
22. Liu Y, Kong C, Gong L, et al. The association of post-stroke cognitive impairment and gut microbiota and its corresponding metabolites. J Alzheimers Dis. 2020;73:1455–66.
23. Hanley DF, Thompson RE, Rosenblum M, et al. Efficacy and safety of minimally invasive surgery with thrombolysis in intracerebral haemorrhage evacuation (MISTIE III): a randomised, controlled, open-label, blinded endpoint phase 3 trial. Lancet. 2019;393:1021–32.
24. Yu X, Zhou G, Shao B, et al. Gut microbiota dysbiosis induced by intracerebral hemorrhage aggravates neuroinflammation in mice. Front Microbiol. 2021;12:647304.
25. Xiao L, Zheng H, Li J, Wang Q, Sun H. Neuroinflammation mediated by NLRP3 inflammasome after intracerebral hemorrhage and potential therapeutic targets. Mol Neurobiol. 2020;57:5130–49.
26. Haak BW, Westendorp WF, van Engelen TSR, et al. Disruptions of anaerobic gut bacteria are associated with stroke and post-stroke infection: a prospective case–control study. Transl Stroke Res. 2021;12:581–92.
27. Sadler R, Cramer JV, Heindl S, et al. Short-chain fatty acids improve poststroke recovery via immunological mechanisms. J Neurosci. 2020;40:1162–73.
28. Zhai Q, Sun T, Sun C, et al. High plasma levels of trimethylamine N-oxide are associated with poor outcome in intracerebral hemorrhage patients. Neurol Sci. 2021;42:1009–16.
29. Li H, Xu H, Li Y, et al. Alterations of gut microbiota contribute to the progression of unruptured intracranial aneurysms. Nat Commun. 2020;11:3218.
30. Shikata F, Shimada K, Sato H, et al. Potential influences of gut microbiota on the formation of intracranial aneurysm. Hypertension. 2019;73:491–6.
31. Sawyer DM, Pace LA, Pascale CL, et al. Lymphocytes influence intracranial aneurysm formation and rupture: role of extracellular matrix remodeling and phenotypic modulation of vascular smooth muscle cells. J Neuroinflammation. 2016;13:185.
32. Ali MS, Starke RM, Jabbour PM, et al. TNF-α induces phenotypic modulation in cerebral vascular smooth muscle cells: implications for cerebral aneurysm pathology. J Cereb Blood Flow Metab. 2013;33:1564–73.
33. Croci DM, Sivanrupan S, Wanderer S, et al. Preclinical and clinical role of interleukin-6 in the development of delayed cerebral vasospasm and neuronal cell death after subarachnoid hemorrhage: towards a potential target therapy? Neurosurg Rev. 2021. Aug 27: https://doi.org/10.1007/s10143-021-01628-9. Epub ahead of print.
34. Jing Y, Bai F, Yu Y. Spinal cord injury and gut microbiota: a review. Life Sci. 2020;266:118865.
35. Cervi AL, Lukewich MK, Lomax AE. Neural regulation of gastrointestinal inflammation: role of the sympathetic nervous system. Auton Neurosci. 2014;182:83–8.
36. O'Connor G, Jeffrey E, Madorma D, et al. Investigation of microbiota alterations and intestinal inflammation post-spinal cord injury in rat model. J Neurotrauma. 2018;35:2159–66.
37. Kigerl KA, Hall JCE, Wang L, Mo X, Yu Z, Popovich PG. Gut dysbiosis impairs recovery after spinal cord injury. J Exp Med. 2016;213:2603–20.
38. Jogia T, Ruitenberg MJ. Traumatic spinal cord injury and the gut microbiota: current insights and future challenges. Front Immunol. 2020;11:2603–20.
39. Myers SA, Gobejishvili L, Saraswat Ohri S, et al. Following spinal cord injury, PDE4B drives an acute, local inflammatory response and a chronic, systemic response exacerbated by gut dysbiosis and endotoxemia. Neurobiol Dis. 2019;124:353–63.

40. Gungor B, Adiguzel E, Gursel I, Yilmaz B, Gursel M. Intestinal microbiota in patients with spinal cord injury. PLoS One. 2016;11:e0145878.
41. Zhang C, Zhang W, Zhang J, et al. Gut microbiota dysbiosis in male patients with chronic traumatic complete spinal cord injury. J Transl Med. 2018;16:353.
42. Lin R, Xu J, Ma Q, et al. Alterations in the fecal microbiota of patients with spinal cord injury. PLoS One. 2020;15:e0236470.
43. Moron R, Galvez J, Colmenero M, Anderson P, Cabeza J, Rodriguez-Cabezas ME. The importance of the microbiome in critically ill patients: role of nutrition. Nutrients. 2019;11:3002.
44. Lubbers T, Kox M, de Haan JJ, et al. Continuous administration of enteral lipid- and protein-rich nutrition limits inflammation in a human endotoxemia model. Crit Care Med. 2013;41:1258–65.
45. Tan M, Zhu JC, Yin HH. Enteral nutrition in patients with severe traumatic brain injury: reasons for intolerance and medical management. Br J Neurosurg. 2011;25:2–8.
46. Cerdó T, Ruíz A, Suárez A, Campoy C. Probiotic, prebiotic, and brain development. Nutrients. 2017;9:1247.
47. Bajaj JS, Salzman NH, Acharya C, et al. Fecal microbial transplant capsules are safe in hepatic encephalopathy: a phase 1, randomized, placebo-controlled trial. Hepatology. 2019;70:1690–703.
48. Rice MW, Pandya JD, Shear DA. Gut microbiota as a therapeutic target to ameliorate the biochemical, neuroanatomical, and behavioral effects of traumatic brain injuries. Front Neurol. 2019;10:875.
49. Vendrik KEW, Ooijevaar RE, de Jong PRC, et al. Fecal microbiota transplantation in neurological disorders. Front Cell Infect Microbiol. 2020;10:98.

Brain–Multiorgan Cross-Talk in Critically Ill Patients with Acute Brain Injury

25

K. Kotfis, D. Siwicka-Gieroba, and W. Dąbrowski

25.1 Introduction

Cross-talk between different organs is a physiological process responsible for the maintenance of whole body homeostasis, which plays a crucial role in several pathologies when breakdown of such homeostasis occurs and pathological influence of one organ dysfunction is deleterious for another. In a multicellular organism, organ cross-talk is mainly based on the physiological response of one or more organs to the acute or chronic pathology in another through activation of different receptors, such as baroreceptors, chemoreceptors, or hormonal response.

The pathophysiology of multiorgan interactions is complex and not well recognized; however, clinicians often observe that the pathology of one organ is associated with severe functional abnormalities or even terminal dysfunction in other organs. The importance of understanding organ-to-organ cross-talk lies in the fact that this bi-directional impact between them may lead to multiple organ dysfunction, when injuries seem to be potentiated rather than merely added.

Brain–multiorgan interactions seem to be the most important of all types of organ-to-organ cross-talk, because the brain is the control center of the mammalian body. These interactions include relationships between the brain and heart, lungs, gut, liver and kidneys, some authors have also suggested a relationship between the brain and skin, muscles, or even bones [1–3]. Extracerebral complications in patients with acute brain injury are frequent and may influence the outcome. Acute

K. Kotfis (✉)
Department of Anesthesiology, Intensive Therapy and Acute Intoxications, Pomeranian Medical University in Szczecin, Szczecin, Poland
e-mail: katarzyna.kotfis@pum.edu.pl

D. Siwicka-Gieroba · W. Dąbrowski
First Department of Anesthesiology and Intensive Therapy, Medical University of Lublin, Lublin, Poland

J.-L. Vincent (ed.), *Annual Update in Intensive Care and Emergency Medicine 2022*, Annual Update in Intensive Care and Emergency Medicine,
https://doi.org/10.1007/978-3-030-93433-0_25

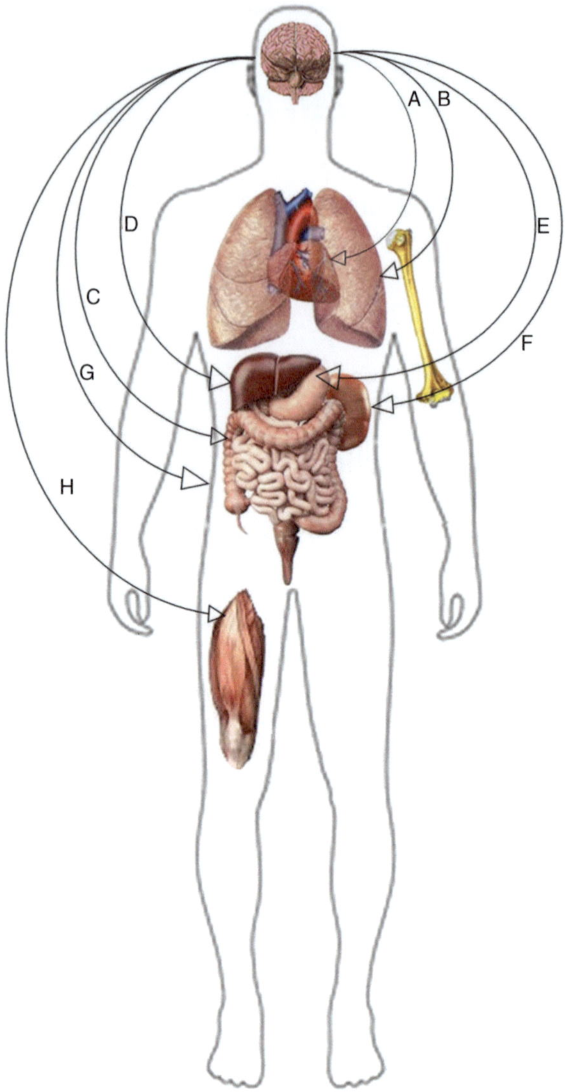

Fig. 25.1 Key areas of brain-multiorgan cross-talk. A: brain–heart cross-talk; B: brain–lung cross-talk; C: brain–microbiome cross-talk; D: brain–liver cross-talk; E. brain–gut cross-talk; F. brain–kidney cross-talk; G. brain–skin and –adipose tissue cross-talk; H. brain–muscle cross-talk. See Table 25.1 for more explanation

brain injury includes a range of central nervous system (CNS) dysfunctions, including encephalopathies of different etiology (e.g., septic, ischemic), acute ischemic stroke, epileptic seizures, subarachnoid hemorrhage (SAH), traumatic brain injury (TBI), intracerebral hemorrhage, or diffuse brain injury in anoxic damage after cardiac arrest.

Coordinated responses of distant organs and organ systems may not only cause a greater burden, leading to profound organ failure, but could also be used as targets for specific, tailor-made interventions to improve outcomes of critically ill patients. The description of brain–other organ cross-talk and potential interventions are shown in Fig. 25.1 and Table 25.1.

Table 25.1 Detailed description of the interactions between organs depicted in Fig. 25.1

	Type of interaction	Potential pathomechanisms	Examples of disorders	Effects on the brain	Potential treatment
A.	Brain–heart	Dysregulation of the autonomic system	EKG abnormalities with life-threatening cardiac arrhythmias	Disorders in cerebral blood flow	Ultra-short-acting and highly selective β-blockers
			Systolic and diastolic dysfunction		Inotropic drugs (dobutamine, levosimendan)
B.	Brain–lung	Systemic inflammatory response	ARDS, VILI, VAP, NPE	Cerebral hypoxia	Levosimendan, caspase-1 inhibitor, dobutamine, sevoflurane, melatonin, lidocaine, selective P2X 7R antagonist, selective CB2R agonist, propofol, stem cell therapy
C.	Brain–microbiome	Systemic inflammatory response	Cognitive dysfunction, neurodegeneration. Increased risk of gastrointestinal dysfunction, nosocomial infection and VAP	Neuroinflammation, increased BBB permeability	Eubiotic therapies (probiotics, microbiota transplant) nutrients, immune modulators, antioxidant, ketamine, statins, melatonin
D.	Brain–liver	Systemic inflammatory response	Hepatic dysfunction. Production and release of neuroactive proteins	Neuroinflammation	Anti-inflammatory and anti-oxidant medications
E.	Brain–gut	Dysregulation of the autonomic system	Gut ischemia, ulcer	Neuroinflammation	Anti-inflammatory and anti-oxidant medications
F.	Brain–kidney	Dysregulation of the autonomic system	Glomerular and tubular apoptosis and fibrogenesis	Neuroinflammation	β-blockers, levosimendan

(continued)

Table 25.1 (continued)

	Type of interaction	Potential pathomechanisms	Examples of disorders	Effects on the brain	Potential treatment
G.	Brain–skin and –adipose tissue	Dysregulation of the autonomic system	Skin dysbiosis Disorders in thermoregulation	Neuroinflammation Disorders in cerebral metabolism	Leptin, resistin and FIAF gene expression silencing techniques, stem cell therapy
H.	Brain–muscle	Motor verve dysfunction	Skeletal muscle immobility	Enhanced neuronal plasticity	Active early mobilization and rehabilitation

ARDS acute respiratory distress syndrome, *BBB* blood–brain barrier, *EKG* electrocardiogram, *FIAF* fasting-induced adipose factor, *NPE* neurogenic pulmonary edema, *VILI* ventilator-induced lung injury, *VAP* ventilator-associated pneumonia

25.2 Brain–Heart Cross-Talk

The interaction between the brain and the heart has been studied for several years, since von Bezold and Hirt and then Jarisch and Richter studied the effects of intravenous injection of veratrum alkaloids on cardiac function before and after cutting the cardiac branches of the vagus nerve [4, 5]. This interaction has been called the Bezold-Jarisch reflex. In general, the brain–heart cross-talk reflects diastolic disorders, impaired cardiac contractility, life-threatening cardiac arrhythmias, cardiac ischemia with impaired myocardial perfusion, and severe electrocardiographic abnormalities [6–10]. Electrocardiographic (EKG) abnormalities are the most frequent and occur in up to 90% of patients treated for isolated severe TBI [6]. These pathologies include significant prolongation of the corrected QT interval, elevation or reduction of the ST-segment, widening of the spatial QRS-T angle and an increased incidence of life-threatening cardiac arrhythmias [6, 7]. Interestingly, more cardiac disorders were observed in patients with severe diffuse brain injury treated with hyperosmolar therapy [6, 8]. Disorders of ventricular repolarization are another pathology developing in patients with TBI. They occur in up to 60% of patients and are commonly associated with changes in the ST-segment [6, 9, 10]. Early systolic dysfunction can occur during the first 24 hours of treatment even in young patients without previous cardiac history, and recovers within the week following trauma [9]. Systolic dysfunction is associated with slight reduction of isovolumetric relaxation time, which reflects impaired diastolic function [10]. Noteworthy, these abnormalities are frequently associated with disorders in the ST-segment and/or corrected QT interval and may result from impaired subendocardial viability [11].

Regardless of clinical manifestation, EKG, and/or echocardiographic abnormalities, two entities of TBI-related pathology have been recognized: stress-induced cardiomyopathy and neurogenic stunned myocardium [12]. Stress-related cardiomyopathy is commonly known as Takotsubo cardiomyopathy or broken heart syndrome and is associated with transient segmental dysfunction of the left ventricle [13, 14]. Neurogenic stunned myocardium is associated with abnormal left ventricular (LV) motion [15]. This dysfunction includes regional global wall motion abnormalities, decreased ejection fraction, and cardiomyopathy, leading to an increased risk of in-hospital mortality [15, 16]. The severity of stunned neurocardiopathy strongly corresponds to plasma norepinephrine concentration following excessive release into the systemic circulation from the over-activated terminals of the sympathetic nerves [16]. However, stress-induced cardiomyopathy and neurogenic stunned myocardium are reversible and in-hospital mortality depends on the age of the patient and the severity of the TBI rather than the TBI-induced cardiac dysfunction [6, 9, 10].

Several medications may improve TBI-induced cardiac dysfunctions. Administration of beta-blockers seems to be the cornerstone treatment of life-threatening arrhythmias resulting from sympathetic hyperactivity [17]. An experimental study documented similar neuroprotective effects when different, low and highly selective beta-blockers were used; however highly-selective and ultra-short-acting beta-blockers appear to be more beneficial due to their minimal effect on blood pressure [18, 19]. Inotropic agents should be preferred over vasopressors in patients with neurologic stunned myocardium. Although dobutamine infusion reverses cerebral vasospasm and increases cerebral blood flow by 50% in TBI patients with stunned myocardium, levosimendan seems to be the agent of choice due to its strong inotropic and vasodilatatory effects and its stimulation of nitric oxide (NO) production [20, 21].

25.3 Brain–Lung Cross-Talk

Respiratory system failure is one of the most common non-neurological complications in brain injured patients. Those with brain trauma often require mechanical ventilation and may develop severe pulmonary injury, including acute respiratory distress syndrome (ARDS), ventilator-induced lung injury (VILI), ventilator-associated pneumonia (VAP), respiratory tract infections, and neurogenic pulmonary edema (NPE) [22]. In addition, pulmonary complications, such as pneumonia or ARDS, are associated with a higher risk of death. Risk factors, such as smoking, tracheostomy, blood transfusion on admission, barbiturate infusion, increased Injury Severity Score (ISS) or head abbreviated injury scale (AIS) all increase the risk of VAP. In addition, VAP *per se* is not associated with increased mortality, but patients with VAP have a longer duration of hospital length of stay [23].

Brain–lung cross-talk has been extensively investigated over recent decades. The hypothesis of brain–lung interaction and lung damage after brain injury, is based on a ‘double hit model’. Activation of inflammatory mediators and release of catecholamines predisposes to systemic innate and adaptive immune responses and activation of different molecular pathways, and causes lungs to be more prone to factors associated with an increase in vascular hydrostatic pressures [24]. Primary brain damage triggers activation of sympathetic pathways, which lead to an increase in capillary permeability and pulmonary vasoconstriction, promoting endothelial dysfunction and molecule infiltrates. One of the major complications – NPE– is observed in up to 20% of patients with TBI. The exact underlying mechanisms of NPE are not clear. The available models, described as neurocardiac model, neurohemodynamic model, blast theory, and pulmonary venule adrenergic hypersensitivity, do not fully explain the mechanism of NPE development. At present, there are no sensitive and specific biological indicators that may be applied to the clinical diagnosis of NPE and many patients are not quickly or accurately diagnosed. Also, the treatment of NPE mainly focuses on reducing intracranial pressure, controlling volume overload, providing hemodynamic optimization, and improving pulmonary capillary permeability. There are currently no specific drugs that are effective against NPE. Recent studies report that drugs such as levosimendan, caspase-1 inhibitor, dobutamine, sevoflurane, melatonin, intrathecal lidocaine, selective P2X 7 receptor antagonists, selective CB2 receptor agonists, and propofol have shown significant effect in treatment of NPE. Thus, it is important to understand the detailed pathophysiological mechanism of NPE to pinpoint novel therapeutic strategies [25].

It is important to mention brain–lung microbiome interactions. Factors determining microbial dysbiosis of the respiratory tract, such as oxygen tension, blood pH, blood flow, alveolar ventilation, temperature, and immune cells, change the physicochemical and metabolic status of the alveoli. Recent studies have shown that hyperoxia causes a selective growth of *Staphylococcus aureus* in critically ill patients, and a change in the composition of the microbiome contributes to the development of pneumonia and ultimately to organ damage [26]. Other mechanisms are the influence of nutritional factors and intercellular signaling influenced by, e.g., glucocorticoids, estrogens, androgens, neurotransmitters (catecholamines, endogenous opioids) and cytokines such as tumor necrosis factor (TNF), interleukin-1 (IL-1), IL-6 and IL-8. Recent research has shown that the lung microbiome is enriched with intestinal microorganisms through the translocation of bacteria facilitated by the increased permeability of the intestines and alveoli that correlates with the increased inflammatory response and may affect the development of ARDS. Early lung dysbiosis in mechanically ventilated patients is associated with increases in the level of inflammatory markers (IL-6 and IL-8), and is strongly associated with the development of late ARDS and, in conjunction with IL-10, with multiple organ dysfunction following TBI [27].

25.4 Brain–Microbiome Cross-Talk

In recent years, microbiome studies have highlighted the crucial role of microbes on human health. The microbiome communities have many functions, including metabolic, barrier and immunological effects. Therefore, understanding of microbiome function is crucial for the generation of future personalized human care, especially in preventing secondary injury after TBI, as it provides insight into different mechanisms of action [28].

Changes in microbiome composition, with a specific exchange of selected commensals may result in dysregulation of fundamental cellular and molecular processes in the CNS, including neuroinflammation, abnormal blood–brain barrier (BBB) permeability, myelination, neurogenesis, immune system responses, microglial activation, and mitochondrial dysfunction [29]. Remarkable changes in the intestinal microbiota observed even 2 h after brain damage affect bacterial translocation, lipopolysaccharide (LPS) exposure, γδ T-cell activation, neutrophil induced release of TNF-α or matrix metallopeptidase (MMP)-9 activation [30]. The intensified microglial activity, neuropathology processes or enhancement of neuroinflammation is the aftermath of the aforementioned imbalance [31]. In addition, activation of nuclear factor-κB (NF-κB) after damage affects up-regulation of intercellular adhesion molecule (ICAM)-1 and increases the production of cytokines like IL-6. These processes reduce the expression of tight junction proteins [32]. Furthermore, expanded brain lesion connect with an elevated number of families of *Firmicutes* bacteria, as *Lactobacillus, Bacillus, Clostridium, Enterococcus* and *Ruminicoccus* and this homeostasis imbalance correlates with the pathophysiology of brain injury [33]. Hence, recent data in an animal model reported that the absence of the gut microbiome amplifies myelination, causes changes in brain neurochemistry, and decreases anxiety, resulting in immune damage of microglial immune response and hyperactivity of the hypothalamic–pituitary–adrenal (HPA) axis.

The microbiome-associated molecular patterns activate Toll-like receptors (TLRs). TLR2 and TLR4 signaling play a significant role in adult neuroplasticity, memory, and learning [34]. In addition, bacterial metabolites, synthesized by intestinal microbiome short-chained fatty acids or secondary bile acids, such as deoxycholic acid, modulate BBB permeability. In experimental models of TBI, administration of sodium butyrate after TBI may prevent BBB breakdown and activate neurogenesis [35]. Another hypothesis is that gut microbiota activate bone marrow-derived cells leading to inflammation and affect the kidney, central and autonomic nervous system (ANS) [36, 37]. Stimulation of the ANS by circulating signals modifies neuronal input to the kidney or intestine. The gut dysbiosis induced by an acute event leads to elevated production and accumulation of p-cresyl and indoxyl sulfates in the intestine finally disrupting the gut barrier and increasing permeability. This mechanism is connected with an influx of endotoxins and uremic toxins into the kidney, which contributes to renal inflammation and dysfunction [38–40]. Therefore, indoxyl sulfate, as a product from tryptophan metabolism, plays a role in neurodegeneration. This nephron vascular toxin significantly contributes to astrocyte inflammation and increases the oxidative stress processes in the CNS via different pathways, such as NF-κB or aryl hydrocarbon receptor (AhR) activation. The indoxyl sulfates reduce neuronal viability and elevated cell death finally predisposes to neurodegeneration and cognitive dysfunction [41]. Yang et al. documented the brain–gut–marrow axis role in blood pressure elevation, where the brain is involved in the gut–kidney axis via the sympathetic nervous system and pathways mentioned above [37]. Evidence for this theory is altered ANS in hypertension in chronic kidney diseases, increased microglial activation, and neuroinflammation in these patients [42].

Finally, there is increasing evidence that the skin microbiome has a neuromodulatory effect and that communication between the skin and the brain is very similar to the gut–brain axis. Skin dysbiosis, mostly observed in patients with chronic wounds, is connected with decreased cognitive function, anxiety and depression, similar to intestinal dysbiosis. In patients with irritable bowel syndrome (IBS), depression severity is positively correlated with an elevation in the number of mast cells infiltrating the cecal mucosa [43]. Similarly, a damaged skin barrier allows molecular and inflammatory compounds such as pathogen-associated molecular patterns (PAMPs) to enter the systemic circulation. There is evidence that skin *Psuedomonas aerugonsa* and *S. aureus* decrease tight junction permeability which decreases the physiological integrity of the skin barrier [44].

Therefore, regulation of the microbiome via eubiotic therapies, such as probiotics, microbiota transplants, and manipulation by nutrients, modulates the immune system and may present beneficial effects and exciting treatment target for TBI. Recent studies have documented that microbiota transplants reduce brain lesion size in animal models of ischemic stroke and repair microglial function [45]. Resolution of microbiome disruption in TBI by probiotics consisting of different butyrate-producing gut bacteria, such as *Bifidobacteria* or *Lactobacilli,* may potentially amplify anti-inflammatory microbiome-gut-brain axis functions and modulate mitochondrial homeostasis, improving bioenergetic function in TBI [46]. Recent preclinical trials showed that control of gut microbiome composition through probiotic supplementation within the first 48 hours following brain injury leads to reduction in gastrointestinal dysfunction, nosocomial infection, and VAP [47]. Eubiotic therapies for patients with TBI may also be beneficial through reduction of antibiotic-induced microbiome disruption, which may worsen outcomes in this group of patients. Brain–microbiome connections may also be modulated by substances with antioxidant, anti-inflammatory properties, such as metformin, baicalein and melatonin. In addition, ketamine and statins interact with gut microbiota [48].

25.5 Brain–Liver Cross-Talk

Brain–liver cross-talk is commonly known as hepatic encephalopathy, which is observed in the end-stage of liver disease. Significant disorders in blood glucose concentration resulting from dramatic liver failure impair metabolic brain function. This liver failure may be induced by brain injury and a general inflammatory response following TBI. Moreover, TBI-related rapid microglial activation results in a massive release of pro-inflammatory cytokines, which can stimulate hepatocytes to produce serum amyloid A and its circulating concentrations can increase up to 1000-fold [49, 50]. An experimental study documented the complex hepatic response to brain injury including neutrophil and macrophage infiltration to the hepatocytes, increase in serum amyloid A production and release, and hepatic cell death [50]. Interestingly, serum amyloid A plays an important role in neuroinflammation and neurodegeneration after brain injury [51]. Clinical observation showed a strong correlation between the severity of intracerebral hemorrhage, clinical condition assessed by the National Institutes of Health Stroke Score (NIHSS), poor outcome and 90-day mortality following hemorrhagic stroke [52]. An anti-inflammatory and anti-oxidative treatment may attenuate the severity of the brain–liver interaction improving outcome and reducing secondary brain injury after trauma.

25.6 Brain–Gut Cross-Talk

Stress-induced gastric ulcer is a well-known complication of TBI, which results from excessive vagus nerve activation. Many clinicians use proton pomp inhibitors and/or H_2 antagonists in the prevention of post-traumatic gastric ulcers. Gastric response effects on the brain in TBI-related stress are associated with the release of different peptides. The stable gastric pentadecapeptide BPC 157 provides the most spectacular neuromodulatory properties [53–55]. It is an anti-ulcer and anti-inflammatory peptide found in human gastric juice, and oral administration is safe [54]. It induces the release of serotonin in specific nigrostriatal regions of the brain, modulating serotoninergic, dopaminergic, GABAergic and opioid systems [55]. Additionally, BPC 157 significantly reduces demyelination and the risk of severe encephalopathy [53]. Its beneficial effects have been observed in stoke and post-traumatic neuroinflammation, somatosensory disorientation, catalepsy, depression, and different behavioral disorders [53, 54]. Therefore, the neuro-beneficial activity of BPC 157 seems to document the link between the brain and the gut and *vice versa*; however the clinical benefit of BPC 157 should be confirmed in large-scale clinical studies.

25.7 Brain–Kidney Cross-Talk

Brain injury may disturb renal function leading to hyponatremia or acute kidney injury (AKI) induced by an overly activated visceral sympathetic nervous system [56, 57]. An experimental study showed that activation of the sympathetic system following right insular cortex infarction due to right-side middle cerebral artery occlusion induced destruction of glomeruli and tubular structure with apoptosis and fibrogenesis [56]. Similar relationships were noted in clinical observations in which patients treated for right insular cortex infarction had a significantly higher risk of AKI [56]. Kidneys are densely innervated by sympathetic nerves. TBI induces release of large amounts of epinephrine and norepinephrine from renal sympathetic nerves, which bind to β1-adrenoreceptor in renal tissue inducing expression of the renin-angiotensin-aldosterone system and leading to renal contraction of afferent arterioles and renal ischemia [57, 58]. This effect seems to be confirmed in experimental studies. Kidney denervation reduces the risk of tubulointerstitial fibrosis, ischemia and inflammation, and local infusion of norepinephrine into denervated kidneys increases transforming growth factor-β1 signaling, interstitial expression of α-smooth muscle actin, and excessive deposition of extracellular collagen matrix, leading to similar pathology to that observed in innervated kidneys [56, 57]. Interestingly, β1-blockade can reduce catecholamine-induced AKI via downregulation of sympathetic activity, attenuation of glomeruli, and tubular apoptosis and fibrogenesis [55]. Therefore ultra-selective β-1 blockers, such as landiolol or esmolol, may reduce the risk of TBI-related AKI; however, this effect should be confirmed in further experimental and clinical observations. Based on the pathomechanisms of TBI-induced AKI, inotropic agents should be preferred over vasopressors. The use of levosimendan significantly reduces the incidence of AKI and the risk of initiation of renal replacement therapy (RRT) in critically ill patients [59]. Due to its beneficial effect on the neurologic stunned heart and cerebral blood flow, levosimendan may be suggested as an agent of choice in the prevention of AKI in TBI patients.

25.8 Brain–Skin and –Adipose Tissue Cross-Talk

Patients with brain injury often present with dermatological symptoms, not visible during their hospital admission. Various causes of dermatological problems have been identified, such as long hospital stay, administration of many different drugs, immobilization, and most importantly the immune status. In addition, stress intensifies chronic skin diseases, such as psoriasis, atopic dermatitis, or alopecia areata [60]. It has been observed in various studies that a neurodermatological association exists between psoriasis and depression, corresponding with immune cell activation, serotonin transporters, and hyperactivity of the HPA [61]. In a group of patients with brain damage, Lee et al. observed mycoses (especially in severe injury), seborrheic dermatitis (as the most frequent manifestation), drug-induced skin eruption, xerosis cutis, irritant contact dermatitis, and pruritus [62].

Current studies show that the CNS and the skin cross talk by various mechanisms. The modern concept of the skin as a neuroimmunoendocrine organ focuses on the interactive connection between the cutaneous peripheral nervous system, the immune system, and the neuroendocrine axis. The CNS and skin are connected directly, via efferent nerves and CNS-derived mediators, and, indirectly, by adrenal glands or immune cells [63]. In turn, the sensory nerve network releases neuropeptides, hormones, proteases, and cytokines, and modulates inflammation, immune response, and cell growth. Sensors from the skin 'talk' to the brain about pain and pruritus, by the contralateral tractus spinothalamicus and afferent sensory nerves. It is worth mentioning the important aspect of cutaneous neurogenic inflammation and the 'axon reflex' resulting in vascular responses, such as the triple response of Lewis, erythema by vasodilatation, and edema by plasma extravasation [64]. The above mentioned interactions determine different physiological effects, such as vasocontraction, vasodilatation, body temperature, barrier function, secretion, cell growth, nerve growth, and pathophysiological effects: inflammation, immunity, apoptosis, or even wound healing. Importantly, direct stimulation, by thermal, mechanical or electrical stimuli, or indirect stimulation by allergens, trauma, stress or inflammation, activates and increases the production of neuropeptides, neurotrophins, neurotransmitters, and oxygen products, such as as NO [65]. This is the reason why brain damage and its treatment predispose to steroid hormone release and alter neuromediators, leading to an abnormal immune response especially in the skin. It is worth remembering that the skin is also an area where millions of bacteria, fungi, and viruses compose the microbiota. In patients with dysbiosis, elevated wound levels of IL-6 and TNF-α were systematically increased and both cytokines were found to increase the BBB permeability and induce neuroinflammatory changes marked by reactive microgliosis [66].

The adipose tissue, which regulates energy balance, bodyweight and thermoregulation is another important puzzle in nervous system functionality. Adipokines, such as leptin, released from white fat tissue play a pivotal role in glucose homeostasis. The hypothalamus controls appetite and metabolism, by recognizing circulating hormones from the gut and adipose tissue. Importantly, activation of sympathetic pathways stimulates white adipose tissue, lipolysis, and release of fatty acids. However, special attention should be placed in the stimulatory effects of leptin on brain protein synthesis and its neuroprotective and trophic functions in the brain [67]. Brown et al. documented that in TBI patients, increasing the central adipokine gene expression may be associated with neuroinflammation and cachexia [68, 69]. In addition, leptin regulates cytokine signaling and immune responses in TBI by autocrine/paracrine pathways. Thus, gene expression silencing techniques, such as leptin, resistin, and fasting-induced adipose factor (FIAF), may become a novel therapeutic method to improve patient recovery after brain damage.

25.9 Brain–Muscle Cross-Talk

Although the CNS plays a crucial role in maintaining muscle integrity, a link between the brain and the muscles is still under investigation and not well understood. TBI significantly reduces skeletal muscle activity. Skeletal muscles secrete approximately 635 proteins including 35 growth factors, 40 cytokines and 36 metallo-peptidases, however, their biological function has been described for only 5% of them [70, 71]. All are called “myokines” or “exercise factors”, and are released into the circulation as a consequence of physical activity. The pathomechanisms of their release are associated with the activation of the calcium signaling pathway in the muscle fibers. Several of them demonstrate strong neuromodulatory activity and play an essential role in normal cerebral function [72]. Studies in humans have documented that regular exercise for a period of 3 months increased the volume of hippocampus and improved memory and learning [72, 73]. Additionally, physical activity reduces the risk of cognitive decline in healthy people and in people with neurodegenerative disorders across the life span [74]. Implementation of physical activity in critically ill patients reduces the risk of delirium and memory dysfunction, and improves muscle activity. Of note, muscular activity is a trigger to release several myokines, such as L-lactate, β-hydroxybutyrate, cathepsin-B, and irisin [70, 72, 75]. All these myokines play important roles in hippocampal neurogenesis, enhancing neuronal plasticity, which corrects memory, sleep, and mood [72]. Thus, active early rehabilitation seems to be a very important potential therapeutic option and target for people with TBI.

25.10 Conclusion

In conclusion, brain–multiorgan cross-talk is an important multidimensional interaction, which, in patients with acute brain injury, may aggravate the primary problem. Despite a large number of studies providing data on different interactions and shedding more light on complex pathomechanisms of these relationships, not all details have been well recognized. Complex interaction between distant organs and organ systems should be used as targets for specific interventions and applications of guided therapies aimed at improving outcomes for critically ill patients. Further studies are needed to explore the underlying molecular pathomechanisms to better understand these fascinating relationships that will, hopefully, lead to an improvement of care for these patients, with lower overall mortality and better functional outcomes.

References

1. Joachim RA, Kuhlmei A, Dinh QT, et al. Neuronal plasticity of the "brain-skin conncetion": stress-triggered up-regulation of neuropeptides in dorsal root ganglia and skin via nerve groeth factor-dependent pathways. J Mol Med. 2007;85:1369–78.
2. Kelly RR, Sidles SJ, LaRue AC. Effects of neurological disorders on bone health. Front Psychol. 2020;11:612366.
3. Delezie J, Handschin C. Endocrine crosstalk between skeletal muscle and the brain. Front Neurol. 2018;9:698.
4. von Bezold AV, Hirt L. Uber die physiologischen wirkungen des essigsauren veratrins. Untersuchungen aus dem Physiologischen Laboratorium Wurzburg. 1867;1:75–156.
5. Jarisch A, Richter H. Die afferenten bahnen des varatrine effekts in den herznerven. Arch Exp Pathol Pharmacol. 1939;193:355–71.
6. Lenstra JJ, Kuznecova-Keppel Hesselink L, la Bastide-van GS, et al. The association of early electrocardiographic abnormalities with brain injury severity and outcome in severe traumatic brain injury. Front Neurol. 2021;11:597737.
7. Dabrowski W, Schlegel TT, Wosko J, et al. Changes in spatial QRS-T angle and QTc interval in patients with traumatic brain injury with or without intra-abdominal hypertension. J Electrocardiol. 2018;51:499–507.
8. Dabrowski W, Siwicka-Gieroba D, Robba C, et al. Plasma hyperosmolality prolongs QTc interval and increases risk for atrial fibrillation in traumatic brain injury patients. J Clin Med. 2020;9:1293.
9. Krishnamoorthy V, Rowhani-Rahbar A, Gibbons EF, et al. Early systolic dysfunction following traumatic brain injury: a cohort study. Crit Care Med. 2017;45:1028–36.
10. Cuisinier A, Maufrais C, Payen JF, Nottin S, Walther G, Bouzat P. Myocardial function at the early phase of traumatic brain injury: a prospective controlled study. Scand J Trauma Resusc Emerg Med. 2016;24:129.
11. Siwicka-Gieroba D, Robba C, Poleszczuk J, et al. Changes in subendocardial viability ratio in traumatic brain injury patients. Brain Connect. 2021;11:349–58.

12. Krishnamoorthy V, Mackensen GB, Gibbons EF, Vavilala MS. Cardiac dysfunction after neurologic injury: what do we know and where are we going? Chest. 2016;149:1325–31.
13. Amin HZ, Amin LZ, Pradipta A. Takotsubo cardiomyopathy: a brief review. J Med Life. 2020;13:3–7.
14. Hurst RT, Prasad A, Askew JW 3rd, Sengupta PP, Tajik AJ. Takotsubo cardiomyopathy: a unique cardiomyopathy with variable ventricular morphology. JACC Cardiovasc Imaging. 2010;3:651–9.
15. Kim W, Choi KS, Lim T, et al. Prognostic value of echocardiography for left ventricular dysfunction after aneurysmal subarachnoid hemorrhage: a systematic review and meta-analysis. World Neurosurg. 2019;126:e1099–111.
16. Sugimoto K, Inamasu J, Kato Y, et al. Association between elevated plasma norepinephrine levels and cardiac wall motion abnormality in poor-grade subarachnoid hemorrhage patients. Neurosurg Rev. 2013;36:259–66.
17. Ibrahim MS, Samuel B, Mohamed W, Suchdev K. Cardiac dysfunction in neurocritical care: an autonomic perspective. Neurocrit Care. 2019;30:508–21.
18. Toru G, Tetsu K, Toshiaki N, Yoshitsugu T, Yoko M. β-Adrenoreceptors antagonists attenuate brain injury after transient focal ischemia in rats. Anesth Analg. 2006;103:658–63.
19. Kawaguchi M, Utada K, Yoshitani K, et al. Effect of a short-acting [beta]1 receptor agonist landiolol on hemodynamics and tissue injury markers in patients with subarachnoid hemorrhage undergoing intracranial aneurysm surgery. J Neurosurg Anesthesiol. 2010;22:230–9.
20. Joseph M, Ziadi S, Nates J, Dannenbaum M, Malkoff M. Increases in cardiac output can reverse flow deficits from vasospasm independent of blood pressure: study useng xenon computed tomographic measurement of cerebral blood flow. Neurosurgery. 2003;53:1044–51.
21. García-Bardon A, Kamuf J, Ziebart A, et al. Levosimendan increases brain tissue oxygen levels after cardiopulmonary resuscitation independent of cardiac function and cerebral perfusion. Sci Rep. 2021;11:14220.
22. Picetti E, Pelosi P, Taccone FS, et al. VENTILatOry strategies in patients with severe traumatic brain injury: the VENTILO survey of the European Society of Intensive Care Medicine (ESICM). Crit Care. 2020;24:158.
23. Li Y, Liu C, Xiao W, Song T, Wang S. Incidence, risk factors, and outcomes of ventilator-associated pneumonia in traumatic brain injury: a meta-analysis. Neurocrit Care. 2020;32:272–85.
24. Mascia L. Acute lung injury in patients with severe brain injury: a double hit model. Neurocrit Care. 2009;11:417–26.
25. Zhao J, Xuan NX, Cui W, Tian BP. Neurogenic pulmonary edema following acute stroke: the progress and perspective. Biomed Pharmacother. 2020;130:110478.
26. Ashley SL, Sjoding MW, Popova AP, et al. Lung and gut microbiota are altered by hyperoxia and contribute to oxygen-induced lung injury in mice. Sci Transl Med. 2020;12:eaau9959.
27. Lee S, Hwang H, Yamal JM, et al. IMPACT probability of poor outcome and plasma cytokine concentrations are associated with multiple organ dysfunction syndrome following traumatic brain injury. J Neurosurg. 2019;131:1931–7.
28. Battaglini D, Siwicka-Gieroba D, Rocco PR, et al. Novel synthetic and natural therapies for traumatic brain injury. Curr Neuropharmacol. 2021;19:1661–87.
29. Braniste V, Al-Asmakh M, Kowal C, et al. The gut microbiota influences blood-brain barrier permeability in mice. Sci Transl Med. 2014;6:263ra158.
30. Lepage P, Leclerc MC, Joossens M, et al. A metagenomic insight into our gut's microbiome. Gut. 2013;62:146–58.
31. Li Z, Zeng G, Zheng X, et al. Neuroprotective effect of formononetin against TBI in rats via suppressing inflammatory reaction in cortical neurons. Biomed Pharmacother. 2018;106:349–54.
32. Hang CH, Shi JX, Li JS, Wu W, Yin HX. Alterations of intestinal mucosa structure and barrier function following traumatic brain injury in rats. World J Gastroenterol. 2003;9:2776–81.
33. Bansal V, Costantini T, Kroll L, et al. Traumatic brain injury and intestinal dysfunction: uncovering the neuro-enteric axis. J Neurotrauma. 2009;26:1353–9.

34. Lathia JD, Okun ET, Griffioen SC, et al. Toll-like receptor 3 is a negative regulator of embryonic neural progenitor cell proliferation. J Neurosci. 2008;28:13978–84.
35. Li H, Sun J, Wang F, et al. Sodium butyrate exerts neuroprotective effects by restoring the blood-brain barrier in traumatic brain injury mice. Brain Res. 2016;1642:70–8.
36. Santisteban MM, Ahmari N, Carvajal JM, et al. Involvement of bone marrow cells and neuroinflammation in hypertension. Circ Res. 2015;117:178–91.
37. Yang TA-O, Richards EM, Pepine CA-OX, Raizada MK. The gut microbiota and the brain-gut-kidney axis in hypertension and chronic kidney disease. Nat Rev Nephrol. 2018;14:442–56.
38. Aronov PA, Luo FJG, Plummer NS, Quan Z, Holmes S, Hostetter TH, Meyer TW. Colonic contribution to uremic solutes. J Am Soc Nephrol. 2011;22:1769–76.
39. Sirich TL, Plummer NS, Gardner CD, Hostetter TH, Meyer TW. Effect of increasing dietary fiber on plasma levels of colon-derived solutes in hemodialysis patients. Clin J Am Soc Nephrol. 2014;9:1603–10.
40. Felizardo RJ, Castoldi A, Andrade-Oliveira V, Câmara NO. The microbiota and chronic kidney diseases: a double-edged sword. Transl Immunol. 2016;5:e86.
41. Sun CY, Li JR, Wang YY, et al. Indoxyl sulfate caused behavioral abnormality and neurodegeneration in mice with unilateral nephrectomy. Aging (Albany NY). 2021;13:6681–701.
42. Shi P, Grobe JL, Desland FA, et al. Direct pro-inflammatory effects of prorenin on microglia. PLoS One. 2014;9:e92937.
43. Piche TSPM, Dainese R, Marine-Barjoan E, et al. Mast cells and cellularity of the colonic mucosa correlated with fatigue and depression in irritable bowel syndrome. Gut. 2008;57:468–73.
44. Bäsler K, Galliano MF, Bergmann S, et al. Biphasic influence of Staphylococcus aureus on human epidermal tight junctions. Ann N Y Acad Sci. 2017;1405:53–70.
45. Singh V, Roth S, Llovera G, et al. Microbiota dysbiosis controls the neuroinflammatory response after stroke. J Neurosci. 2016;36:7428–40.
46. Ma Y, Liu T, Fu J, et al. Lactobacillus acidophilus exerts neuroprotective effects in mice with traumatic brain injury. J Nutr. 2019;149:1543–52.
47. Zhao J, Li LQ, Chen CY, Zhang GS, Cui W, Tian BP. Do probiotics help prevent ventilator-associated pneumonia in critically ill patients? A systematic review with meta-analysis. ERJ Open Res. 2021;7:00302–2020.
48. Dabrowski W, Siwicka-Gieroba D, Kotfis K, Zaid S, Terpilowska S, Robba C, Siwicki AK. The brain-gut axis-where are we now and how can we modulate these connections? Curr Neuropharmacol. 2021;19:1164–77.
49. Jensen LE, Whitehead AS. Regulation of serum amyloid a protein expression during the acute-phase response. Biochem J. 1998;334:489–503.
50. Villapol S, Kryndushkin D, Balarezo MG, et al. Hepatic expression of serum amyloid A1 is induced by traumatic brain injury and modulated by telmisartan. Am J Pathol. 2015;185:2641–52.
51. Wicker E, Benton L, George K, Furlow W, Villapol S. Serum amyloid a protein as a potential biomarker for severity and acute outcome in traumatic brain injury. Biomed Res Int. 2019;2019:5967816.
52. Huangfu XQ, Wang LG, Le AD, Tao B. Utility of serum amyloid a as a potential prognostic biomarker of acute primary basal ganglia hemorrhage. Clin Chim Acta. 2020;505:43–8.
53. Sikiric P, Seiwerth S, Rucman R, et al. Stress in gastrointestinal tract and stable gastric pentadecapeptide BPC 157. Finally, do we have a solution? Curr Pharm Des. 2017;23:4012–28.
54. Vukojevic J, Milavic M, Perovic D, Ilic S, Cilic AZ, Duran N. Pentadecapeptide BPC 157 and the central nervous system. Neural Regen Res. 2022;17:482–7.
55. Sikiric P, Jelovac N, Jelovac-Gjeldum A, et al. Pentadecapeptide BPC 157 attenuates chronic amphetamine-induced behaviour disturbances. Acta Pharmacol Sin. 2002;23:412–22.
56. Cai Y, Lu X, Cheng X, Lv Q, Xu G, Liu X. Increased renal dysfunction, apoptosis and fibrogenesis through sympathetic hyperactivity after focal cerebral infarction. Transl Stroke Res. 2021. May 12. https://doi.org/10.1007/s12975-021-00900-w. Epub ahead of print.

57. Jang HS, Kim J, Padanilam BJ. Renal sympathetic nerve activation Vis alpha2-adrenergic receptors in chronic kidney progression. Kidney Res Clin Pract. 2019;38:6–14.
58. Kim J, Padanilam BJ. Renal denervation prevents long-term sequele of ischemic renal injury. Kidney Int. 2015;87:350–8.
59. Bove T, Matteazzi A, Belletti A, et al. Beneficial impact of levosimendan in critically ill patients with or at risk for acute renal failure: a meta-analysis of randomized control trials. Heart Lung Vessel. 2015;7:35–46.
60. Pondeljak N, Lugović-Mihić L. Stress-induced interaction of skin immune cells, hormones, and neurotransmitters. Clin Therap. 2020;42:757–70.
61. Maqbool S, Ihtesham A, Langove MN, Jamal S, Jamal T, Safian HA. Neuro-dermatological association between psoriasis and depression: an immune-mediated inflammatory process validating skin-brain axis theory. AIMS Neurosci. 2021;8:340–54.
62. Lee J, Hwang S-H, Park J-H, Kim W-S. Dermatological conditions in patients with brain damage. Dermatol Sin. 2014;32:133–6.
63. Slominski A. Neuroendocrine system of the skin. Dermatology. 2005;211:199–208.
64. Roosterman D, Goerge T, Schneider SW, Bunnett NW, Steinhoff M. Neuronal control of skin function: the skin as a neuroimmunoendocrine organ. Physiol Rev. 2006;86:1309–79.
65. Basso L, Serhan N, Tauber M, Gaudenzio N. Peripheral neurons: master regulators of skin and mucosal immune response. Eur J Immunol. 2019;49:1984–97.
66. Zhang J, Sadowska GB, Chen X, et al. Anti-IL-6 neutralizing antibody modulates blood-brain barrier function in the ovine fetus. FASEB J. 2015;29:1739–53.
67. Dicou E, Attoub S, Gressens P. Neuroprotective effects of leptin in vivo and in vitro. Neuro Rep. 2001;12:3947–51.
68. Wilkinson M, Brown R, Imran SA, Ur E. Adipokine gene expression in brain and pituitary gland. Neuroendocrinology. 2007;86:191–209.
69. Brown R, Thompson HJ, Imran SA, Ur E, Wilkinson M. Traumatic brain injury induces adipokine gene expression in rat brain. Neurosci Lett. 2008;432:73–8.
70. Henningsen J, Rigbolt KT, Blagoev B, Pedersen BK, Kratchmarova I. Dynamics of the skeletal muscle secretome during myoblast differentiation. Mol Cell Proteomics. 2010;9:2482–96.
71. Khan SU, Ghafoor S. Myokines: discovery challenges and therapeutic impediments. J Pak Med Assoc. 2019;69:1014–7.
72. Delezie J, Handschin C. Endocrine crosstalk between skeletal muscle and the brain. Front Neurol. 2018;24:698.
73. Pajonk FG, Wobrock T, Gruber O, et al. Hippocampal plasticity in response to exercise in schizophrenia. Arch Gen Psychiatry. 2010;67:133–43.
74. Voss MW, Nagamatsu LS, Liu-Ambrose T, Kramer AF. Exercise, brain and cognition across the life span. J Appl Physiol. 2011;111:1505–13.
75. Tipping CJ, Harrold M, Holland A, Romero L, Nisbet T, Hodgson CL. The effect of active mobilisation and rehabilitation in ICU on mortality and function: a systematic review. Intensive Care Med. 2017;43:171–83.

The Importance of Neuromonitoring in Non Brain Injured Patients

26

D. Battaglini, P. Pelosi, and C. Robba

26.1 Introduction

The use of non-invasive neuromonitoring in patients without brain injury has increased over the past decades [1]. Most common clinical applications of non-invasive neuromonitoring in the non-neurological setting include the study of patients without primary brain injury but with a potential for neurological derangement. These clinical conditions include liver failure, post-cardiac arrest syndrome, severe respiratory failure with or without extracorporeal membrane oxygenation (ECMO) or extracorporeal carbon dioxide removal ($ECCO_2R$), polytrauma, stroke, sepsis, pregnancy, pediatric population, and the surgical population in the perioperative period [1]. In recent years, a growing literature has suggested the use of non-invasive techniques in this population, and these are becoming increasingly popular among general critical care physicians for daily and bedside patient management [1, 2]. The aim of this chapter is to provide anesthesiologists and intensivists with an up-to-date view of the most frequent clinical conditions with potential for neurological complications in patients without brain injury, and to describe the role of non-invasive multimodal neuromonitoring in the early identification and management of these complex scenarios.

D. Battaglini
Anesthesia and Critical Care, San Martino Policlinico Hospital, IRCCS for Oncology and Neuroscience, Genoa, Italy

Department of Medicine, University of Barcelona, Barcelona, Spain

P. Pelosi · C. Robba (✉)
Anesthesia and Critical Care, San Martino Policlinico Hospital, IRCCS for Oncology and Neuroscience, Genoa, Italy

Department of Surgical Science and Integrated Diagnostics, University of Genoa, Genoa, Italy
e-mail: chiara_robba@unige.it

J.-L. Vincent (ed.), *Annual Update in Intensive Care and Emergency Medicine 2022*, Annual Update in Intensive Care and Emergency Medicine,
https://doi.org/10.1007/978-3-030-93433-0_26

26.2 Basics of Neuromonitoring in Anesthesia and Critical Care

In this paragraph, we will introduce the most commonly used non-invasive neuromonitoring tools in anesthesia and in the critical care settings. However, a detailed description of each neuromonitoring system is beyond the aim of the present manuscript, and the reader should refer to the dedicated literature.

Table 26.1 presents the methodology, strengths, and limitations of the main neuromonitoring techniques (electroencephalography [EEG], processed EEG [pEEG], somatosensory evoked potentials [SSEPs] and motor-sensory potentials [MEPs], transcranial Doppler [TCD], optic nerve sheath diameter [ONSD], pupillometry, and near-infrared spectroscopy [NIRS]).

26.3 Clinical Applications

26.3.1 Neuromonitoring in the Operating Room

Intraoperative and postoperative neurological complications, such as delirium, postoperative cognitive decline, stroke, spinal cord ischemia, and postoperative visual loss, are frequently underestimated [2]. These complications have the potential to increase mortality and morbidity and should therefore be promptly identified and prevented [2]. Some types of surgery are more susceptible than others to cerebral complications. In major vascular surgery, registries have reported an intra/postoperative stroke rate of 7% after carotid stenting and of 3.2% after endarterectomy [3]. During aortic procedures, the T4-T8 segment is particularly susceptible to reduced blood perfusion, because of the variable location of the radiculomedullary arteries and of the artery of Adamkiewicz; this may influence pathological processes and the metabolic state of the tissue during aortic surgery, thus causing paralysis in the worst cases [3]. During thoracic aorta surgery, following the circulatory arrest with consequent transient ischemia, an early phase of parenchymal hypoperfusion is present, with consequent systemic inflammation and possible reperfusion injury. This results in a potential for severe temporary or permanent neurologic dysfunction including possible ischemic stroke, prolonged obtundation, disorientation, Parkinson-like movements, and loss of cognitive function [3, 4].

Similarly, in cardiac surgery, neuronal and vascular damage, inflammation, and embolism may result in inadequate oxygen delivery to the brain and altered cerebral autoregulation, predisposing to neurological complications [4]. Indeed, neurocognitive dysfunction, including postoperative delirium, effects up to 50% of patients after cardiac surgery, with stroke affecting 2%, and postoperative neurocognitive dysfunction up to 42% [4].

In addition, neurological complications can also occur following non-high-risk surgery. Some trials have revealed that use of adequate neuromonitoring during anesthesia can prevent or limit the occurrence of adverse effects [2]. Standard monitoring during anesthesia includes mainly hemodynamic and respiratory parameters

Table 26.1 Basic functioning of different neuromonitoring devices

Type	Methodology	Strengths (S) and limitations (L)	Action of medications
EEG	EEG gives information about cortical activity Global information Scalp electrodes	S: Global information of cerebral activity L: EEG trace needs experienced operators for interpretation	Ketamine increases the activity of excitatory neurons and high frequency oscillations Nitrous oxide increases the amplitude of high frequency activity Dexmedetomidine causes slow oscillations with deeper sedation but easily awakened patient Propofol increases theta, alpha, spindle beta power, slow waves and delta activity
pEEG	Translation between analogic signal of EEG to digital (numeric). Awake status = 100; general anesthesia = 40–60; suppressed EEG = 0 Regional information Adhesive pads DSA is a colored trace obtained from EEG frequencies and transformed into decibels of bi-hemispheric activity that can change from red (more frequent) to blue (rare)	S: Bedside application S: Easy interpretation S: Availability L: Muscle artifact L: Translation between analogic signal of EEG to digital L: Delay between event and measure L: Cerebral activity in limited area (frontal) L: Several noisy elements can interfere with the signal L: Effects of medications L: Validation in non-older adults	Ketamine increases the activity of excitatory neurons and high frequency oscillations Nitrous oxide increases the amplitude of high frequency activity Dexmedetomidine causes slow oscillations with deeper sedation but easily awakened patient Propofol induces slow waves, until suppressed pEEG with increases in dosage Sevoflurane effects on BIS are unclear

(continued)

Table 26.1 (continued)

Type	Methodology	Strengths (S) and limitations (L)	Action of medications
SSEPs	SSEPs measured by stimulating a peripheral sensory nerve and recording the signal transmitted to the sensory cortex Bedside application	S: Bedside application S: Availability L: Interference with electric devices L: Interpretation by expert	Ketamine increases cortical SSEP amplitude Dexmedetomidine affects amplitude minimally Propofol has minimal effects on SSEPs. Sevoflurane affects SSEPs in a dose-dependent way Barbiturates increase latency and decrease amplitude of SSEPs Benzodiazepines reduce amplitude and increase latency. Opioids do not significantly affect SSEPs, but remifentanil prolongs SSEP latency
MEPs	MEPs measured by transcranial stimulation of the cortex and recording the signal at the spinal cord level, peripheral motor nerves, or the muscles	S: Bedside application S: Availability L: Interference with electric devices L: Interpretation by expert equipment	Ketamine increases amplitude at increased frequency of MEPs Dexmedetomidine causes a decrease in MEP amplitude Propofol has excitatory effects on MEPs Sevoflurane has a depressant effect on MEPs Benzodiazepines attenuate MEPs
TCD	Investigation of local blood flow and velocities in the circle of Willis 2 mHz probe placed in acoustic windows (i.e., transtemporal) Measure of nICP and eCPP Cerebral autoregulation Critical closing pressure Diastolic closing margin Midline shift Emboli, obstruction, stenosis	S: Bedside application S: Availability L: Need for experienced operators L: Availability of windows	Ketamine may affect cerebral hemodynamics Propofol decreases the tone of the venous capacitance vessels and decreases cerebral metabolism Remifentanil reduces cerebral blood flow velocity despite constant perfusion pressure Thiopental decreases CBF velocities Benzodiazepines decrease CBF velocity

ONSD	Measure of nICP and eCPP	S: Bedside application S: Easy interpretation S: Availability	ONSD is larger with propofol in comparison to sevoflurane
Pupillometry	Pupillometry measures the diameter of the pupils and the pupillary light reflex NPi is an algorithm using parameters to determine pupillary light response, with a scale 0–5, <3 is abnormal Maximum and minimum pupil diameter (mm) refers to diameter at rest and peak constriction Latency is the time (seconds) delay between light stimulus and pupillary constriction CV is the distance (mm) of constriction divided by duration (seconds) of constriction Dilation velocity is the distance (mm) of re-dilation divided by duration (seconds) of re-dilation	S: Bedside application S: Easy interpretation S: Availability L: Agitated or confused patients can be difficult to evaluate L: Patients with scleral edema, periorbital edema, intraocular lens replacement prior ocular surgical procedures can limit assessment with pupillometry L: Ambient light can influence the measure L: Expensive	Remifentanil determines miosis and reduces PLR Propofol determines miosis and reduces CV Barbiturate titrated to burst suppression reduces CV Droperidol causes miosis and reduces PDR Metoclopramide causes miosis and reduces PDR

(continued)

Table 26.1 (continued)

Type	Methodology	Strengths (S) and limitations (L)	Action of medications
NIRS	NIRS measures cerebral oxygen saturation by using a near-infrared light passing through adhesive pads and tissues. The light is therefore adsorbed by oxyhemoglobin and deoxyhemoglobin, thus obtaining a value reflecting the local amount of oxygen within the frontal region A decrease of 20% from baseline can be associated to the reduction of CBF, hypoperfusion and neurologic symptoms Regional measure Adhesive pads Various devices are available with different algorithms and components, including Masimo (Masimo Corp., Irvine, CA), INVOS (Medtronic, Minneapolis, USA)	S: Bedside application S: Easy interpretation S: Availability L: Regional evaluation of cerebral oximetry that may not reflect global changes in hemodynamics L: Bias with skin color and gender L: Variations due to systemic extracranial perfusion L: Elimination of oxygen degradation products in patients with liver diseases that can alter the absorption of light	Propofol and dexmedetomidine equally preserve cerebral oxygenation and do not affect neurological outcome Cerebral oxygenation may be better preserved with sevoflurane than propofol Midazolam and morphine may alter cerebral oxygenation and hemodynamics

EEG electroencephalogram, *pEEG* processed EEG, *BIS* Bispectral index, *DSA* density spectral array, *ONSD* optic nerve sheath diameter, *CBF* cerebral blood flow, *SSEPs* somatosensory evoked potentials, *MEPs* motor sensory evoked potentials, *TCD* transcranial Doppler, *nICP* non-invasive intracranial pressure, *eCPP* estimated cerebral perfusion pressure, *CV* constriction velocity, *NPi* Neurological Pupil index, *PLR* pupillary light reflex, *PRD* pupillary reflex dilation among essential minimum monitoring data [5]. However, the primary targets of anesthetics and analgesics are the central and peripheral nervous systems [2]. It seems logical to assume that this ironic clinical gap in standards of monitoring during anesthesia deserves further revision, or at least should be individualized and implemented in case of predisposing comorbidities, perioperative events, and high-risk procedures [2].

In this section, we describe the most common clinical scenarios for potential of brain injury in the operating room and the utility of each neuromonitoring system in the early identification of such devasting complications. Table 26.2 resumes the most common clinical applications of neuromonitoring in the operating room.

Table 26.2 Clinical application of neuromonitoring in the operating room

Type of surgery/procedure	Neurological complications	Neuromonitoring	Evidence
Major vascular surgery	Stroke, delirium, cognitive decline, paralysis	EEG or pEEG	Beta bands, slow background, reduction of amplitude on EEG, reduction of BIS on pEEG are signs of ischemia (carotid surgery)
		Evoked potentials	Abnormalities in the SSEPs of median and tibial nerves if hypoperfusion (carotid surgery). MEPs correlate with NIRS
		TCD	TCD can allow detection of stenosis, turbulence, and emboli (carotid surgery)
		NIRS	Cerebral $rSO_2 < 70\%$ is indicative of possible hypoperfusion (carotid surgery), lumbar $rSO_2 < 75\%$ for 15 min can cause spinal cord injury (aortic repair)
Cardiac surgery	Delirium, cognitive dysfunction, stroke	EEG or pEGG	Long-term EEG burst suppression is associated with cognitive dysfunction and delirium. Decrease in alpha and beta waves is indicative of tissue hypoperfusion
		Evoked potentials	Help in the detection of ischemia, not specific
		TCD	TCD can detect changes in CBF, microemboli, flow asymmetries
		NIRS	An rSO_2 value which falls by 10–20% or < 50% is associated with postoperative complications. The threshold of $rSO_2 > 80\%$ prevents complications
Abdominal surgery	Neurological deterioration, intracranial hypertension	TCD	TCD can allow non-invasive calculation of ICP, identification of changes in CBF due to high ICP or carbon-dioxide vasodilatation
Orthopedic surgery	Cerebral deoxygenation	NIRS	Cerebral rSO_2 monitoring can prevent cerebral deoxygenation and neurological complications

EEG electroencephalogram, *pEEG* processed EEG, *TCD* transcranial Doppler; *NIRS* near infrared spectroscopy, *BIS* Bispectral index, *rSO_2* regional saturation of oxygen, *MEPs* motor evoked potentials, *SSEPs* sensory evoked potentials, *CBF* cerebral blood flow, *ICP* intracranial pressure

26.3.1.1 Electroencephalography

pEEG monitoring was primarily introduced into the operating room to reduce the risk of awareness during surgery, to optimize anesthetic titration, and to individualize the depth of anesthesia [6]. The main raw traces identified by pEEG are shown in Fig. 26.1, panel A, while an example of a density spectral array (DSA) trace is presented in Fig. 26.1, panel B. In 2017, the European Society of Anesthesiology (ESA) produced a consensus suggesting that all patients undergoing surgery should have anesthesia depth monitored [7]. EEG responses to anesthesia depend on the interaction between surgical stimulus, sedatives, and anesthetic plane. The phase of induction of anesthesia is characterized by an increase in beta activity (13–30 Hz), followed by the maintenance phase which is characterized by an increase of alpha (8–12 Hz) and delta (0–4 Hz) activities, while during the emergence phase, a reverse order of frequencies appears. A numeric index between 40–60, which is the result of the integration of the raw signals, is recommended to avoid awareness and excessive sedation [2].

The use of pEEG devices has been validated to reduce awareness in patients receiving volatile anesthetics with a minimum alveolar concentration (MAC) value <0.7, and during total intravenous anesthesia [2]. Moreover, pEEG may reduce drug consumption, thus reducing the incidence of postoperative nausea and vomiting and facilitating extubation and earlier discharge [2]. The intraoperative use of pEEG has been shown to reduce the incidence of delirium, cognitive dysfunction, and ischemic stroke in the postoperative period [2].

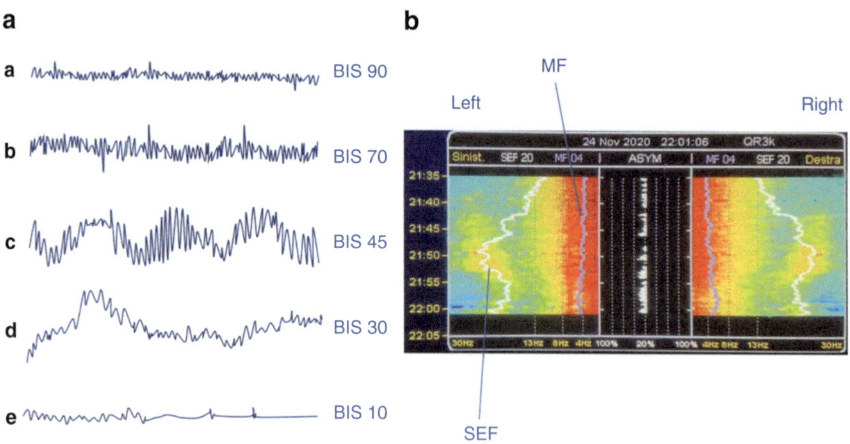

Fig. 26.1 Processed electroencephalography (pEEG). The main raw traces identified by pEEG are shown in Panel A: (**a**) small amplitude, fast frequency wave (patient awake), (**b**) moderate sedation, (**c**) large amplitude, slow frequency wave (general anesthesia), (**d**) slow oscillations (deep anesthesia), (**e**) isoelectric trace and burst suppression. The density spectral array (DSA), a colored trace obtained from EEG and transformed into decibels of bi-hemispheric activity that can change from red (highest powers) to blue (lowest powers), is shown in Panel B. The white line in the DSA represents the spectral edge frequency (SEF) (in Hertz); 95% of the power of the brain resides below that line. The purple line in the DSA in the median frequency (MF). *BIS* bispectral index

In major vascular surgery settings, the presence of beta bands, a decrease of more than 50% of background activity, a reduction in amplitude of 60%, an increase in delta and slow wave activities, or a complete loss of signal is highly suggestive for ischemic complications [8]. Of note, during carotid endarterectomy, changes in cerebral blood flow (CBF) frequently reflect on the EEG within 20–30 s after clamping [3]. When using pEEG, a reduction in bispectral index (BIS) value has also been correlated to ischemia and neurological deficit [9].

In cardiac surgery, long-term EEG burst suppression has been associated with postoperative neurocognitive dysfunction and delirium [4], while decreased alpha and beta waves can be indicative of a CBF < 22 ml/100 g brain tissue/minute, and further reduction to 7-to-15 ml/100 g/min can result in an isoelectric EEG [4]. However, a recent large randomized controlled trial (RCT) did not support the use of EEG-guided anesthetic administration for the prevention of postoperative delirium in major surgery [10]. EEG or pEEG monitoring might also be useful to detect and avoid periods of burst suppression, which have been associated with postoperative delirium. However, evidence is still lacking on this topic [4].

26.3.1.2 Evoked Potentials

Evoked potentials are restricted to specific procedures, since their use often requires dedicated equipment and training. During carotid endarterectomy, hypoperfusion of the middle cerebral and anterior cerebral arteries could be detected by abnormalities in the SSEP signal at the median and tibial nerves [3]. Information from evoked potentials has the advantage of being objective and providing quantitative information on neurological complications, but during surgery the signal may be modified by general anesthetics, and in particular volatile agents. SSEPs may also have high false-positive rates (40–67%) and a moderate false-negative (13%) rate, and a delayed response for spinal cord ischemia. Indeed, during aortic surgery, the blood flow is more often compromised in the anterior motor tract than in the sensory dorsal column, and the limited ability of evoked potentials to detect altered motor function during ischemia in case of isolated spinal injury becomes even more worrisome [11].

26.3.1.3 Transcranial Doppler

TCD flows of the main intracranial arteries are shown in Fig. 26.2. There are still no clear indications for TCD in the perioperative setting, but some authors have suggested its use during liver transplant for the detection of cerebral complications and in particular brain edema [12]. During pneumoperitoneum and the Trendelenburg position, TCD can also be considered for the detection of episodes of high intracranial pressure (ICP) [13] following increases in carbon dioxide (CO_2) that can result in cerebral vasodilatation [14].

The beach chair position is a technique used for shoulder surgery, which has shown to put the patient at risk of neurological complications as it may decrease cerebral perfusion due to blood pressure fall [15]. Moreover, major orthopedic surgery is a discipline at high risk of microembolic complications and TCD may help in the early diagnosis of embolic stroke in the perioperative period [16].

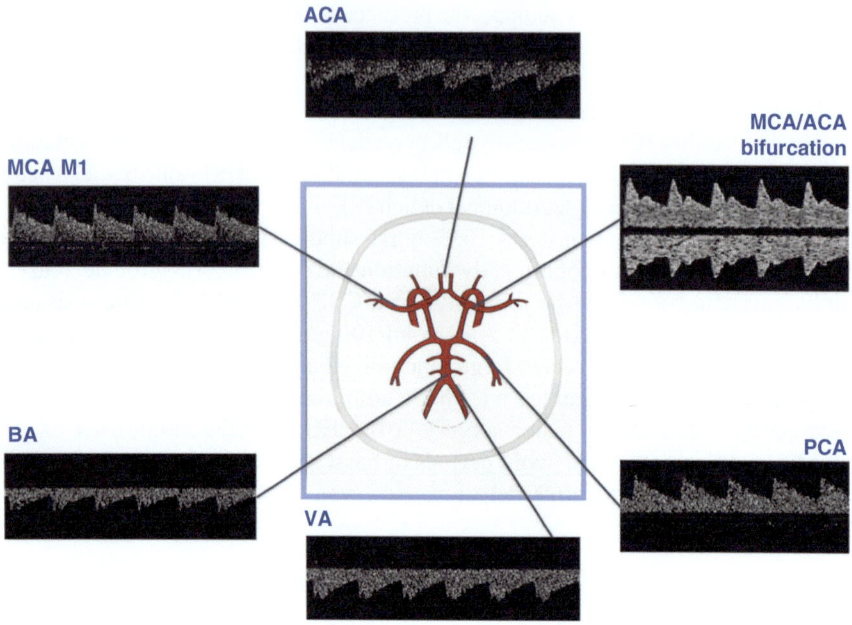

Fig. 26.2 Transcranial Doppler monitoring. The circle of Willis is represented in red with specific transcranial color Doppler sonographic images for each intracranial artery. *MCA* mean cerebral artery, *PCA* posterior cerebral artery, *ACA* anterior cerebral artery, *VA* vertebral artery, *BA* basilar artery

TCD in major vascular surgery can detect isolated arterial stenosis, which results in focal velocity increase and turbulence, inadequate collateral flow after proximal carotid cross-clamping by detecting compromised flow, and high-intensity signals at the Doppler spectral waveforms that can be indicative of emboli [17].

Finally, TCD is frequently used in cardiac surgery to detect changes in flow velocities and flow asymmetries and can be a valid option to assess anterograde cerebral perfusion during aortic arch surgery and for the detection of high-intensity signals related to microemboli [18, 19].

26.3.1.4 Near-Infrared Spectroscopy

NIRS can provide important information on changes in cerebral oxygenation during the perioperative period, but NIRS signals can be modified by anesthetics and sedatives. In orthopedic surgery, NIRS has been used together with TCD during the beach chair position to prevent cerebral deoxygenation with good effect [16], but its use is specifically recommended in major vascular and cardiac surgery [4, 20].

In carotid surgery, a regional cerebral oxygen saturation (rSO_2) of <70% (50 to 75%) has been suggested as a possible indicator of hypoperfusion, and in patients undergoing aortic repair, a lumbar rSO_2 of <75% for 15 min predicted the

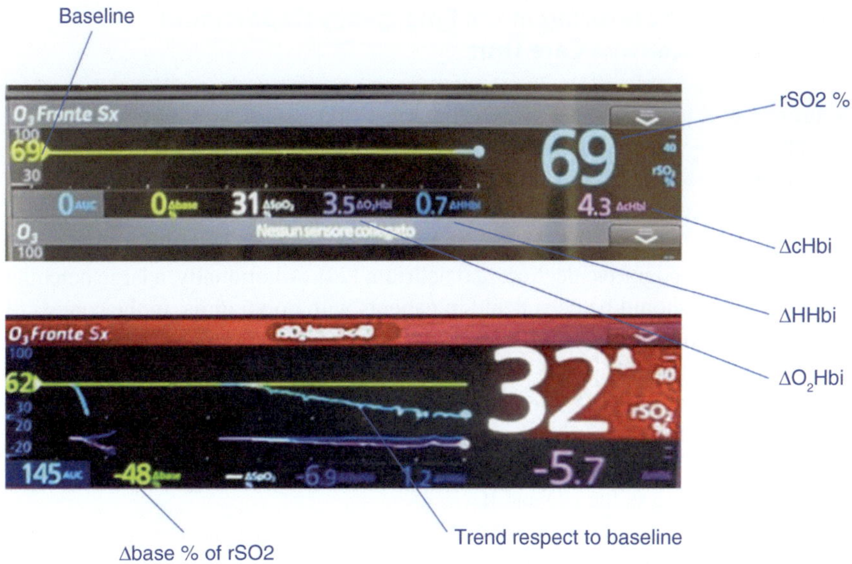

Fig. 26.3 Near infrared spectroscopy. This figure represents two possible traces, one with normal values and the other with abrupt decrease in regional oxygen saturation (rSO_2) values. *ΔO_2Hbi* index associated with variation of the oxygenated component of the hemoglobin in the total calculation of rSO_2 (arterial component of rSO_2), *ΔHHbi* an index associated with variation of the deoxygenated component of hemoglobin within the total calculation of rSO_2 (venous component of rSO_2), *ΔcHbi* is the sum of $\Delta HHbi+\Delta O_2Hbi$. SpO_2 - rSO_2 is the difference between the value of peripheral saturation of oxygen (SpO_2) and rSO_2

development of spinal cord injury [4, 20]. The sensitivity of NIRS in detecting cerebral ischemia is 60–100% with good specificity (94–98%) [20], although neurological monitoring and awake anesthesia remain the gold standard [21].

NIRS has also been recommended in cardiac surgery, both in the preoperative and intraoperative periods, to detect patients at higher risk of neurological complications and to identify episodes of acute cerebral hypoperfusion, which are common in these settings [22]. Cerebral oximetry should be cautiously interpreted, considering the baseline values and its trend, as well as preoperative patient status [22]. A recent meta-analysis assessing preoperative rSO_2 values in cardiac surgery found a reference range of between 51% and 82%, with a mean baseline value of 66% [23]. According to the literature, intervention is needed when the rSO_2 values decrease by 10–20% from baseline or below the absolute value of 50%; moreover, the time spent with $rSO_2 < 50\%$ is significantly associated with the occurrence of postoperative delirium during coronary artery bypass graft surgery [23].

Fig. 26.3 shows an example of cerebral oximetry using the Masimo (Masimo Corp., Irvine, CA) device.

26.3.2 Neuromonitoring in the Emergency Department and Intensive Care Unit

Neuromonitoring in the emergency department (ED) and ICU might be a valuable complement to clinical diagnosis and diagnostic images in patients without primary brain injury who are at risk of cerebral hemodynamic impairment [24]. Neurological impairment is common in patients admitted to the ED and ICU with sepsis, metabolic, renal, or hepatic diseases, and intoxication as these conditions can cause encephalopathy, cognitive decline, and delirium [24]. Additionally, a large potential for brain injury should be considered in patients with polytrauma, in the context of focused assessment with sonography in trauma (FAST) [25, 26].

Despite the diagnostic and prognostic potentiality of non-invasive multimodal neuromonitoring in the ED, use of these techniques is still limited in these settings, and they are currently more frequently adopted in post-emergency settings after ICU admission. Table 26.3 resumes some of the most common clinical applications of neuromonitoring in the ED and ICU.

26.3.2.1 Electroencephalography

EEG is mainly used in the ED for the early diagnosis of first-time seizures that are often caused by non-primary brain injury, such as with systemic fever and metabolic disturbances [27]. The utility of pEEG in the ED has been poorly investigated, but it may potentially be used in patients who need sedation for various reasons, to assess the occurrence of burst suppression, to help in the induction of anesthesia, and to monitor brain activity for any causes [9, 28, 29].

In the ICU setting, in addition to the detection of seizures or status epilepticus, one of the main applications of EEG is in the assessment of patient prognosis [30], in particular with the detection of a suppressed EEG in case of vegetative state and electrocerebral silence in brain death [31]. This is particularly useful in cardiac arrest patients [31].

In patients receiving ECMO, EEG has shown to be useful in the identification of patients at risk for neurological complications and to predict poor outcome, by the identification of specific patterns, such as suppression [32] and absence of EEG reactivity [33]. Abnormal background abnormalities have also been demonstrated to be common EEG features of patients with coronavirus disease 2019 (COVID-19), with an incidence of 96%, while epileptiform discharges were present in 20% of patients [34].

26.3.2.2 Evoked Potentials

Evoked potentials are frequently used for neuroprognostication in specific diseases (e.g., traumatic brain injury [TBI], cardiac arrest) as part of multimodality algorithms that include clinical examination, electrophysiologic testing, imaging, and laboratory markers (e.g., serum enolase) [31]. Following cardiac arrest, SSEPs are still considered a cornerstone of prognostic algorithms, especially when delayed 48–72 after cardiac arrest [31]. Typical patterns of SSEPs in the median nerve following cardiac arrest include: bilaterally negative N20, which is indicative of death

Table 26.3 Clinical application of neuromonitoring in the emergency department and intensive care unit

Setting	Neurological complications	Neuromonitoring	Evidence
Cardiac arrest	Neurological outcome	EEG or pEEG	Prognostication after cardiac arrest
		Evoked potentials	Prognostication after cardiac arrest (SSEPs) after 48–72 h
		TCD	Detection of CBF abnormalities and intracranial hypertension
		Pupillometry	Prognostication after cardiac arrest
Brain death	Diagnosis	EEG or pEGG	Electrocerebral silence
		TCD	Detection of flow inversion, intracranial hypertension. Ancillary test
		Pupillometry	No response
ECMO	Neurological outcome	EEG or pEGG	Prognostication in patients receiving ECMO
		TCD	CBF alterations, stroke
		NIRS	Association with neurological injury
ARDS and COVID-19 ARDS	Neurological complications, delirium	EEG or pEGG	Typical EEG includes abnormal background, epileptiform discharges in only 20%
		TCD	Pulmonary shunt, microemboli, CBF alterations, cerebral autoregulation
		NIRS	To detect brain deoxygenation, and responses to hemodynamic and respiratory maneuvers
		Pupillometry	Inconclusive evidence
Liver diseases	Encephalopathy	TCD	High resistances on TCD, CBF alterations
		NIRS	Association with outcome
		Pupillometry	Pupillary abnormalities are associated with neurological complications
Kidney disease	Encephalopathy	TCD	CBF alterations
		NIRS	Association with outcome
Sepsis	Encephalopathy	TCD	High resistances on TCD, altered CBF, high PI. Association between PI and delirium
		NIRS	Association with outcome
		Pupillometry	Pupillary abnormalities are associated with neurological complications

EEG electroencephalogram, *pEEG* processed EEG, *TCD* transcranial Doppler, *NIRS* near infrared spectroscopy, *BIS* Bispectral index, *rSO2* regional saturation of oxygen, *SSEPs* sensory evoked potentials, *CBF* cerebral blood flow, *ICP* intracranial pressure, *PI* pulsatility index, *ARDS* acute respiratory distress syndrome, *COVID-19* coronavirus disease 2019, *ECMO* extracorporeal membrane oxygenation

or vegetative state and poor prognosis; presence of N20 potentials and absent mismatch negativity, which is diagnostic of indeterminate prognosis; and presence of N20 with mismatch negativity, which represents a 95% chance of recovery with good neurological function [31]

26.3.2.3 Transcranial Doppler

TCD has considerable diagnostic potential in the ED and the ICU. Hepatic encephalopathy is a complication which occurs in up to 70% of patients with liver cirrhosis, and that manifests with psychomotor, attentive, and executive alterations [35]. Higher vascular resistances and pulsatility index in the middle and posterior cerebral arteries of cirrhotic patients have been reported in comparison to controls, with 74% accuracy of the middle cerebral artery resistive index for discriminating the presence of hepatic encephalopathy [35].

Alterations in CBF have also been found in patients with uremia and chronic kidney disease, typically with a decrease in CBF observed after hemodialysis [36].

Sepsis-associated encephalopathy is considered as an independent risk factor for mortality [37] that is characterized by a decrease in the density of cerebral microvessels that can alter cerebrovascular resistances, with potential for inadequate oxygen supply and cerebral dysfunction. On TCD, the pulsatility index was higher in septic patients than in controls [38], and high pulsatility index values on the first day of sepsis diagnosis were associated with a positive CAM-ICU delirium assessment [39].

TCD after cardiac arrest has been extensively studied, and includes four different features: pulsatility index <0.6 (very low resistance), associated with possible hyperemia, vasospasm or stenosis; pulsatility index 1.2–1.6 (high resistance) with possible microangiopathy or mild intracranial hypertension; pulsatility index 1.7–1.9 (very high resistance) with severe intracranial hypertension; and pulsatility index ≥2 with cerebral hypoperfusion. In patients who remain comatose >20 min after return of spontaneous circulation the main pattern described is a high pulsatility index [40].

In patients with polytrauma admitted to the ED at risk for intracranial hypertension or with contraindications to invasive ICP placement, TCD and ONSD can be a valid option for the assessment of high ICP and for excluding extracranial hypertension [25, 26].

In mechanically ventilated patients with acute respiratory distress syndrome (ARDS) (including COVID-19 ARDS), TCD has been extensively used and has the potential to indicate the effect of mechanical ventilation strategies on cerebral function, to detect secondary brain dysfunction, and to assess cerebral autoregulation during hemodynamic and respiratory rescue maneuvers [41–43].

26.3.2.4 Near Infrared Spectroscopy

The use of NIRS is gaining increasing interest in the ED and ICU settings to detect microcirculatory changes in patients with septic or metabolic alterations. Although the majority of studies have been conducted in the ICU, some studies in the ED have concluded that NIRS may correlate with severity of illness, especially after cardiac arrest, with variable association between rSO_2 values and outcome [44, 45].

NIRS has been also used for the evaluation of cerebral complications and outcome in sepsis, with a rSO_2 cut-off of 75% as predictor of neurological sequelae [46]. Similarly, an increase in rSO_2 during hospitalization, and lower tissue oxygen extraction rates detected using NIRS, have been shown to be associated with improved survival in polytrauma patients [47].

Finally, in mechanically ventilated patients with ARDS (and COVID-19 ARDS), NIRS has been shown to be useful in assessment of the effect of hemodynamic and respiratory maneuvers on brain oxygenation and cerebral hemodynamics [42, 43, 48].

26.3.2.5 Automated Pupillometry

In the critical care setting, pupillary size and reactivity to light may provide information about intracranial disease, including elevated ICP and altered perfusion, sedation and analgesia, delirium assessment, brain metabolic derangements, and prognostication [49, 50]. Some studies have used pupillometry to assess the pupillary response to a light stimulus before painful procedures in order to assess adequacy of analgesia. In addition, pupillometry has been shown to be useful to assess the level of sedation, with a good correlation with BIS values [50].

Metabolic disorders can impair the sympathetic system and affect pupillary light reactivity. This can also be observed in patients with sepsis or liver-associated encephalopathy, and neurological disorders. Some authors have suggested that patients with a delayed recovery of pupillary reflexes developed demyelinating encephalopathy or dementia, suggesting that pupillary abnormalities may be associated with potential neurological derangements [49, 50].

Automated pupillometry is also gaining interest as part of the prognostication algorithms adopted after cardiac arrest [49]. A pupillary light reflex <6%, neurologic pupillary index (NPi) of 0 at 6 h from the cardiac arrest, and a pupillary light response <13% have shown to be predictive of poor outcome [49]. Pupillary light reactivity, when used in combination with EEG and SSEP has also been shown to improve sensitivity to 100% for the prediction of outcome after cardiac arrest [49].

Intracranial hypertension can also occur in non-primary brain injured patients. Automated pupillometry can detect and even predict elevated ICP. For example, unilateral pupillary dilation and loss of reactivity can be detected as a sign of transtentorial herniation [49]. An altered constriction velocity has been identified during and before ICP elevation, and improvement in constriction velocity has been described after osmotic treatment to reduce brain edema [49].

At present, no consensus exists concerning the routine use of automated pupillometry in ED and ICU settings, although recent research supports its use to obtain objective information on pupillary function compared with manual pupillary examination [49, 50].

26.4 Conclusion

Increasing evidence suggests that the use of brain monitoring –EEG, evoked potentials, TCD, and NIRS– is gaining popularity even in non-neurocritical care settings, e.g., in the perioperative setting, ED, and ICU, to improve patient care. Neuromonitoring devices can be non-invasive, low-cost, safe tools available at the bedside, with a great potential for both diagnosis and monitoring of patients at risk of brain insult.

Further clinical and research developments, training and teaching programs are urgently needed to support implementation of neuromonitoring in daily clinical practice.

References

1. Robba C, Goffi A, Geeraerts T, et al. Brain ultrasonography: methodology, basic and advanced principles and clinical applications. A narrative review. Intensive Care Med. 2019;45:913–27.
2. Bonatti G, Iannuzzi F, Amodio S, et al. Neuromonitoring during general anesthesia in non-neurologic surgery. Best Pract Res Clin Anaesthesiol. 2021;35:255–66.
3. So VC, Poon CCM. Intraoperative neuromonitoring in major vascular surgery. Br J Anaesth. 2016;117:ii13–25.
4. Milne B, Gilbey T, Gautel L, Kunst G. Neuromonitoring and neurocognitive outcomes in cardiac surgery: a narrative review. J Cardiothorac Vasc Anesth. 2021. Jul 21. https://doi.org/10.1053/j.jvca.2021.07.029. Epub ahead of print.
5. Checketts MR, Alladi R, Ferguson K, et al. Recommendations for standards of monitoring during anaesthesia and recovery 2015 : Association of Anaesthetists of Great Britain and Ireland. Anaesthesia. 2016;71:85–93.
6. Romagnoli S, Franchi F, Ricci Z. Processed EEG monitoring for anesthesia and intensive care practice. Minerva Anestesiol. 2019;85:1219–30.
7. Aldecoa C, Bettelli G, Bilotta F, et al. European Society of Anaesthesiology evidence-based and consensus-based guideline on postoperative delirium. Eur J Anaesthesiol. 2017;34:192–214.
8. Roseborough GS. Pro: routine shunting is the optimal management of the patient undergoing carotid endarterectomy. J Cardiothorac Vasc Anesth. 2004;18:375–80.
9. Estruch-Pérez MJ, Barberá-Alacreu M, Ausina-Aguilar A, Soliveres-Ripoll J, Solaz-Roldán C, Morales-Suárez-Varela MM. Bispectral index variations in patients with neurological deficits during awake carotid endarterectomy. Eur J Anaesthesiol. 2010;27:359–63.
10. Wildes TS, Mickle AM, Ben Abdallah A, et al. Effect of electroencephalography-guided anesthetic administration on postoperative delirium among older adults undergoing major surgery. JAMA. 2019;321:473.
11. Sloan TB, Edmonds HL, Koht A. Intraoperative electrophysiologic monitoring in aortic surgery. J Cardiothorac Vasc Anesth. 2013;27:1364–73.
12. Cardim D, Robba C, Schmidt E, et al. Transcranial Doppler non-invasive assessment of intracranial pressure, autoregulation of cerebral blood flow and critical closing pressure during orthotopic liver transplant. Ultrasound Med Biol. 2019;45:1435–45.
13. Robba C, Bacigaluppi S, Cardim D, et al. Intraoperative non invasive intracranial pressure monitoring during pneumoperitoneum: a case report and a review of the published cases and case report series. J Clin Monit Comput. 2016;30:527–38.
14. Citerio G, Vascotto E, Villa F, Celotti S, Pesenti A. Induced abdominal compartment syndrome increases intracranial pressure in neurotrauma patients: a prospective study. Crit Care Med. 2001;29:1466–71.
15. Aguirre JA, Märzendorfer O, Brada M, Saporito A, Borgeat A, Bühler P. Cerebral oxygenation in the beach chair position for shoulder surgery in regional anesthesia: impact on cerebral blood flow and neurobehavioral outcome. J Clin Anesth. 2016;35:456–64.
16. Kietaibl C, Engel A, Horvat Menih I, et al. Detection and differentiation of cerebral microemboli in patients undergoing major orthopaedic surgery using transcranial Doppler ultrasound. Br J Anaesth. 2017;118:400–6.
17. Sloan MA. Prevention of ischemic neurologic injury with intraoperative monitoring of selected cardiovascular and cerebrovascular procedures: roles of electroencephalography, somatosensory evoked potentials, transcranial doppler, and near-infrared spectroscopy. Neurol Clin. 2006;24:631–45.

18. Messerotti Benvenuti S, Zanatta P, Valfrè C, Polesel E, Palomba D. Preliminary evidence for reduced preoperative cerebral blood flow velocity as a risk factor for cognitive decline three months after cardiac surgery: an extension study. Perfusion. 2012;27:486–92.
19. Ono M, Joshi B, Brady K, et al. Risks for impaired cerebral autoregulation during cardiopulmonary bypass and postoperative stroke. Br J Anaesth. 2012;109:391–8.
20. Stilo F, Spinelli F, Martelli E, et al. The sensibility and specificity of cerebral oximetry, measured by INVOS - 4100, in patients undergoing carotid endarterectomy compared with awake testing. Minerva Anesth. 2012;78:1126–35.
21. Guay J, Kopp S. Cerebral monitors versus regional anesthesia to detect cerebral ischemia in patients undergoing carotid endarterectomy: a meta-analysis. Can J Anesth. 2013;60:266–79.
22. Thiele RH, Shaw AD, Bartels K, et al. American Society for Enhanced Recovery and Perioperative Quality Initiative Joint Consensus Statement on the role of Neuromonitoring in perioperative outcomes: cerebral near-infrared spectroscopy. Anesth Analg. 2020;131:1444–55.
23. Chan MJ, Chung T, Glassford NJ, Bellomo R. Near-infrared spectroscopy in adult cardiac surgery patients: a systematic review and meta-analysis. J Cardiothorac Vasc Anesth. 2017;31:1155–65.
24. de Azevedo DS, Salinet ASM, de Lima Oliveira M, Teixeira MJ, Bor-Seng-Shu E, de Carvalho Nogueira R. Cerebral hemodynamics in sepsis assessed by transcranial Doppler: a systematic review and meta-analysis. J Clin Monit Comput. 2017;31:1123–32.
25. Rasulo FA, Bertuetti R, Robba C, et al. The accuracy of transcranial Doppler in excluding intracranial hypertension following acute brain injury: a multicenter prospective pilot study. Crit Care. 2017;21:44.
26. Robba C, Pozzebon S, Moro B, Vincent J-L, Creteur J, Taccone FS. Multimodal non-invasive assessment of intracranial hypertension: an observational study. Crit Care. 2020;24:379.
27. Yigit O, Eray O, Mihci E, Yilmaz D, Arslan S, Eray B. The utility of EEG in the emergency department. Emerg Med J. 2012;29:301–5.
28. Fritz BA, Kalarickal PL, Maybrier HR, et al. Intraoperative electroencephalogram suppression predicts postoperative delirium. Anesth Analg. 2016;122:234–42.
29. Crepeau AZ, Rabinstein AA, Fugate JE, et al. Continuous EEG in therapeutic hypothermia after cardiac arrest: prognostic and clinical value. Neurology. 2013;80:339–44.
30. Choi WJ, Lee JH, Kim SH. Neurological prognostication using raw EEG patterns and spectrograms of frontal EEG in cardiac arrest patients. J Clin Neurophysiol. 2021. Sep 28. https://doi.org/10.1097/WNP.0000000000000787. Epub ahead of print.
31. Koenig MA, Kaplan PW. Clinical applications for EPs in the ICU. J Clin Neurophysiol. 2015;32:472–80.
32. Peluso L, Rechichi S, Franchi F, et al. Electroencephalographic features in patients undergoing extracorporeal membrane oxygenation. Crit Care. 2020;24:629.
33. Cho S-M, Choi CW, Whitman G, et al. Neurophysiological findings and brain injury pattern in patients on ECMO. Clin EEG Neurosci. 2019;52:462–9.
34. Kubota T, Gajera PK, Kuroda N. Meta-analysis of EEG findings in patients with COVID-19. Epilepsy Behav. 2021;115:107682.
35. Ponziani FR, Funaro B, Lupascu A, et al. Minimal hepatic encephalopathy is associated with increased cerebral vascular resistance. A transcranial doppler ultrasound study. Sci Rep. 2019;9:15373.
36. Olguín-Ramírez L, Hernández-Guajardo D, Celis-Jasso J, et al. Difference of cerebral flows in uremia as a cause of encephalopathy. Follow-up by transcranial Doppler. Neurology. 2020;94:5413.
37. Mazeraud A, Righy C, Bouchereau E, Benghanem S, Bozza FA, Sharshar T. Septic-associated encephalopathy: a comprehensive review. Neurotherapeutics. 2020;17:392–403.
38. Szatmári S, Végh T, Csomós Á, et al. Impaired cerebrovascular reactivity in sepsis-associated encephalopathy studied by acetazolamide test. Crit Care. 2010;14:R50.
39. Pierrakos C, Attou R, Decorte L, et al. Transcranial Doppler to assess sepsis-associated encephalopathy in critically ill patients. BMC Anesthesiol. 2014;14:45.

40. Lemiale V, Huet O, Vigué B, et al. Changes in cerebral blood flow and oxygen extraction during post-resuscitation syndrome. Resuscitation. 2008;76:17–24.
41. Battaglini D, Santori G, Chandraptham K, et al. Neurological complications and noninvasive multimodal neuromonitoring in critically ill mechanically ventilated COVID-19 patients. Front Neurol. 2020;11:602114.
42. Robba C, Messina A, Battaglini D, et al. Early effects of passive leg-raising test, fluid challenge, and norepinephrine on cerebral autoregulation and oxygenation in COVID-19 critically ill patients. Front Neurol. 2021;12:674466.
43. Robba C, Ball L, Battaglini D, et al. Early effects of ventilatory rescue therapies on systemic and cerebral oxygenation in mechanically ventilated COVID-19 patients with acute respiratory distress syndrome: a prospective observational study. Crit Care. 2021;25:111.
44. Macdonald SPJ, Brown SGA. Near-infrared spectroscopy in the assessment of suspected sepsis in the emergency department. Emerg Med J. 2015;32:404–8.
45. Takegawa R, Hayashida K, Rolston DM, et al. Near-infrared spectroscopy assessments of regional cerebral oxygen saturation for the prediction of clinical outcomes in patients with cardiac arrest: a review of clinical impact, evolution, and future directions. Front Med. 2020;7:587930.
46. Macdonald SPJ, Kinnear FB, Arendts G, Ho KM, Fatovich DM. Near-infrared spectroscopy to predict organ failure and outcome in sepsis: the assessing risk in sepsis using a tissue oxygen saturation (ARISTOS) study. Eur J Emerg Med. 2019;26:174–9.
47. Donati A, Damiani E, Domizi R, Pierantozzi S, Calcinaro S, Pelaia P. Near-infrared spectroscopy to assess tissue oxygenation in patients with polytrauma: relationship with outcome. Crit Care. 2015;19:P308 (abst).
48. Khan I, Rehan M, Parikh G, et al. Regional cerebral oximetry as an indicator of acute brain injury in adults undergoing veno-arterial extracorporeal membrane oxygenation–a prospective pilot study. Front Neurol. 2018;9:993.
49. Bower MM, Sweidan AJ, Xu JC, Stern-Neze S, Yu W, Groysman LI. Quantitative pupillometry in the intensive care unit. J Intensive Care Med. 2021;36:383–91.
50. Phillips SS, Mueller CM, Nogueira RG, Khalifa YM. A systematic review assessing the current state of automated pupillometry in the neuroICU. Neurocrit Care. 2019;31:142–61.

Part IX

Artificial Intelligence

Artificial Intelligence in Critical Care Medicine

27

J. H. Yoon, M. R. Pinsky, and G. Clermont

27.1 Introduction

The clinical outcome of critically ill patients has improved significantly and to an unprecedented level as standards of care have improved [1]. However, conventional critical care practice still has limitations in understanding the complexity of acuity, handling extreme individual heterogeneity, anticipating deterioration, and providing early treatment strategies before decompensation. Critical care medicine has seen the arrival of advanced monitoring systems and various non-invasive and invasive treatment strategies to provide timely intervention for critically-ill patients. Whether the mergence of such systems represents the next step in improving bedside care is an existing, yet unproven possibility.

The simplified concept of artificial intelligence (AI) is to allow computers to find patterns in a complex environment of multidomain and multidimensional data, with the prerequisite that such patterns would not be recognized otherwise. Previously, applying the concept in real life required a tremendous amount of computing time and resources. This could only be done in limited fields, including physics or astronomy. However, with recent exponential growth in computing power and portability, the power of AI became available to many fields, including critical care medicine where data are vast, abundant, and complex [2]. More and more clinical investigations are being performed using AI-driven models to leverage the data in the intensive care unit (ICU), but our understanding of the power and utility of AI in critical care medicine is still quite rudimentary. In addition, there are many obstacles and

J. H. Yoon (✉)
Division of Pulmonary, Allergy, and Critical Care Medicine, Department of Medicine, University of Pittsburgh, Pittsburgh, PA, USA
e-mail: yoonjh@upmc.edu

M. R. Pinsky · G. Clermont
Department of Critical Care Medicine, University of Pittsburgh, Pittsburgh, PA, USA

J.-L. Vincent (ed.), *Annual Update in Intensive Care and Emergency Medicine 2022*, Annual Update in Intensive Care and Emergency Medicine,
https://doi.org/10.1007/978-3-030-93433-0_27

pitfalls for AI to overcome before becoming a core component of our daily clinical practice.

In this chapter, we seek to introduce the roles of AI with the potential to change the landscape of our conventional practice patterns in the ICU, describe its current strengths and pitfalls, and consider future promise for critical care medicine.

27.2 Applications of AI in Critical Care

27.2.1 Disease Identification

Oftentimes, finding the root cause of clinical deterioration from the exhaustive list of differential diagnoses is challenging, because of the insidious characteristic of early disease progression or the presence of co-existing conditions masking the main problem (Fig. 27.1). More than anything, the underlying context should be deciphered correctly, often a challenging task. For example, pulmonary infiltrates cannot simply be assumed to represent excessive alveolar fluid. They could indicate pulmonary edema from a cardiac cause, pleural effusion, parapneumonic fluid from inflammation or infection, or in some cases collections of blood as a result of trauma. Without clinical context and further testing, adequate and timely management could be delayed. AI could assist in such cases by obtaining a more precise diagnosis, given advanced text and image processing capability. The presence of congestive heart failure (CHF) could be differentiated from other causes of lung disease using a machine learning model [3], and amounts of pulmonary edema secondary to the CHF could be quantified with semi-supervised machine learning

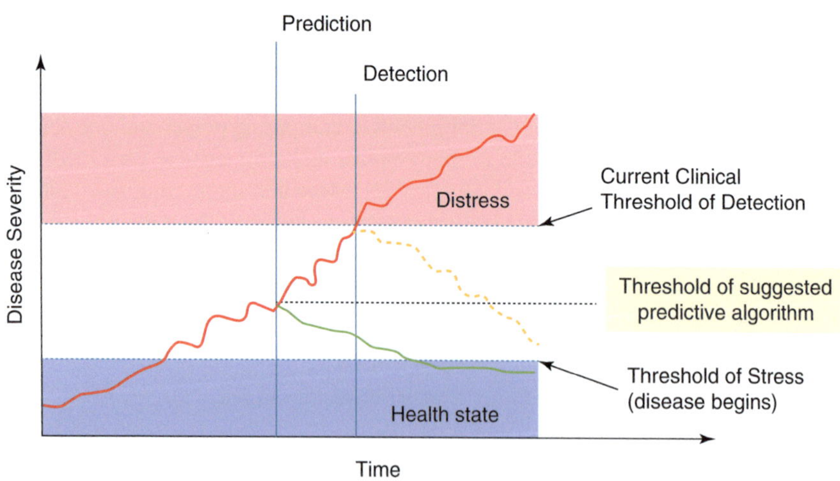

Fig. 27.1 Conceptual role of artificial intelligence (AI)-driven predictive analytics on disease progression. The AI model enables timely detection or prediction of disease enabling clinicians to manage critically ill patients earlier (green line) than conventional strategy (yellow dotted line)

using a variational autoencoder [4]. During the severe acute respiratory syndrome coronavirus 2 (SARS-CoV-2) pandemic, imaging data from patients admitted to hospital were processed to detect coronavirus disease 2019 (COVID-19) using an AI model [5]. With recent efforts in image segmentation and quantification of lesions by convolutional neural networks, a type of algorithm particularly apt at interpreting images, the presence of traumatic brain injury (TBI) on head computed tomography (CT) could be evaluated with higher accuracy than manual reading [6]. Similarly, traumatic hemoperitoneum was quantitatively visualized and measured using a multiscale residual neural network [7].

27.2.2 Disease Evolution Prediction

Disease detection and prediction of disease evolution is one of the holy grails for critically ill patients. Given that the disease process is a continuum, instability of clinical condition can take various paths, even prior to ICU admission [8]. In a series of step-down unit patients who experienced cardiorespiratory instability (defined as hypotension, tachycardia, respiratory distress, or a desaturation event using numerical thresholds), a dynamic model using a random forest classification showed that a personalized risk trajectory predicted deterioration 90 minutes ahead of the crisis [9].

In the ICU, rapid clinical deterioration is common, and the result can be irreversible and even lead to mortality if detected late. Thus, efforts are being made to predict such hemodynamic decompensation. Tachycardia, one of the most commonly observed deviations from normality prior to shock, was predicted 75 minutes prior to development using a normalized dynamic risk score trajectory with a random forest model [10]. Hypotension, a manifestation of shock, was also predicted in the operating room [11]. The utility of a machine learning model in reducing intraoperative hypotension was further confirmed in a randomized controlled trial in patients having intermediate and high-risk surgery, with hypotension occurring in 1.2% of patients managed with an AI driven intervention, versus 21.5% using conventional methods [12]. Hypotension events have also been predicted in the ICU where vital sign granularities are lower and datasets contain more noise. Using electronic health record (EHR) as well as physiologic numeric vital sign data, clinically relevant hypotension events were predicted with a random forest model, achieving a sensitivity of 92.7%, with the average area under the curve (AUC) of 0.93 at 15 minutes before the actual event [13].

Hypoxia and respiratory distress have also been major targets for prediction, the roles of which have expanded during the recent coronavirus pandemic. In the first few months of the pandemic, AI-driven models were used to predict the progression of COVID-19, using imaging, biological, and clinical variables [14]. Cardiac arrest has also been predicted using an electronic Cardiac Arrest Risk Triage (eCART) score from EHR data, showing non-inferior scores compared to conventional early warning scoring systems [15]. Sepsis has also been predicted, with an AUC of 0.85 using Weibull-Cox proportional hazards model on high-resolution vital sign time series data and clinical data [16]. Other clinical outcomes may be predicted using AI models, including mortality after TBI [17] or mortality of COVID-19 patients with different risk profiles [18].

27.2.3 Disease Phenotyping

Critical illness is complex and its manifestations can rarely be reduced to typical presentations. Rather, critical illness manifests in a lot of different ways (inherent heterogeneity), and carries significant risks for organ dysfunction that can subsequently complicate the underlying disease process or recovery processes. Such syndromes should not be treated blindly without careful consideration of underlying etiologies or clinical conditions for a given individual. Moreover, the complex critical states change over time, such that clinicians cannot rely on assessments from even a few hours earlier. Yet, evidence-based guidelines should be followed whenever these exist. With its strong capability of pattern recognition from complex data, AI could delineate distinctive phenotypes or endotypes that could reflect influences from the critical state and hence open up avenues to personalize management, integrated into existing guidelines.

Sepsis, one of the most common ICU conditions, is a highly heterogenous syndrome, and has been a favorite target of AI algorithms. Recently, using different clinical trial cohorts, sepsis was clustered into four phenotypes (α, β, γ, and δ) by consensus K-means clustering, a type of unsupervised machine learning model. The phenotypes had distinctive demographic characteristics, different biochemical presentations, correlated to host-response patterns, and were eventually associated with different clinical outcomes [19]. Such phenotypes are of a descriptive nature, are useful in describing case-mix, and could represent targets for predictive enrichment of clinical trials. However, they are not at this juncture based in mechanism and thus are not therapeutically actionable. Nevertheless, further explorations using richer data might allow a greater degree of actionability.

In the acute respiratory distress syndrome (ARDS), latent class analysis (LCA) revealed two subtypes (hypo- and hyper-inflammatory subtypes) linked with different clinical characteristics, treatment responses, and clinical outcomes [20]. A parsimonious model was developed and achieved similar performance to the initial LCA using a smaller set of classifier variables (interleukin [IL]-6, -8), protein C, soluble tumor necrosis factor (TNF) receptor 1, bicarbonate, and vasopressors). This result was validated in a secondary analysis of three different randomized clinical trials [21]. This machine learning-driven ARDS phenotyping has expanded our knowledge in assessing and treating complex disease, and become one of the criteria for predictive enrichment of future clinical trials.

Dynamic phenotyping for prediction of clinical deterioration can be performed on time series data. Using analysis of 1/20 Hz granular physiologic vital sign data, several unique phenotypes, including persistently high, early onset, and late onset deterioration, were identified prior to overt cardiorespiratory deterioration, using K-means clustering (Fig. 27.2) [9]. Time-series of images can be clustered for dynamic phenotyping, as performed using transesophageal echocardiographic

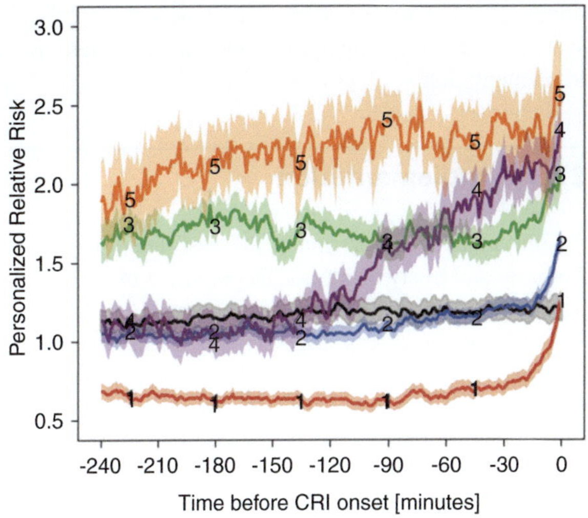

Fig. 27.2 Dynamic, personal risk trajectory prior to cardiorespiratory instability (CRI). Black line represents control subjects. Orange line (5) indicates 'persistent high', purple line (4) indicates 'early rise', and green (3), blue (2), and red (1) lines indicate 'late rise' to CRI. Adapted from [9] with permission of the American Thoracic Society. Copyright © 2021 American Thoracic Society.

monitoring images in patients with septic shock: using a hierarchical clustering method, septic shock was clustered into three cardiac deterioration patterns and two responses to interventions, which were linked with clinical outcome with different day 7 and ICU mortality rates [22].

27.2.4 Guiding Clinical Decisions

For a complex problem, one-size-fits-all solutions do not work well. Over the last decade, research has failed to improve the outcome of septic shock with different treatment guidelines [23, 24]. The extreme heterogeneity of septic shock, various underlying conditions, and different host-responses could be at least partially addressed by AI to provide individualized solutions using reinforcement learning. The algorithm in reinforcement learning is designed to detect numerous variables in a given state to build an action model, which then learns from the reward or penalty from the results of the action. Applying this to the sepsis population, reinforcement learning could provide optimal sequential decision-making solutions for sepsis treatment, showcasing the potential impact of AI to generate personalized solutions [25]. In patients receiving mechanical ventilation, time series data with 44 features were extracted and reinforcement learning (Markov Decision Process) resulted in better results compared to physicians' standard clinical care, with target outcomes of 90-day and ICU mortality [26]. These examples demonstrate the role AI may have in guiding important decision-making for critically ill patients. The notion of AI's therapeutic utility could be more pronounced and provocative in different clinical environments, such as critical case scenarios in remote areas where clinicians are not available and patient transfer is not possible, or resource-limited settings where treatment options are limited. Because the optimality of such treatment recommendations is computed from retrospective and observational datasets, it is imperative that recommendation sequences or policies originating from such AI systems be fully analyzed and then tested prospectively before clinical implementation.

27.3 Implementation

An important consideration in successful deployment of AI at the bedside is system usability and trustworthiness. Deployment of such systems should involve all stakeholders, including clinicians and patients (end users), researchers (producers), and hospital administrators (logistics and management). In a specific research project, an implementation strategy entails creating models with adequate amounts of information (not a 'flood' of information with alarms), delivered with understandable (interpretable) logics, and placed on a visually appealing vehicle or dashboard - a graphic user interface. These systems, when deployed as alerting tools, must be accurate enough and parsimonious enough to prevent alarm fatigue, which leads to delays in detecting, and intervening for, developing crises [27]. In recent work on prediction of hypotension in the ICU, researchers found that AI-generated alerts could be reduced tenfold while maintaining sensitivity, when they used a stacked random forest model, or a model checking on another model before generating alerts [13].

Understanding AI-derived predictions and recommendations is arguably an important component of AI acceptance at the bedside. Although complex models can be thought of as 'black-boxes', an enormous effort is underway to enhance model interpretability and explainability. For example, in a recent report on hypoxia detection, researchers adopted concepts from game theory to differentially weight predictive physiological readouts during surgery, as an attempt to interpret the clinical drivers of hypoxic alarming from an AI system [28]. Creating the graphic user interface is necessary not only for the AI output to be delivered to the bedside, but also to improve hospital workflow and alleviate nursing burden. As shown in recent work, deep learning could be used to analyze fiducial points from the face, postures, and action of patients, and from environmental stimuli to discriminate delirious and non-delirious ICU patients [29]. Future ICU design should embrace the functionalities of AI solutions to enable clinicians to react earlier to any potential deterioration, and researchers to build models that perform better using more comprehensive data, and presented in such a way that it will be readily available, highly accurate, and trusted by bedside clinicians.

27.4 Pitfalls of AI in Critical Care

As much as the power of the AI model changes the current landscape of data analysis and plays an important role in assisting early diagnosis and management, there are many road blocks that should not be overlooked when introducing AI models for critically ill patients.

27.4.1 Explainability and Interpretability

Many AI models have complex layers of nodes that enable the characteristics of input data to be more meaningful in revealing hidden patterns. While the model may produce seemingly accurate output through that process, oftentimes the rationale of the computation cannot be provided to the end users. In the clinical environment, this can create strong resistance to accepting AI models into daily practice, as clinicians fear that performing unnecessary interventions or changing a treatment strategy without supporting scientific evidence could easily violate the first rule of patient care, *primum non nocere*. In critical care medicine, such a move could be directly and rapidly associated with mortality. On the other hand, many novel treatments did not have enough evidence when first introduced in the history of medicine, and 'black-box' models do not need to be completely deciphered, advocating the use of inherently interpretable AI [30]. Another recent approach argues that providing detailed methodologies for the model validation, robustness of analysis, history of successful/unsuccessful implementations, and expert knowledge could alleviate epistemological and methodological concerns and gain reliability and trust [31].

Multiple efforts have been introduced to overcome the complexity of deep learning models. Explaining feature contribution on a dynamic time series dataset became possible by leveraging game theory into measuring feature importance, when predicting near-term hypoxic events during surgery [32]. In that report, contributing features explained by SHapley Additive exPlanation (SHAP) showed consistency with the literature and prior knowledge from anesthesiologists for upcoming hypoxia risks. Moreover, anesthesiologists were able to make better clinical decisions to prevent intraoperative hypoxia when assisted by the explainable AI model.

27.4.2 Lack of Robustness

The readiness of AI for the real-life clinical environment is limited by the lack of adequate clinical experiments and trials, with a disappointingly low rate of reproducibility and prospective analyses. In a recent review of 172 AI-driven solutions created from routinely collected chart data, the clinical readiness level for AI was low. In that study, the maturity of the AI was classified into nine stages corresponding to real world application [33]. Strikingly, around 93% of all analyzed articles remained below stage 4, with no external validation process, and only 2% of published studies had performed prospective validation. Thus, current AI models in critical care medicine have largely been generated using retrospective data, without external validation or prospective evaluation.

Reproducibility of AI solutions is not guaranteed and no clear protocols exist to examine this thoroughly. As mentioned above, AI solutions already have limitations in terms of data openness and almost inexplicable algorithmic complexity, so the lack of reproducibility on top of these factors could significantly impact the fidelity of the AI model. A recent study attempted to reproduce 38 experiments for 28 mortality prediction projects using the Medical Information Mart for Intensive Care (MIMIC-III) database, and reported large sample size differences in about a half the experiments [34]. This problem highlights the importance of accurate labeling, understanding the clinical context to create the study population, as well as precise reporting methods including data pre-processing and featurization.

Adherence to reporting standards and risks of bias is also sub-optimal, as a study that analyzed 81 non-randomized and 10 randomized trials using deep learning showed only 6 of 81 non-randomized studies had been tested in a real-world clinical setting and 72% of studies showed high risks of bias [35]. Hence, considering the scientific rigor of conventional randomized controlled trials needed to prove scientific hypothesis, the maturity and robustness of AI-driven models would be even less convincing for everyday practice.

More complex and sophisticated AI models, like reinforcement learning are also not free from challenges, as such intricate models require a lot of computational resources and are difficult to test on patients in order to train or test the models in a clinical environment. Inverse reinforcement learning, which infers information about rewards, could be a new model-agnostic reinforcement learning approach to constructing decision-making trajectories, because this approach alleviates the stress of manually designing a reward function [36]. With those algorithmic advances, decision-assisting engines can be more robust and reliable when input data varies, which may be a great asset to critical care data science where work is conducted with enormous quantity and extreme heterogeneity of data.

27.4.3 Ethical Concerns

Use of AI in critical care is still a new field to most researchers and clinicians. We will not really appreciate what ethical issues we will encounter until AI becomes more widely used and apparent in the development pipeline and bedside applications. However, given the nature of AI characteristics and current AI-driven solutions, a few aspects can be discussed to look around the corner into likely ethical dilemmas of AI models in critical care. The first issue is in data privacy and sharing. Innovation in data science allows us to collect and manipulate data to find hidden patterns, during which course collateral data leakage could pose threats, especially in its pre-processing and in external validation steps towards generalization. It is very hard to remove individual data points from the dataset once they are already being used by the AI model. De-identification and parallel/distributive computing could provide some solutions to data management, and novel models, including federated learning, might minimize data leakage and potentially speed up the multicenter validation process.

A second issue in ethics is safety of the AI model at the bedside. To semi-quantitatively describe the safety of the model, the analogous maturity metric used by self-driving cars was used for clinical adaptability of AI-driven solutions, with 6 levels [37]: 0 (no automation) to 2 (partial automation) represent situations where the human driver monitors the environment; 3 (conditional automation) to 5 (full automation) represent situations where the system is monitoring the environment rather than any human involvement. According to this scale, if used in real life, most of the AI-driven solutions developed would fall into categories 1 or 2. This concept signifies that the safety and accountability of the AI model cannot be blindly guaranteed, and decision making by clinicians remains an integral part of patient care. Also, the autonomy of individual patients has never been more important, including generating informed consent or expressing desire to be treated in life-threatening situations – here the AI recommendations might not be aligned with those of the patient. Recognition of such ethical issues and preparing for potential solutions to overcome limitations of AI, as well as understanding more about patient perspectives could allow researchers and clinicians to develop more practical and ethical AI solutions.

27.5 Future Tasks of AI in Critical Care

27.5.1 Data De-identification/Standardization/Sharing Strategy

Like any other clinical research, AI solutions need validation from many different angles. External validation, which uses input data from other environments, is one of the most common ways to generalize a model. Although external validation and prospective study designs certainly require collaborative data pools and concerted efforts, creating such a healthy ecosystem for AI research in critical care demands considerable groundwork.

De-identification of the healthcare data is probably the first step to ascertain data privacy and usability. The Society of Critical Care Medicine (SCCM)/European Society of Intensive Care Medicine (ESICM) Joint Data Science Task Force team has published the process to create a large-scale database from different source databases, including the following steps: (1) using an anonymization threshold, personal data are separated from anonymous data; (2) iterative, risk-based process to de-identify personal data; (3) external review process to ensure privacy and legal considerations to abide within the European General Data Protection Regulation (GDPR) [38]. Such a de-identification process would ascertain safe data transfer and could further facilitate high-quality AI model training.

Other important groundwork for the multi-center collaboration is data standardization. Individual hospital systems have developed numerous different data labeling strategies in different EHR layers. Even within the same hospital system, small discrepancies, including the number of decimals, commonly used abbreviations, and data order within the chart, could be stumbling blocks for systematic data standardization. In addition, data with higher granularity, including physiologic waveform data, are even harder to standardize, as there are no distinctive labels to express the values in a structured way. To address this, international researchers have developed a standardized format to facilitate efficient exchange of clinical and physiologic data [39]. In this Hierarchical Data Format-version 5 (HDF5)-based critical care data exchange format, multiparameter data could be stored, compressed, and streamed real time. This type of data exchange format would allow integration of other types of large-scale datasets as well, including imaging or genomics.

While one cannot completely remove the data privacy and governance concerns, rapid collaboration can be facilitated when those are less of an issue. An example is federated learning, where models can be designed to be dispatched to local centers for training, instead of data from participating centers collected to one central location for model training. While the data are not directly exposed to the outside environment, the model could still be trained by outside datasets with comparable efficacy and performance [40]. Federated learning could be even more useful when the data distribution among different centers is imbalanced or skewed, demonstrating the real-world collaboration environment [41]. A comprehensive federated learning project was performed during the COVID-19 pandemic. Across the globe, 20 academic centers collaborated to predict clinical outcomes from COVID-19 by constructing federated learning within a strong cloud computing system [42]. During the study phase, researchers developed an AI model to predict the future oxygen requirements of patients with symptomatic COVID-19 using chest X-ray data, which was then dispatched to participating hospitals. The trained model was calibrated with shared partial-model weights, then the averaged global model was generated, while privacy was preserved in each hospital system. In that way, the AI model achieved an average AUC > 0.92 for predicting 24- to 72-h outcomes. In addition, about a 16% improvement in average AUC, with a 38% increase in generalizability was observed when the model was tested with federated learning compared to the prediction model applied to individual centers. This report exemplifies the potential power of a federated learning-based collaborative approach, albeit the source data (chest X-ray and other clinical data) are relatively easy to standardize for the federated learning system to work on.

27.5.2 Novel AI Models and Trial Designs

Labeling target events for AI models is a daunting, labor-intensive task, and requires a lot of resources. To make the task more efficient, novel AI models, such as weakly supervised learning, have been introduced. Weakly supervised learning can build desired labels with only partial participation of domain experts, and may potentially preserve resource use. One example was provided by performing weakly supervised classification tasks using medical ontologies and expert-driven rules on patients visiting the emergency department with COVID-19 related symptoms [43]. When ontology-based weak supervision was coupled with pretrained language models, the engineering cost of creating classifiers was reduced more than for simple weakly supervised learning, showing an improved performance compared to a majority vote classifier. The results showed that this AI model could make unstructured chart data available for machine learning input, in a short period of time, without an expert labeling process in the midst of a pandemic.

Future clinical trials could also be designed with AI models, especially to maximize benefits and minimize risks to participants, as well as to make the best use of limited resources. One example of such an innovative design is the REMAP-CAP (Randomized Embedded Multifactorial Additive Platform for Community-Acquired Pneumonia), which adopted a Bayesian inference model. In detail, this multicenter clinical trial allows randomization with robust causal inference, creates multiple intervention arms across multiple patient subgroups, provides response-adaptive randomization with preferential assignment, and provides a novel platform with perpetual enrollment beyond the evaluation of the initial treatments [44]. The platform, initially developed to identify optimal treatment for community-acquired pneumonia, continued to enroll throughout the COVID-19 pandemic, and has contributed to improved survival among critically ill COVID-19 patients [45, 46].

27.5.3 Real-Time Application

To establish a valuable AI system in the real-life setting, the model should be able to deliver important information in a timely manner. In critically ill patients, the feedback time should be extremely short, sometimes less than a few minutes. Prediction made too early would have enough time to formulate the model, but have less predictive power, and prediction made very close to target events would have higher performance, with no time to curate the input data and run the model for output.

To be used in the real-life environment, a real time AI model should be equipped with a very fast data pre-processing platform, and able to parsimoniously featurize to update the model with new input data simultaneously. The output should also be delivered to the bedside rapidly. In that strict sense of real time, almost no clinical studies have accomplished real-time prediction. A few publications claim real-time prediction, but most of them used retrospective data, and failed to demonstrate continuous real-time data pre-processing without time delay. Using a gradient boosting tree model, one study showed dynamic 'real-time' risks of the onset of sepsis from a large retrospective dataset. The duration of ICU stay was divided into three periods (0–9 h, 10–49 h, and more than 50 h of ICU stay), partitioned to reflect different sepsis onset events, and resulted in different utility scores in each phase [47]. While this provides valuable information on different performances of the AI model for different durations of ICU stay, use of continuous real-time pre-processing without a time delay was not demonstrated. Another study using a recurrent neural network on postoperative physiologic vital sign data produced a high positive predictive value of 0.90 with sensitivity of 0.85 in predicting mortality, and was superior to the conventional metric to predict mortality and other complications [48]. The study also showed that the predictive difference between the AI solution and conventional methods was evident from the beginning of the ICU stay. However, prediction from the earliest part of the ICU stay also does not qualify as true real-time prediction. Although this is a challenging task for current technology, application of the real-time AI model to the critical care environment could yield significant benefit in downstream diagnostic or therapeutic options without time delay.

27.5.4 Quality Control after Model Deployment

Once the AI model achieves high performance and is deemed to be useful in a real-life clinical setting, implementation strategies as well as quality assessment efforts should follow. Anticipating such changes in the clinical/administrative landscape, the National Academy of Medicine of the United States has published a white paper on AI use in healthcare, in which the authors urge the development of guidelines and legal terms for safer, more efficacious, and personalized medicine [49]. In particular, for the maturity of AI solutions and their integration with healthcare, the authors suggested addressing implicit and explicit bias, contextualizing a dialogue of transparency and trust, developing and deploying appropriate training and educational tools, and avoiding over-regulation or over-legislation of AI solutions.

27.6 Conclusion

Rapid development and realization of AI models secondary to an unprecedented increase in computing power has invigorated research in many fields, including medicine. Many research topics in critical care medicine have employed the concept of AI to recognize hidden disease patterns among the extremely heterogeneous and noise-prone clinical datasets. AI models provide useful solutions in disease detection, phenotyping, and prediction that might alter the course of critical diseases. They may also lead to optimal, individualized treatment strategies when multiple treatment options exist. However, at the current stage, development and implementation of AI solutions face many challenges. First, data generalization is difficult without proper groundwork, including de-identification and standardization. Second, AI models are not robust, with sub-optimal adherence to reporting standards, a high risk of bias, lack of reproducibility, and without proper external validation with open data and transparent model architecture. Third, with the nature of the obscurity and probabilistic approach, AI models could lead to unforeseen ethical dilemmas. For the successful implementation of AI into clinical practice in the future, collaborative research efforts with plans for data standardization and sharing, advanced model development to ascertain data security, real-time application, and quality control are required.

References

1. Zimmerman JE, Kramer AA, Knaus WA. Changes in hospital mortality for United States intensive care unit admissions from 1988 to 2012. Crit Care. 2013;17:R81.
2. Yoon JH, Pinsky MR. Predicting adverse hemodynamic events in critically ill patients. Curr Opin Crit Care. 2018;24:196–203.
3. Seah JCY, Tang JSN, Kitchen A, Gaillard F, Dixon AF. Chest radiographs in congestive heart failure: visualizing neural network learning. Radiology. 2019;290:514–22.
4. Horng S, Liao R, Wang X, Dalal S, Golland P, Berkowitz SJ. Deep learning to quantify pulmonary edema in chest radiographs. Radiol Artif Intell. 2021;3:e190228.

5. Li L, Qin L, Xu Z, et al. Using artificial intelligence to detect COVID-19 and community-acquired pneumonia based on pulmonary CT: evaluation of the diagnostic accuracy. Radiology. 2020;296:E65–e71.
6. Monteiro M, Newcombe VFJ, Mathieu F, et al. Multiclass semantic segmentation and quantification of traumatic brain injury lesions on head CT using deep learning: an algorithm development and multicentre validation study. Lancet Digit Health. 2020;2:e314–e22.
7. Dreizin D, Zhou Y, Fu S, et al. A multiscale deep learning method for quantitative visualization of traumatic hemoperitoneum at CT: assessment of feasibility and comparison with subjective categorical estimation. Radiol Artif Intell. 2020;2:e190220.
8. Vincent JL. The continuum of critical care. Crit Care. 2019;23(Suppl 1):122.
9. Chen L, Ogundele O, Clermont G, Hravnak M, Pinsky MR, Dubrawski AW. Dynamic and personalized risk forecast in step-down units. Implications for monitoring paradigms. Ann Am Thorac Soc. 2017;14:384–91.
10. Yoon JH, Mu L, Chen L, et al. Predicting tachycardia as a surrogate for instability in the intensive care unit. J Clin Monit Comput. 2019;33:973–85.
11. Wijnberge M, Geerts BF, Hol L, et al. Effect of a machine learning-derived early warning system for intraoperative hypotension vs standard care on depth and duration of intraoperative hypotension during elective noncardiac surgery: the HYPE randomized clinical trial. JAMA. 2020;323:1052–60.
12. Joosten A, Rinehart J, Van der Linden P, et al. Computer-assisted individualized hemodynamic management reduces intraoperative hypotension in intermediate- and high-risk surgery: a randomized controlled trial. Anesthesiology. 2021;135:258–72.
13. Yoon JH, Jeanselme V, Dubrawski A, Hravnak M, Pinsky MR, Clermont G. Prediction of hypotension events with physiologic vital sign signatures in the intensive care unit. Crit Care. 2020;24:661.
14. Lassau N, Ammari S, Chouzenoux E, et al. Integrating deep learning CT-scan model, biological and clinical variables to predict severity of COVID-19 patients. Nat Commun. 2021;12:634.
15. Bartkowiak B, Snyder AM, Benjamin A, et al. Validating the electronic cardiac arrest risk triage (eCART) score for risk stratification of surgical inpatients in the postoperative setting: retrospective cohort study. Ann Surg. 2019;269:1059–63.
16. Nemati S, Holder A, Razmi F, Stanley MD, Clifford GD, Buchman TG. An interpretable machine learning model for accurate prediction of sepsis in the ICU. Crit Care Med. 2018;46:547–53.
17. Raj R, Luostarinen T, Pursiainen E, et al. Machine learning-based dynamic mortality prediction after traumatic brain injury. Sci Rep. 2019;9:17672.
18. Banoei MM, Dinparastisaleh R, Zadeh AV, Mirsaeidi M. Machine-learning-based COVID-19 mortality prediction model and identification of patients at low and high risk of dying. Crit Care. 2021;25:328.
19. Seymour CW, Kennedy JN, Wang S, et al. Derivation, validation, and potential treatment implications of novel clinical phenotypes for sepsis. JAMA. 2019;321:2003–17.
20. Calfee CS, Delucchi KL, Sinha P, et al. Acute respiratory distress syndrome subphenotypes and differential response to simvastatin: secondary analysis of a randomised controlled trial. Lancet Respir Med. 2018;6:691–8.
21. Sinha P, Delucchi KL, McAuley DF, O'Kane CM, Matthay MA, Calfee CS. Development and validation of parsimonious algorithms to classify acute respiratory distress syndrome phenotypes: a secondary analysis of randomised controlled trials. Lancet Respir Med. 2020;8:247–57.
22. Geri G, Vignon P, Aubry A, et al. Cardiovascular clusters in septic shock combining clinical and echocardiographic parameters: a post hoc analysis. Intensive Care Med. 2019;45:657–67.
23. Rivers E, Nguyen B, Havstad S, et al. Early goal-directed therapy in the treatment of severe sepsis and septic shock. N Engl J Med. 2001;345:1368–77.
24. Rowan KM, Angus DC, Bailey M, et al. Early, goal-directed therapy for septic shock - a patient-level meta-analysis. N Engl J Med. 2017;376:2223–34.

25. Komorowski M, Celi LA, Badawi O, Gordon AC, Faisal AA. The artificial intelligence clinician learns optimal treatment strategies for sepsis in intensive care. Nat Med. 2018;24:1716–20.
26. Peine A, Hallawa A, Bickenbach J, et al. Development and validation of a reinforcement learning algorithm to dynamically optimize mechanical ventilation in critical care. NPJ Digit Med. 2021;4:32.
27. Hravnak M, Pellathy T, Chen L, et al. A call to alarms: current state and future directions in the battle against alarm fatigue. J Electrocardiol. 2018;51:S44–s8.
28. Thorsen-Meyer HC, Nielsen AB, Nielsen AP, et al. Dynamic and explainable machine learning prediction of mortality in patients in the intensive care unit: a retrospective study of high-frequency data in electronic patient records. Lancet Digit Health. 2020;2:e179–e91.
29. Davoudi A, Malhotra KR, Shickel B, et al. Intelligent ICU for autonomous patient monitoring using pervasive sensing and deep learning. Sci Rep. 2019;9:8020.
30. Rudin C. Stop explaining black box machine learning models for high stakes decisions and use interpretable models instead. Nat Mach Intell. 2019;1:206–15.
31. Durán JM, Jongsma KR. Who is afraid of black box algorithms? On the epistemological and ethical basis of trust in medical AI. J Med Ethics. 2021;47:329–35.
32. Lundberg SM, Nair B, Vavilala MS, et al. Explainable machine-learning predictions for the prevention of hypoxaemia during surgery. Nat Biomed Eng. 2018;2:749–60.
33. Fleuren LM, Thoral P, Shillan D, Ercole A, Elbers PWG. Machine learning in intensive care medicine: ready for take-off? Intensive Care Med. 2020;46:1486–8.
34. Johnson AEW, Pollard TJ, Mark RG. Reproducibility in critical care: a mortality prediction case study. PMLR. 2017;68:361–76.
35. Nagendran M, Chen Y, Lovejoy CA, et al. Artificial intelligence versus clinicians: systematic review of design, reporting standards, and claims of deep learning studies. BMJ. 2020;368:m689.
36. Fu J, Luo K, Levine S. Learning robust rewards with adversarial inverse reinforcement learning. arXiv preprint 2017:1710.11248.
37. Topol EJ. High-performance medicine: the convergence of human and artificial intelligence. Nat Med. 2019;25:44–56.
38. Thoral PJ, Peppink JM, Driessen RH, et al. Sharing ICU patient data responsibly under the Society of Critical Care Medicine/European Society of Intensive Care Medicine Joint Data Science Collaboration: the Amsterdam university medical centers database (AmsterdamUMCdb) example. Crit Care Med. 2021;49:e563–e77.
39. Laird P, Wertz A, Welter G, et al. The critical care data exchange format: a proposed flexible data standard for combining clinical and high-frequency physiologic data in critical care. Physiol Meas. 2021;42:065002.
40. Rieke N, Hancox J, Li W, et al. The future of digital health with federated learning. NPJ Digit Med. 2020;3:119.
41. Lee GH, Shin SY. Federated learning on clinical benchmark data: performance assessment. J Med Internet Res. 2020;22:e20891.
42. Dayan I, Roth HR, Zhong A, et al. Federated learning for predicting clinical outcomes in patients with COVID-19. Nat Med. 2021;27:1735–43.
43. Fries JA, Steinberg E, Khattar S, et al. Ontology-driven weak supervision for clinical entity classification in electronic health records. Nat Commun. 2021;12:2017.
44. Angus DC, Berry S, Lewis RJ, et al. The REMAP-CAP (randomized embedded multifactorial adaptive platform for community-acquired pneumonia) study. Rationale and design. Ann Am Thorac Soc. 2020;17:879–91.
45. Angus DC, Derde L, Al-Beidh F, et al. Effect of hydrocortisone on mortality and organ support in patients with severe COVID-19: the REMAP-CAP COVID-19 corticosteroid domain randomized clinical trial. JAMA. 2020;324:1317–29.
46. Gordon AC, Mouncey PR, Al-Beidh F, et al. Interleukin-6 receptor antagonists in critically ill patients with Covid-19. N Engl J Med. 2021;384:1491–502.
47. Li X, Xu X, Xie F, et al. A time-phased machine learning model for real-time prediction of sepsis in critical care. Crit Care Med. 2020;48:e884–e8.

48. Meyer A, Zverinski D, Pfahringer B, et al. Machine learning for real-time prediction of complications in critical care: a retrospective study. Lancet Respir Med. 2018;6:905–14.
49. Matheny ME, Whicher D, Thadaney IS. Artificial intelligence in health care: a report from the National Academy of Medicine. JAMA. 2020;323:509–10.

Artificial Intelligence in Infection Management in the ICU

28

T. De Corte, S. Van Hoecke, and J. De Waele

28.1 Introduction

Research and development of data-driven artificial intelligence (AI), so-called machine learning, in the intensive care unit (ICU) is at an all-time high. Data scientists and physicians are exploring the potential of machine learning in a vast range of domains, including infection management. From both a data science and a medical point of view, infection management in the ICU is an attractive yet challenging research topic: it is a highly complex area where information from several different medical specialties and sources has to be integrated for a single patient. At the same time, there is an urgent need to optimize infection management in the ICU, both for the individual patient – as timely and adequate treatment determines a patient's survival – and for society – as rising antimicrobial resistance and inadequate treatment results in increased morbidity and mortality and hence increased costs [1]. Evidence-based, data-generated, and automated AI support is expected to help ICU clinicians and antimicrobial stewardship teams take the next step in tackling these problems. Although the main focus of AI research in the ICU has been occurrence of sepsis and its outcome prediction as well as, more recently, almost every aspect of coronavirus disease 2019 (COVID-19), important progress has been made in the infection management field as well [2–4]. In this chapter, we provide an overview of the current stance of AI/machine learning research in different areas of antimicrobial infection management, the barriers that hinder clinical adaptation, and pitfalls for bedside use.

T. De Corte (✉) · J. De Waele
Department of Internal Medicine and Pediatrics, Faculty of Medicine and Health Sciences, Ghent University, Ghent, Belgium

Department of Intensive Care Medicine, Ghent University Hospital, Ghent, Belgium
e-mail: Thomas.decorte@ugent.be

S. Van Hoecke
IDLab, Ghent University – imec, Zwijnaarde, Belgium

J.-L. Vincent (ed.), *Annual Update in Intensive Care and Emergency Medicine 2022*, Annual Update in Intensive Care and Emergency Medicine,
https://doi.org/10.1007/978-3-030-93433-0_28

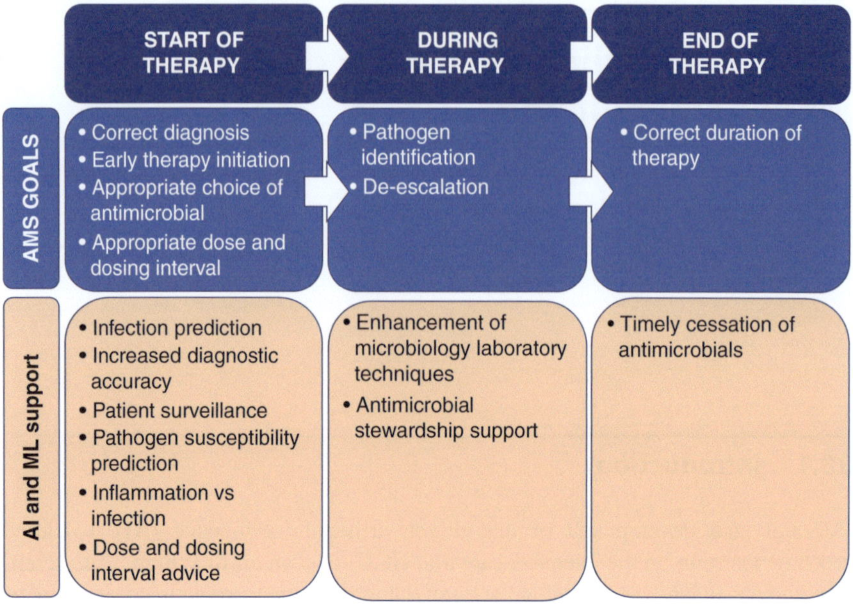

Fig. 28.1 The antimicrobial stewardship (AMS) cycle. *AI* artificial intelligence, *ML* machine learning

To this end, we have written a narrative review that takes a pragmatic approach using the antimicrobial stewardship cycle as a framework (Fig. 28.1).

28.2 Start of Antimicrobial Therapy

28.2.1 Predicting Infection

A significant number of AI/machine learning models have been developed that try to predict the occurrence of an event in advance, commonly termed 'forecasting'. Ventilator associated pneumonia (VAP), central-line associated blood stream infections (CLABSI), as well as the risk of colonization/infection with a multidrug resistant pathogen (MDR) are just a few examples for which prediction models have been developed [5–8]. The forecasting of sepsis and/or septic shock has, however, dominated this domain, as illustrated by the no more than 15 retrospective papers and 1 prospective interventional study carried out solely in the ICU that were identified by Fleuren et al. in their recent systematic review [9]. In these and other prediction models, inference of the future risk is made by developing machine learning models on (most often) routinely collected healthcare data (e.g., medical history, clinical parameters, biochemistry results, etc.) from retrospective databases. The rationale behind prediction models is the idea that the clinical course can be altered if the physician is aware of the imminent event. As some predictions can be seen as

28.2.2.2 Differentiating Inflammation from Bacterial Infection

From an antimicrobial stewardship point of view, probably the most difficult but also most impactful distinction to make is whether the patient actually has an infection or rather has systemic inflammation without any infection involved. Differentiating between these two disease states requires integration of different types of data, none of which are highly sensitive or specific since abnormal values for these variables is common in both disease states and highly discriminative tests are currently lacking. Lamping et al. however have demonstrated that a machine learning approach, based on random forests using eight routinely available parameters, outperforms currently available biomarkers to discriminate infectious versus non-infectious states in critically ill children [14]. When identification of 100% of sepsis cases was targeted, the model correctly categorized 28% of non-infectious cases. If external validation and clinical trials confirm the validity of the model, it could be associated with a significant reduction in unnecessarily prescribed antimicrobials. A more recent example, where differentiating between inflammation and bacterial infection proved to be burdensome, was the COVID-19 pandemic during which the diagnosis of co-infection of bacterial origin was very difficult to make. This led Rawson et al. to develop machine learning models that support the diagnosis of bacterial infection using only routinely available blood test results [15]. Prospective evaluation of the algorithms is underway, but a preliminary area under the receiver operator curve (AUROC) of 0.96 on 54 patients is encouraging.

28.2.3 Initiating Antimicrobial Therapy

Today, antimicrobials are either prescribed on an empirical basis or complemented with information from surveillance cultures when available. In either case, the causative pathogen is unknown. In addition, the antimicrobial susceptibility of the causative pathogen is only known long after antimicrobial therapy has been initiated. Ideally, rapid diagnostics would lead to the identification of the pathogen and antimicrobial susceptibility directly from clinical samples within approximately 30 min as this would greatly diminish the need for empirical treatment or allow adjustments to the antimicrobial therapy to be made before a second dose is administered, thereby leading to more timely and more appropriate therapy [16]. Also for this domain, researchers have shown that AI/machine learning can play a role.

28.2.3.1 Enhancing Available Techniques

Machine learning applications have been investigated to enhance currently available phenotypic and genotypic pathogen and resistance identification techniques. Roux-Dalvai et al. for example developed a proteomics library for the 15 most prevalent bacterial species in urinary tract infections (making up 84% of all urinary tract infections) using a liquid chromatography with tandem mass spectrometry technique combined with machine learning, which enables detection of the presence of one of these 15 species within 4 h without the need for bacterial culture [17]. In another study, Feretzakis et al. tested multiple machine learning models that only needed limited information (including source of specimen, presumed site of infection, Gram stain of the pathogen, and previous susceptibility data) to predict susceptibility to a specific antibiotic with 72.6% accuracy in patients admitted to the ICU [18]. But the most promising study from a clinical point of view was by Ho et al. who combined Raman spectroscopy on blood samples and deep learning to develop a base classification model for the 30 most common bacterial and yeast isolate classes in the ICU worldwide [19]. Not only does their method achieve a very high performance in pathogen and resistance identification while only needing ten bacterial cells to function, they also demonstrated that their initial model could be continuously improved with the addition of new Raman spectrums. As the authors state that this technique can process blood, sputum, or urine samples in a few hours without the need for an incubation period, this technique has the potential to greatly diminish the time to pathogen and antimicrobial resistance identification while providing a very high accuracy for certain infections.

28.2.3.2 Susceptibility Prediction

Although drastically reducing the time to identification, the above mentioned techniques still require sampling and sample processing, and hence will not be able to guide the choice of antimicrobial therapy at the time of initiation. Alternatively, models that can aid in predicting the causative organism and/or antimicrobial resistance at sampling time are also under investigation. Prediction models have been developed, mostly using supervised machine learning, on routinely collected and readily available healthcare data, collected at or before sampling time. A variety of sample types, pathogens of interest, and antimicrobials of concern have already been investigated using this approach with variable degrees of success [20–24]. An advantage of some models is their implementation potential in low and middle income countries. For example, a study performed by Oonsivilai et al. in a Cambodian children's hospital tested multiple machine learning models to predict the result of the Gram stain and the susceptibility of the pathogen to ampicillin and gentamicin, ceftriaxone or none of the former using only variables derived from clinical and demographic data as well as information regarding their living conditions [24]. Their best performing model had fair predictive performance with an area under the curve (AUC) of 0.71 for the Gram stain result, 0.8 for ceftriaxone susceptibility, 0.74 for ampicillin and gentamicin susceptibility, and 0.85 for resistance to the afore mentioned antimicrobials.

28.2.3.3 Antimicrobial Dose and Dosing Interval

Pharmacometrics has historically led dose and dosing intervals by means of linear regression, population pharmacokinetic models, and Bayesian forecasting. Developed models are mostly still in the research phase, trying to find their way into the wards as dosing software, but wide implementation in clinical practice is lacking [25, 26]. Introduction of machine learning into pharmacometrics is still in its infancy although the potential of a partnership is increasingly being recognized [27]. At the same time, machine learning research is ongoing to improve antimicrobial dosing, as is illustrated by the vancomycin dose prediction model using XGBoosting developed by Huang et al. [28]. However, more research is needed here as the error is rather high to have potential in clinical practice.

28.3 During Antimicrobial Therapy

28.3.1 Machine Learning and the Microbiology Laboratory

By contrast to the pharmacometrics domain, machine learning applications are being explored in all aspects of the microbiology laboratory. For an in-depth review on this topic we refer to the article by Peiffer-Smadja et al. [29]. From microscopic images over spectroscopy data and transcriptomics to gene sequences, no stone is being left unturned. In general, the goal of most of these models is microorganism identification/quantification and evaluation of antimicrobial resistance with the purpose of reducing the turnaround time. As an example, Inglis et al. demonstrated that supervised machine learning could expedite the identification of antimicrobial resistance by using data generated through flow-cytometer-assisted antimicrobial susceptibility testing [30]. Their prototype was able to generate a predictive inhibitory concentration within 3 h of identification of a positive blood culture, where standard methods take approximately 24 h after culture positivity. By combining machine learning with infrared spectroscopy, Lechowicz et al. were able to bring the turnaround time even further down to 30 min, but it should be noted that their machine learning models, based on artificial neural networks, did not achieve perfect classification results [31].

28.3.2 Antimicrobial Stewardship Support

In recent years, a lot of effort has gone into the development and maintenance of hospital tailored antimicrobial stewardship programs. Implementation of these antimicrobial stewardship programs has already had a significant impact on the length of stay and antimicrobial expenditure [1]. One essential element in most of these plans is antimicrobial prescription review and prescriber feedback, where several key parameters for prescribed antimicrobials (e.g., indication, dosage, route of administration, duration) are evaluated. Suggestions are made by the reviewer if adaptations are deemed necessary. Since this is a time-consuming job, computerized systems are often used to help identify patients where a review is warranted. It should however be noted that these clinical decision support systems (CDSS) often have an expert and rule-based knowledge base, which mandates that development and maintenance of these systems to changing guidelines are also time and resource intensive. In addition, resource constraints lead to certain antibiotics of interest being singled out instead of evaluating all prescribed antibiotics. To overcome these shortcomings, Bystritsky et al. tried to develop linear regression and boosted-tree models using routinely available health care data to identify patients that could possibly benefit from prescription review and prescriber feedback [32]. Although the discriminatory power of these retrospectively developed models was only fair and the number of patients that needed to be reviewed by the model to identify one patient who required an intervention was high, the premise that all patients with a prescribed antimicrobial could be evaluated in an automated way could yield a large advantage. Another approach could be to combine the currently available CDSS systems for antimicrobial stewardship with machine learning. Researchers from the Université de Sherbrooke demonstrated that their supervised learning module could identify clinically relevant new rules complementing the rules already in their knowledge base by evaluating past recommendations from clinical pharmacists [33]. Although promising, incorporating new rules, learned through machine learning, into the already available knowledge base and automating rule maintenance remains an important challenge.

28.4 End of Antimicrobial Therapy

At present, sometimes empiric antimicrobials are prescribed for patients who do not need it, or they are not stopped in a timely manner. Eickelberg et al. investigated whether machine learning could help identify patients at low risk for bacterial infection and hence suitable for antimicrobial discontinuation [34]. Different machine learning models were investigated, using clinical parameters and characteristics, blood gas and laboratory results, as well as certain administered medications, to evaluate the bacterial infection risk at three time points after initiation of empirical antimicrobial therapy: 24 h, 48 h and 72 h. Interestingly, there was little variation in performance between the 24 h and the 72 h models. The best performing models identified patients with a low risk of bacterial infection with a negative predictive value of more than 93%.

28.5 Future Directions

28.5.1 From Research to Clinical Practice

Based on the information provided above, AI and machine learning research are more and more intertwining with every aspect of the antimicrobial stewardship cycle, albeit to varying degrees. However, clinical implementation has only sporadically been realized as most models are still in the design/prototype phase, or have only been tested on internal clinical data [35, 36]. Validation of these models, prior to implementation on external datasets and in clinical trials, will be paramount and adequately designing these trials will be a challenge. Choosing the correct reference standard as a comparator for models for which the ground truth is objective (e.g., prediction of an antimicrobial concentration) is more straightforward than determining this standard for a task where human interpretation and hence subjectivity is involved (e.g., the diagnosis of VAP) [37]. At the same time, a decision will have to be made as to what level of performance we, as clinicians, deem sufficient for a model to be put into clinical practice depending on the given task. Expecting flawlessness from machine learning models is a utopian dream as long as we are not able to incorporate variables that resemble the complete causal pathophysiological process. And even then it is unlikely that models will be flawless, as for even the most objective ground truth, repeated measurements can vary owing to the measurement method used (e.g., the between-run and within-run imprecision of high-performance liquid chromatography with tandem mass spectrometry for antimicrobial concentration determination).

Other aspects that need to be solved are the ethical and legal responsibilities when, for example, clinicians follow off-label dosing suggestions, or follow the advice of a model that later turns out to be flawed. Closely linked to this aspect is the need to educate physicians to critically appraise and evaluate model capabilities and associated studies. As clinicians will be the end-users of these AI systems, education is needed, not only to ensure appropriate usage, but also to empower physicians to identify and report emerging problems.

Finally, all models mentioned in this paper have a standalone design and are focused on one particular aspect of antimicrobial stewardship. Incorporating and managing the variety of engineered models into everyday practice in a meaningful way so that the whole domain of antimicrobial stewardship is supported while not chaining the physician to a screen might pose the greatest challenge of all.

28.5.2 Post-Implementation Surveillance of Machine Learning Models

Since deployment of machine learning models into clinical practice is foreseeable in the very near future, governance of these models will be a new task that will have to be taken up by clinicians, at the very least partially. As end-users, clinicians will become the first line of defense to identify circumstances where AI fails to perform reliably. This possibility of failure is not unrealistic, as was recently demonstrated by Finlayson et al. for the proprietary Epic Sepsis prediction model that suffered from a phenomenon called dataset shift [38]. Dataset shift occurs when a machine learning system underperforms after it is deployed because of a mismatch between the data/context it was developed for and the data/context it is deployed in [39]. Translated to clinical practice, this means that any difference or change in patient demographics or delivery of care between the patients the model was developed upon and the actual patients for which the model is asked to give a suggestion, can flaw the suggestion of the model. These differences or changes can be readily identifiable (e.g., evolving antimicrobial resistance epidemiology, or introduction of a new first-line antimicrobial) but can also be very subtle (e.g., behavioral changes of the clinicians induced by the AI system after its implementation, or change of a diagnostic test, which alters the reference values). As clinical practice is changing more rapidly than ever before, keeping models accurate and up to date will be an undertaking in which clinicians will have to take a key role within a medicine-transcendent multidisciplinary team to ensure patient safety. Machine learning solutions such as online learning might prove to be of use in this area as well.

28.5.3 Emerging Research Possibilities

28.5.3.1 Personalization through the 'Internet of Things'

The diagnostic process of infection is often triggered by a change in clinical parameters (e.g., body temperature) or laboratory results (e.g., increase in C-reactive protein). For the latter category, increases above a set threshold value as well as trends over time are typically used in clinical practice. For the former category, however, current guidelines use hard thresholds to differentiate a pathological from a normal state, which obviously does not hold true for all patients. For example, fever in adult patients is often defined as a temperature ≥ 38 °C, whereas, depending on the measurement method and age of the patient, the normal population range varies between 35.61 °C and 37.76 °C [40]. Often, older patients do not experience fever while they are having an infection. By integrating information from currently widespread used wearables through the 'internet of things', new research opportunities arise to determine –at an individual level– which thresholds should be used to identify significant changes in physiological parameters. Disclosing these baseline physiological characteristics to the physician could help to personalize treatment at a patient level and may also help in the development of machine learning models to do the same. Several companies and healthcare systems have already taken initiatives to enable integration of wearable health technology data into the electronic health record (EHR), but actual clinical impact has not yet been demonstrated [41].

28.5.3.2 Omics

In addition to AI and machine learning, different types of omics are also being intensively researched in every aspect of healthcare, as it is believed that omics might provide the tools necessary to advance clinical practice toward precision medicine [42]. A difficulty in omics research, however, is the amount of generated data that has to be analyzed and the computational power needed to do so. As AI and machine learning are capable of handling these kinds of issues, combining the two domains might create new insight by integrating information from different omics research fields, as has been illustrated by the ShockOmics research project [43].

28.6 Conclusion

AI and machine learning research for antimicrobial stewardship in the ICU is at an all-time high, but to date, implementation into clinical practice has only been sporadic. Internal validation results are promising, so an increase in external validation studies and randomized controlled clinical trials is to be expected in the coming years. Providing the prerequisites to safely validate and implement these models will be necessary for bedside clinical deployment in the near future. Within new beyond-the-borders-of-medicine multidisciplinary teams, bedside clinicians will have an important role in facilitating this process.

References

1. Nathwani D, Varghese D, Stephens J, Ansari W, Martin S, Charbonneau C. Value of hospital antimicrobial stewardship programs [ASPs]: a systematic review. Antimicrob Resist Infect Control. 2019;8:35.
2. Goh KH, Wang L, Yeow AYK, Poh H, Li K, Yeow JJL, Tan GYH. Artificial intelligence in sepsis early prediction and diagnosis using unstructured data in healthcare. Nat Commun. 2021;12:711.
3. van Doorn WPTM, Stassen PM, Borggreve HF, Schalkwijk MJ, Stoffers J, Bekers O, Meex SJR. A comparison of machine learning models versus clinical evaluation for mortality prediction in patients with sepsis. PLoS One. 2021;16:e0245157.
4. Adamidi ES, Mitsis K, Nikita KS. Artificial intelligence in clinical care amidst COVID-19 pandemic: a systematic review. Comput Struct Biotechnol J. 2021;19:2833–50.
5. Giang C, Calvert J, Rahmani K, et al. Predicting ventilator-associated pneumonia with machine learning. Medicine (Baltimore). 2021;100:e26246.
6. Tacconelli E, Górska A, De Angelis G, et al. Estimating the association between antibiotic exposure and colonization with extended-spectrum β-lactamase-producing gram-negative bacteria using machine learning methods: a multicentre, prospective cohort study. Clin Microbiol Infect. 2020;26:87–94.
7. Mora-Jiménez I, Tarancón-Rey J, Álvarez-Rodríguez J, Soguero-Ruiz C. Artificial intelligence to get insights of multi-drug resistance risk factors during the first 48 hours from ICU admission. Antibiotics. 2021;10:239.
8. Parreco JP, Hidalgo AE, Badilla AD, Ilyas O, Rattan R. Predicting central line-associated bloodstream infections and mortality using supervised machine learning. J Crit Care. 2018;45:156–62.
9. Fleuren LM, Klausch TLT, Zwager CL, et al. Machine learning for the prediction of sepsis: a systematic review and meta-analysis of diagnostic test accuracy. Intensive Care Med. 2020;46:383–400.
10. Shimabukuro DW, Barton CW, Feldman MD, Mataraso SJ, Das R. Effect of a machine learning-based severe sepsis prediction algorithm on patient survival and hospital length of stay: a randomised clinical trial. BMJ Open Respir Res. 2017;4:e000234.
11. Hwang EJ, Park S, Jin KN, et al. Development and validation of a deep learning–based automated detection algorithm for major thoracic diseases on chest radiographs. JAMA Netw Open. 2019;2:e191095.
12. Chen CY, Lin WC, Yang HY. Diagnosis of ventilator-associated pneumonia using electronic nose sensor array signals: solutions to improve the application of machine learning in respiratory research. Respir Res. 2020;21:45.
13. de Bruin JS, Adlassnig K-P, Blacky A, Koller W. Detecting borderline infection in an automated monitoring system for healthcare-associated infection using fuzzy logic. Artif Intell Med. 2016;69:33–41.
14. Lamping F, Jack T, Rübsamen N, et al. Development and validation of a diagnostic model for early differentiation of sepsis and non-infectious SIRS in critically ill children - a data-driven approach using machine-learning algorithms. BMC Pediatr. 2018;18:112.
15. Rawson TM, Hernandez B, Wilson RC, et al. Supervised machine learning to support the diagnosis of bacterial infection in the context of COVID-19. JAC Antimicrob Resist. 2021;3:dlab002.
16. Burnham C-AD, Leeds J, Nordmann P, O'Grady J, Patel J. Diagnosing antimicrobial resistance. Nat Rev Microbiol. 2017;15:697–703.
17. Roux-Dalvai F, Gotti C, Leclercq M, et al. Fast and accurate bacterial species identification in urine specimens using LC-MS/MS mass spectrometry and machine learning. Mol Cell Proteomics. 2019;18:2492–505.

18. Feretzakis G, Loupelis E, Sakagianni A, et al. Using machine learning techniques to aid empirical antibiotic therapy decisions in the intensive care unit of a general hospital in Greece. Antibiotics (Basel). 2020;9:E50.
19. Ho CS, Jean N, Hogan CA, et al. Rapid identification of pathogenic bacteria using Raman spectroscopy and deep learning. Nat Commun. 2019;10:4927.
20. Roimi M, Neuberger A, Shrot A, Paul M, Geffen Y, Bar-Lavie Y. Early diagnosis of bloodstream infections in the intensive care unit using machine-learning algorithms. Intensive Care Med. 2020;46:454–62.
21. Van Steenkiste T, Ruyssinck J, De Baets L, Decruyenaere J, De Turck F, Ongenae F, Dhaene T. Accurate prediction of blood culture outcome in the intensive care unit using long short-term memory neural networks. Artif Intell Med. 2019;97:38–43.
22. Moran E, Robinson E, Green C, Keeling M, Collyer B. Towards personalized guidelines: using machine-learning algorithms to guide antimicrobial selection. J Antimicrob Chemother. 2020;75:2677–80.
23. Goodman KE, Lessler J, Harris AD, Milstone AM, Tamma PD. A methodological comparison of risk scores versus decision trees for predicting drug-resistant infections: a case study using extended-spectrum beta-lactamase (ESBL) bacteremia. Infect Control Hosp Epidemiol. 2019;40:400–7.
24. Oonsivilai M, Mo Y, Luangasanatip N, et al. Using machine learning to guide targeted and locally-tailored empiric antibiotic prescribing in a children's hospital in Cambodia. Welcome Open Res. 2018;3:131.
25. Roggeveen LF, Fleuren LM, Guo T, et al. Right dose right now: bedside data-driven personalized antibiotic dosing in severe sepsis and septic shock — rationale and design of a multicenter randomized controlled superiority trial. Trials. 2019;20:745.
26. Chai MG, Cotta MO, Abdul-Aziz MH, Roberts JA. What are the current approaches to optimising antimicrobial dosing in the intensive care unit? Pharmaceutics. 2020;12:638.
27. Koch G, Pfister M, Daunhawer I, Wilbaux M, Wellmann S, Vogt JE. Pharmacometrics and machine learning partner to advance clinical data analysis. Clin Pharmacol Ther. 2020;107:926–33.
28. Huang X, Yu Z, Wei X, et al. Prediction of vancomycin dose on high-dimensional data using machine learning techniques. Exp Rev Clin Pharmacol. 2021;14:761–71.
29. Peiffer-Smadja N, Dellière S, Rodriguez C, Birgand G, Lescure FX, Fourati S, Ruppé E. Machine learning in the clinical microbiology laboratory: has the time come for routine practice? Clin Microbiol Infect. 2020;26:1300–9.
30. Inglis TJJ, Paton TF, Kopczyk MK, Mulroney KT, Carson CFY. Same-day antimicrobial susceptibility test using acoustic-enhanced flow cytometry visualized with supervised machine learning. J Med Microbiol. 2020;69:657–69.
31. Lechowicz L, Urbaniak M, Adamus-Białek W, Kaca W. The use of infrared spectroscopy and artificial neural networks for detection of uropathogenic Escherichia coli strains' susceptibility to cephalothin. Acta Biochim Pol. 2013;60:713–8.
32. Bystritsky RJ, Beltran A, Young AT, Wong A, Hu X, Doernberg SB. Machine learning for the prediction of antimicrobial stewardship intervention in hospitalized patients receiving broad-spectrum agents. Infect Control Hosp Epidemiol. 2020;41:1022–7.
33. Beaudoin M, Kabanza F, Nault V, Valiquette L. Evaluation of a machine learning capability for a clinical decision support system to enhance antimicrobial stewardship programs. Artif Intell Med. 2016;68:29–36.
34. Eickelberg G, Sanchez-Pinto LN, Luo Y. Predictive modeling of bacterial infections and antibiotic therapy needs in critically ill adults. J Biomed Inform. 2020;109:103540.
35. van de Sande D, van Genderen ME, Huiskens J, Gommers D, van Bommel J. Moving from bytes to bedside: a systematic review on the use of artificial intelligence in the intensive care unit. Intensive Care Med. 2021;47:750–60.
36. Fleuren LM, Thoral P, Shillan D, et al. Machine learning in intensive care medicine: ready for take-off? Intensive Care Med. 2020;46:1486–8.

37. Chen PHC, Mermel CH, Liu Y. Evaluation of artificial intelligence on a reference standard based on subjective interpretation. Lancet Digit Health. 2021;3:e693–5.
38. Finlayson SG, Subbaswamy A, Singh K, et al. The clinician and dataset shift in artificial intelligence. N Engl J Med. 2021;385:283–6.
39. Subbaswamy A, Saria S. From development to deployment: dataset shift, causality, and shift-stable models in health AI. Biostatistics. 2020;21:345–52.
40. Geneva II, Cuzzo B, Fazili T, Javaid W. Normal body temperature: a systematic review. Open forum. Infect Dis. 2019;6:ofz032.
41. Dinh-Le C, Chuang R, Chokshi S, Mann D. Wearable health technology and electronic health record integration: scoping review and future directions. JMIR Mhealth Uhealth. 2019;7:e12861.
42. Chen R, Snyder M. Promise of personalized omics to precision medicine. Wiley Interdiscip Rev Syst Biol Med. 2013;5:73–82.
43. Aushev A, Ripoll VR, Vellido A, et al. Feature selection for the accurate prediction of septic and cardiogenic shock ICU mortality in the acute phase. PLoS One. 2018;13:e0199089.

Part X

Quality of Care

Acute Medical Rehabilitation in Intensive Care

29

H. M. Buyruk, Y. Buyruk, and C. Ince

29.1 Introduction

From the first day (acute phase) on the intensive care unit (ICU), rehabilitation of the patient should start with a multidisciplinary approach [1, 2]. Weekly meetings of the rehabilitation team are advised, including active specialists playing a role in the treatment of the patient, ICU specialists, physical medicine and rehabilitation specialist, nurses, and therapists. The purpose of this brief chapter is to present a possible alternative approach, which we refer to as 'acute rehabilitation', for rehabilitation of the patient in the ICU. It has been shown that such acute medical rehabilitation can result in a shorter ICU stay for children [1–3].

During the patient's admission into the ICU, a rehabilitation plan should be made and care givers, such as doctors and therapists, should be determined. ICU rehabilitation is much more complicated than the patient in a rehabilitation center, normal hospital room, or at home. There are many catheters, vascular access tubes, or sensors connected to the patient. Many medical conditions, such as fractures, exist that require immobilization of the patient or their limbs. Although some connections can be temporarily removed, initiating exercise, manipulations, and positioning require specialized skills, training and experience from the therapist. Physiotherapists,

H. M. Buyruk (✉)
Department of Intensive Care, Erasmus MC, University Medical Center, Rotterdam, The Netherlands

VitalMed Rehab Center, Bodrum, Muğla, Turkey
e-mail: hmuzafferbuyruk@hotmail.com

Y. Buyruk
Department of Anesthesiology and Intensive Care, American Hospital, Bodrum, Muğla, Turkey

C. Ince
Department of Intensive Care, Erasmus MC, University Medical Center, Rotterdam, The Netherlands

J.-L. Vincent (ed.), *Annual Update in Intensive Care and Emergency Medicine 2022*, Annual Update in Intensive Care and Emergency Medicine,
https://doi.org/10.1007/978-3-030-93433-0_29

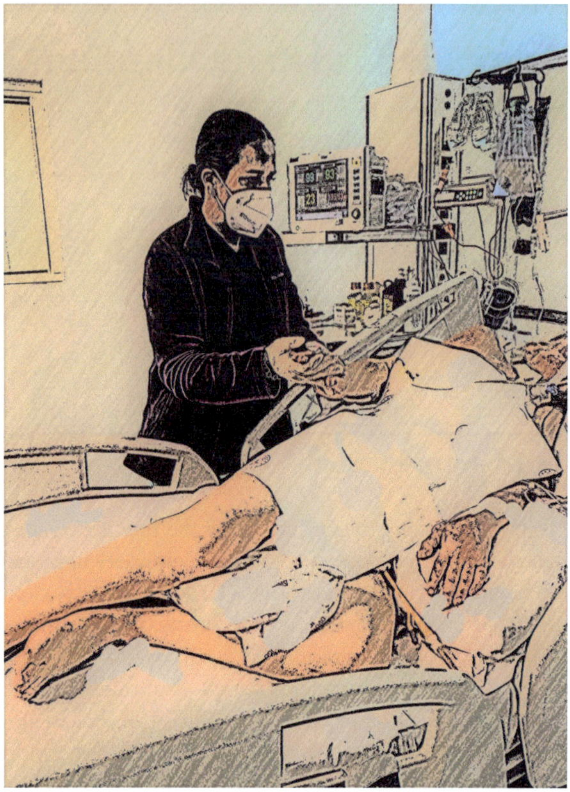

Fig. 29.1 Rehabilitation in the intensive care unit (ICU)

occupational therapists, psychotherapists, speech therapists, orthotic and prosthetic technicians, rehabilitation nurses, dieticians, and social workers can all deliver services in the ICU (Fig. 29.1, Table 29.1).

The ICU stay should be as short as possible, since the human body is exceedingly resilient in its ability to renew itself during daily function. If it is not overloaded, the human body can renew itself continuously, especially when it is in the vertical position. Daily regular exercise including the whole body, using joints and muscles for about 45 min is enough for daily body maintenance. The human body is not a mechanical machine where broken parts can be replaced with spare ones (e.g., hip and knee joint prosthetics) if it is not necessary to treat the patient within a short period of time. There are different levels of cell regeneration of tissues such as bones, cartilage, muscle, ligaments and internal organs and even neurons. Some parts of the body, such as cartilage, lack a blood supply since they have no blood vessels in them, but they do supply the chondrocytes with nutrients. Nutrients diffuse through a dense connective tissue surrounding the cartilage (called the perichondrium) and into the core of the cartilage. In unsheathed tendons, vessels may pass through the surrounding tissue into the tendon at any point along the tendon. Sheathed tendons have better blood supply; the blood vessels enter the tendon only at specific points along the tendon. Ligaments are very similar to tendons with limited blood supply and regeneration capacity. Poor or no blood supply can be a

Table 29.1 Acute medical rehabilitation team

Team member	Function in the team
Intensive care specialist	• Primary care giver • Determines the patient's need for rehabilitation • ICU medical therapy
Physical medicine and rehabilitation (PMR) specialist	• Designs the rehabilitation program • Communication between the external doctors and therapists • Regular consultations for the follow up
Consulting doctor	• Medical therapy for trauma, cardiac, neurologic etc. • Executing the necessary interventions, surgical and medical
Physiotherapist	• Daily exercise program, active or passive • Stretching the contractures, muscles, ligaments • Passive and ROM exercises for patients under sedation
Occupational therapist	• Checking the bed conditions for the patient • Choosing wheelchair or other assistive devices after intensive care • Designing hospital room according to the patient's need
Psychotherapist	• Controlling cognitive functions and mental status
Rehabilitation nurse	• Treating the wounds, decubitus ulcers, amputations
Speech therapist	• Following speech and swallowing problems and training
Prosthetic technician	• Splints and casts for contracture prevention • Temporary prostheses for amputations • Assistive devices for different musculoskeletal pathologies
Social worker	• Regulating the problems in legal, family, professional and social life
Nutritionist	• Special diets for major pathology or side pathologies

ROM range of motion

special disadvantage to some structures in the musculoskeletal system. Therefore, a sufficient amount of full range joint motion is required daily to regenerate the cells and protect the system.

Long periods of bed rest, especially in the horizontal position, with inactivity loses about 1–5% of muscle mass per day secondary to age-related decreases in growth hormone. Patients with limited joint mobility will see muscle shortening and atrophy, osteoporosis, ligament and tendon shortening, and cartilage degeneration, therefore joint contractures. Such muscle atrophy has been associated with increased risk of organ failure [4]. This is the reason why rehabilitation of the patient has to start in the acute phase of the ICU admission to ensure shortened recovery [1, 2] .

The general global perception is that the rehabilitation period is a medical intervention that is relevant for the post-clinic and chronic phase. The usual ICU approach is that if the patient survives the critical period in the ICU, a plan is drawn up for rehabilitation in the hospital ward. Yet before many planned surgeries, the pre-rehabilitation, ICU rehabilitation, and postoperative rehabilitation should be planned to ensure fast recovery.

Physiotherapy is an integral part of patient management in the ICU of hospitals in industrialized countries. Physiotherapy can result in metabolic and hemodynamic changes. The importance and safety of physiotherapy treatment in the ICU has also recently been highlighted and there is growing evidence for the role of exercise rehabilitation beginning in the ICU and extending to beyond ICU discharge [5–9].

29.2 Admission to the Intensive Care Unit

At admission, the patient's blood pressure, electrocardiogram, oxygen saturation, and heart rhythm is checked. Hemodynamic stability is provided by peripheral vascular access or central catheter. If there is arrhythmia, correction is initiated. If there is no contraindication, nasogastric and urinary catheters are placed. The patient is monitored continuously from admission to discharge. An informed consent form should be signed by the patient or one of the close relatives.

All the pathologies and conditions mentioned above require acute medical rehabilitation [1, 2]. Intervention should commence from ICU admission or as soon as all conditions are suitable for rehabilitation. The general condition of the patient can decline rapidly, especially the musculoskeletal system if the patient is immobilized. The patient's motivation for recovery plays an important role in shortening this period. Sometimes full recovery never happens due to lack of motivation. That is why acute medical rehabilitation needs to be initiated as early as possible.

29.3 Cardiac Patients

Although in some countries cardiac rehabilitation has been standard practice for more than 30 years, it is rarely started at the very early stage of the postoperative period. Most cardiac patients have a sedentary life dealing with low cardiac output. ICU admission also has a negative contribution to the patient's heart condition. The rehabilitation of cardiac patients should be according to cardiac rehabilitation protocols. Cardiac rehabilitation protocols should be the same as general ones even if they are started during the ICU stay. An early start is important for successful cardiac rehabilitation.

According to the European Society of Cardiology, cardiovascular rehabilitation is a multi-factorial and comprehensive intervention in secondary prevention, supervised and carried out by adequately trained health professionals, aimed at obtaining clinical stabilization, limiting the physiological and psychological effects of cardiovascular disease, managing symptoms and reducing the risk of future cardiovascular events [10]. Cardiovascular rehabilitation is traditionally divided into three phases: *Phase I* is typically an inpatient service including the acute phase in the ICU, which consists of early mobilization, becoming aware of the illness, trusting one's own body again, the rehabilitation, risk factor management and planning, training of the patient and the family. *Phase II* is a supervised outpatient program after discharge. *Phase III* is a heart maintenance program where the aim is to diminish the risks and install a less sedentary lifestyle and promote training. It is important to continue the exercise lifelong. Active but not excessive activities are advised.

The goals of cardiac rehabilitation include reducing smoking and alcohol, more active life with less depression, better diet, diminished use of medical drugs, daily exercise, training for healthy life, behavioral changes from the earlier life style. In many institutions where cardiac surgery is done, the postoperative ICU is a separate unit from other ICUs. Patient care is more specific to the patient's condition. After surgery, more parameters of the patient are followed in the ICU and more device connections are present. Therapists should be trained for cardiac surgery complications and be aware of the whole process [11–13].

29.4 Stroke Patients

The rehabilitation of stroke patients depends on the type –infarct, bleeding or both, or transient ischemic attack (TIA)– on the pathology, and on the extent of the brain injury. Timely splinting is important for contracture prevention. Repositioning the patient is required to prevent pressure sores and deep vein thrombosis. The patient's progression to rehabilitation in the ICU is dependent on: a stable condition medically, sitting with good balance, standing with or without walker, and walking with a walker, parallel bar, tripod, walking stick, or without helping device.

Occupational therapists evaluate the wheelchair, walking assist devices, and house and workplace adaptations. Speech therapists evaluate aphasia and swallowing, and provide the tools for communication. The neuropsychologist evaluates symptoms of depression, anxiety, post-traumatic stress disorder, or a combination of these. Cognitive impairment, memory loss, and poor attention are also checked. The nutritionist should check for stroke risk factors, such as high blood pressure, excess weight, and unhealthy cholesterol levels [14, 15].

29.5 Trauma Patients

Trauma, especially multi-trauma, needs special care dependent on the extent and the parts of the body that are damaged. In the Emergency Department, the airway is checked and, if needed intubated, hemodynamics are established by vascular access or catheterization, and X-rays and computerized tomography are performed on potentially injured areas. Consultation by specialists is requested if necessary. Emergency surgery, or later elective surgery, is performed if necessary.

In case of multiple fractures, if possible, splinting should be preferred over full casting. If casting is necessary for treatment, cutting the cast in half from both sides is advised to sustain joint mobility for exercise. Rehabilitation interventions are much easier with splints than with casts. This important joint saving strategy should be applied to all broken bones and neighboring joints. Bone fractures are important but they can be corrected in multiple ways, such as re-breaking, cutting, using osteosynthetic materials and bone grafts, without loss of function. Once the joint is damaged by contracture, joint surface deformation, calcification and ligament rupture make it very hard to regain the original function. Splinting gives care givers more freedom for easy removal and for initiation of a joint protection program. Nerve and vascular repairs, unstable vertebral fractures are an obstacle for easy therapy in the ICU. Internal organ operations, such as with open abdominal interventions, are also a limiting factor, since exercise can increase intraabdominal pressure. Therapists should perform isometric exercises for the patient in whom mobility is dangerous for the damaged body parts [16].

29.6 Patients with Cancer

Acute medical rehabilitation should be planned for cancer patients even if the life expectancy is not very long [1, 2]. Even though the patient's laboratory findings may not be optimal, rehabilitation therapies should be realized. Daily maintenance of the patient is much easier if the patient is mobile and cooperating with the caregiver. Psychologic support is important for the cancer patient. The feeling that something is being done for his or her illness has a positive effect for the stress of the disease since diminishing general stress supports the immune system.

Rehabilitation may vary dependent on the type of the cancer and a program should be planned by the rehabilitation specialist, tailor-made for every patient. An easy rehabilitation program is advised for patients with short life expectancy in order to keep them mobile as long as possible and promote a feeling of well-being for the patient.

29.7 Patients with Spinal Cord Injury

Rehabilitation interventions and plans change according to the spinal cord injury level. Partial or complete cord compression is important for prognostic estimates and the length of rehabilitation. The spinal cord begins under the foremen magnum of the occipital bone and finishes at L1–2 level. There are 31 bilateral nerve roots, 8 cervical, 12 thoracic, 5 lumbar, 5 sacral, and 1 coccygeal nerve. The spinal cord and bone levels are different, since the spinal cord ends with the cauda equina. According to whether the injury happens at the upper (spinal cord), with spasticity developing after spinal shock, or lower (cauda equina) neuron, with flaccid muscles, specialized plans are needed.

Rehabilitation starts at the very early stage when the medical treatment of the patient is arranged and the patient stable. The expected recovery and the usual complications should be evaluated properly by the rehabilitation team. The American Spinal Injury Association (ASIA) impairment scale determines the damage and recovery expectations. Preparation of the family and the patient to arrange new living conditions, which may be temporary or lifelong, can already start in the ICU [17, 18].

Achievements of rehabilitation are dependent on the spinal cord injury level:

- C2-C3: respiratory muscles and diaphragm are paralyzed, respiratory support and phrenic nerve stimulators are required, complete dependency for all activities
- C4: Diaphragm, upper cervical para-spinal muscles, sternocleidomastoid, trapezius are spared. Complete dependency for all activities
- C5: Elbow flexion and shoulder activity partly exists; patients can perform personal care with special orthoses.
- C6: Elbow flexion, shoulder activity and wrist extension exists. Using tenodesis, grasp of the hand can be improved, thus patients can manage personal care such as brushing teeth and eating.
- C7: Finger flexors and extensors and triceps exist. Patients are independent with transfers.
- C8-T1: Self washing is possible; independent including transfers, wheelchair use and communication
- T2-T10: Orthoses for standing and ambulation
- T11-L2: With the use of long leg braces and crutches moves independently and wheel chair for outdoors
- L3–S3: Without wheelchair ambulates inside and outside with short leg braces

29.8 Patients with Chronic Diseases

Chronic disease involves having a poor physical condition in combination with many other altered body parameters. Age, life style, and the type of disease (progressive or regressive) are important. These patients mostly have a worsening general condition and once the threshold values are exceeded resulting in organ failure, ICU admission is compulsory. A patient's condition may worsen due to their disease, but a lack of motivation can also be an important factor. Low mood resulting from the long sickness period may demotivate patients to change their lifestyle, especially in older patients. Psychological intervention is important for the ICU patient when motivation is needed for change (diet, nutrition, weight control, daily exercise, social contacts, not smoking, alcohol consumption and drugs etc.) after discharge [1, 2].

29.9 Chronic Neurologic Diseases

Amyotrophic lateral sclerosis, Alzheimer's disease, dementia, epilepsy, restless leg syndrome, malignant migraine attacks, multiple sclerosis are some of the chronic neurologic diseases where intensive care may be necessary. A good memory is essential for good rehabilitation. Coma patients or sedated patients or patients with dementia can receive passive exercise programs, decubitus prevention, positioning, range of motion exercises, and rehabilitation nursing. Cognitive functions, including time, place and person, and mental status need to be remembered [1, 2].

29.10 Anoxic Encephalopathy

Drowning is one of the leading causes of anoxic encephalopathy. The clinical prognosis of drowning is related to the duration of being under water. The Glasgow Coma Scale, unreactive pupils, intracranial pressure, lack of motor response to pain, duration of cardiopulmonary resuscitation are also determining factors for prognosis. Existence of voluntary movements is a sign of better neurologic recovery. Anoxic encephalopathy develops into spasticity and joint contractures. The rehabilitation goal for this group of patients is prevention of contractures and complications rather than recovery [19, 20].

29.11 Pressure Sores

The prevention of pressure sores is a major target on admission of the patient. Pressure sores develop as the external pressure exceeds the capillary pressure of the tissue. When the blood supply to the area is diminished, delivery of oxygen and nutrients vital to cell survival is diminished. Localized hypoxia, cellular death, and injury to the surrounding tissue result in the development of a pressure sore. Pressure sores most commonly involve head, sacrum and heels. In the supine position, sacrum, occiput, and heels are the areas under risk of ulceration. Other areas of pressure sore development include the ischium, spinous processes, scapula, trochanter, and malleolus of the ankle. Areas under risk of pressure sore development in various positions are shown in Fig. 29.2.

Pressure sores are graded according to the depth and extent of the tissue damage. The four stages of the pressure sores are:

Stage I: Non-blanchable erythema

Stage II: Partial skin loss

Stage III: Full-thickness loss of skin and subcutaneous tissue

Stage IV: Full-thickness skin loss, extending to the muscle, bone

Repositioning of the patients every 2–4 h and placement of support surfaces to decrease pressure are the first preventive measures. Caregivers should be careful during repositioning not to cause friction injuries. Elimination of the risk factors and intensive care is of primary importance. As a daily routine, skin care should be performed (not too dry, not too wet, friction avoided) and devices, e.g., tracheostomy and splints, should be cleaned regularly.

Healthcare workers may be unwilling to move the patients after spinal stabilization procedures. Surgery, sepsis, or other life-threatening problems may further lengthen the duration of immobilization of the patient. Patients may be mobilized by stabilization and avoiding rotation with more than two care givers.

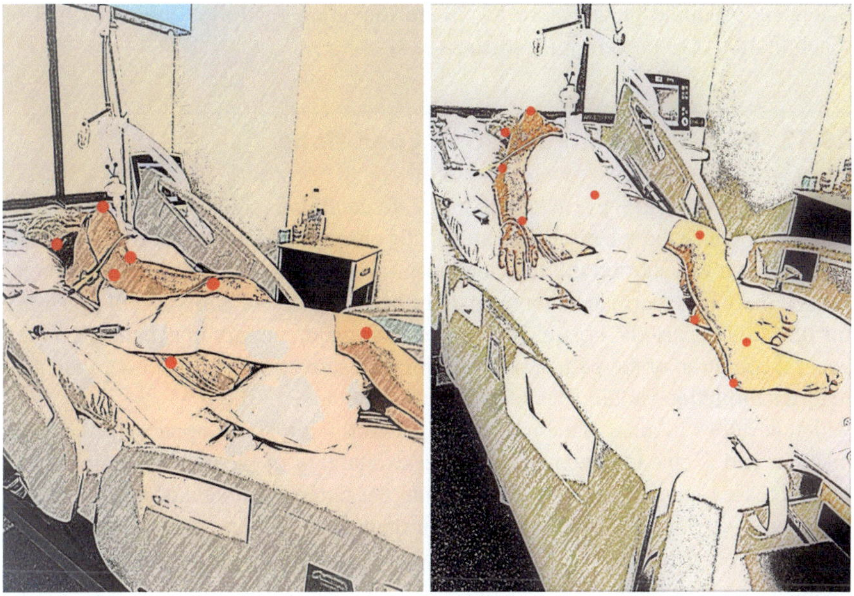

Fig. 29.2 Areas at risk of pressure sore development in various positions are shown with red dots

Many pressure reduction surfaces (egg-crate and foam-mattress overlays, gel pads, and specialty beds) have been associated with a reduction in the development of pressure sores. Repositioning of tubing, masks, and probes reduces the risk of device-related breakdown.

For wound irrigation, sterile water and saline can be used without aggressive cleaning or rubbing. Antiseptic solutions may damage the skin. Debriding necrotic tissue and treating infections with creams and antibiotics is essential [21–23].

Continuous rotation therapy, 40° on each side with 6–8 turns an hour, is provided by specialized beds providing mechanical turning of the patient from side to side; in order to prevent airway atelectasis, obstruction, and infection.

29.12 Heterotopic Ossification

Heterotopic ossification is new bone production around joints. Unilateral or bilateral bone formation is trabecular and forms only at the soft tissue around the joint. In order to protect the range of motion in the joint, diagnosis and treatment is important to maintain joint mobility. Long bone fractures, coma longer than 2 weeks, spasticity, acute respiratory distress syndrome (ARDS), trauma, and burns can result in heterotopic ossification specifically in the large joints like the hip and knee. Range of motion limitation and pain are common. Heterotopic ossification can trigger erythema and swelling. X-rays and three phase scintigraphy are used for diagnosis. Alkaline phosphatase levels are important for follow up. The goal of rehabilitation is to prevent joint stiffness [24].

29.13 Miscellaneous Pathologic Conditions

Diseases involving kidney, liver, and lungs are conditions frequently requiring ICU admission. Since these pathologies are mostly chronic, a rapid start to the rehabilitation program can shorten the ICU and hospital stay. Intoxications are short admissions if there is no permanent damage in the body and rehabilitation is not necessary for these short periods. Postoperative care after major surgery is dependent on the general condition of the patient. If the estimated recovery period is longer than normal, rehabilitation should start early during the course of the ICU stay. Spasticity, which develops in many patients with spinal cord injury, is an upper motor neuron disorder and is characterized by the hyper-excitability of the muscle stretch reflex and increased tendon reflexes. Burns, acute neuromuscular weakness, spinal cord disorders, anterior horn cell disorders, neuromuscular junction disorders, and critical illness polyneuromyopathy are pathologies that are common and need acute medical rehabilitation [1, 2]. Viral infections and coronavirus disease 2019 (COVID-19) are a new challenge for care givers and the rehabilitation team in the ICU. Further research should be done to identify the advantages of acute medical rehabilitation in new diseases such as COVID-19.

Many acute medical rehabilitation principals are similar for many pathologies that require ICU admission. For example, starting exercises late can increase the possibility of emboli from thromboses that develop during an inactive period over the first few days of the ICU stay [1, 2, 25–39].

29.14 Conclusion

An extended ICU stay results in muscle atrophy, accelerated bone demineralization, shortening and decrease in collagen, thrombosis in different parts of the body, nerve entrapments, joint contractures, decreased bowel peristalsis, postural abnormalities, and impairment in cognitive function and memory due to medication. All the complications named above are major treatment areas of rehabilitation. Early intervention reduces ICU and hospital stays. Mobilization of the patient and physiotherapy while in the intensive care bed are not easy and may be risky due to the tubes and cables connected to the patients. Restoring independency in activities of daily living is a primary target in the ICU. When the patient is stabilized and no longer needs to be monitored, they can be discharged to the hospital ward.

References

1. Stam HJ, Buyruk HM, Melvin J, Stucki G. Acute medical rehabilitation textbook, vol. I. Bodrum: VitalMed Book Publishing; 2012. p. 1–450.
2. Stam HJ, Buyruk HM, Melvin JL, Ward AN. Acute medical rehabilitation textbook, vol. II. Bodrum: VitalMed Book Publishing; 2019. p. 1–407.
3. Hopkins RO, Choong K, Zebuhr CA, Kudchadkar SR. Transforming PICU culture to facilitate early rehabilitation. J Pediatr Intensive Care. 2015;4:204–11.
4. Puthucheary ZA, Rawal J, McPhail M, et al. Acute skeletal muscle wasting in critical illness. JAMA. 2013;310:1591–600.
5. Yatao P, Hongling L, Long Z, Chunxia Z. An established early rehabilitation therapy demonstrating higher efficacy and safety for care of intensive care unit patients. Med Sci Monit. 2019;25:7052–8.
6. Brummel NE, Jackson JC, Girard TD, et al. A combined early cognitive and physical rehabilitation program for people who are critically ill: the activity and cognitive therapy in the intensive care unit (ACT-ICU) trial. Phys Ther. 2012;92:1580–92.
7. Fuke R, Hifumi T, Kondo Y, et al. Early rehabilitation to prevent postintensive care syndrome in patients with critical illness: a systematic review and meta-analysis. BMJ Open. 2018;5:e019998.
8. Castro-Avila AC, Serón P, Fan E, Gaete M, Mickan S. Effect of early rehabilitation during intensive care unit stay on functional status: systematic review and meta-analysis. PLoS One. 2015;10:e0130722.
9. Hopkins RO, Spuhler VJ. Strategies for promoting early activity in critically ill mechanically ventilated patients. AACN Adv Crit Care. 2009;20:277–89.
10. Corrà U, Piepoli MF, Carré F. Secondary prevention through cardiac rehabilitation: physical activity counselling and exercise training: key components of the position paper from the cardiac rehabilitation section of the European Association of Cardiovascular Prevention and Rehabilitation. Eur Heart J. 2010;31:1967–74.
11. Anderson L, Thompson DR, Oldridge N, et al. Exercise-based cardiac rehabilitation for coronary heart disease. Cochrane Database Syst Rev. 2016;2016:CD001800.
12. Long L, Mordi IR, Bridges C, et al. Exercise based cardiac rehabilitation for adults with heart failure. Cochrane Database Syst Rev. 2019;1:CD003331.
13. Salzwedel A, Jensen K, Rauch B, et al. Effectiveness of comprehensive cardiac rehabilitation in coronary artery disease patients treated according to contemporary evidence-based medicine: update of the cardiac rehabilitation outcome study (CROS-II). Eur J Prev Cardiol. 2020;27:1756–74.
14. Alamri MS, Waked IS, Amin FM, Al-quliti KW, Manzar MD. Effectiveness of an early mobility protocol for stroke patients in intensive care unit. Neurosciences (Riyadh). 2019;24:81–8.
15. Yen HC, Jeng JS, Chen WS, et al. Early mobilization of mild-moderate intracerebral hemorrhage patients in a stroke center: a randomized controlled trial. Neurorehabil Neural Repair. 2020;34:72–81.
16. Higgins SD, Erdogan M, Coles SJ. Green RS. Early mobilization of trauma patients admitted to intensive care units: a systematic review and meta-analyses. Injury. 2019;50:1809–15.
17. Zidek K, Srinivasan R. Rehabilitation of a child with spinal cord injury. Semin Pediatr Neurol. 2003;10:140–50.
18. Little JW, Mickleson P, Umlauf R, Britell C. Lower extremity manifestations of spasticity in chronic spinal cord injury. Am J Phys Med Rehabil. 1989;68:32–6.
19. Meyer RJ, Theodorou AA, Berg RA. Childhood drowning. Pediatr Rev. 2006;27:163–8.
20. Zandbergen EG, de Haan RJ, Stoutenbeek CP, Koelman JH, Hijdra A. Systematic review of early prediction of poor outcome in anoxic-ischemic coma. Lancet. 1998;352:1808–12.
21. Bernabe KQ. Pressure ulcers in the pediatric patient. Curr Opin Pediatr. 2012;24:352–6.

22. Schindler CA, Mikhailov TA, Kuhn EM, et al. Protecting fragile skin: nursing interventions to decrease development of pressure ulcers in pediatric intensive care. Am J Crit Care. 2011;20:26–34.
23. Allen C, Glasziou P, Del Mar C. Bed rest: a potentially harmful treatment needing more careful evaluation. Lancet. 1999;354:1229–33.
24. Hurvitz EA, Mandac BR, Davidoff G, Johnson JH, Nelson VS. Risk factors for heterotopic ossification in children and adolescents with severe traumatic brain injury. Arch Phys Med Rehabil. 1992;73:459–62.
25. Aissaoui N, Martins E, Mouly S, Weber S, Meune C. A meta-analysis of bed rest versus early ambulation in the management of pulmonary embolism, deep vein trombosis, or both. Int J Cardiol. 2009;137:37–41.
26. Haining R, Taggart P. Chapter 17. Rehabilitation of burn injuries. In: Molnar GE, Alexander MA, editors. Pediatric rehabilitation. 3rd ed. Philadelphia: Hanley&Belfus Inc.; 1999. p. 269–88.
27. Krach LE, Kriel RL. Chapter 13. Traumatic brain injury. In: Molnar GE, Alexander MA, editors. Pediatric rehabilitation. 3rd ed. Philadelphia: Hanley&Belfus Inc.; 1999. p. 245–68.
28. Clini E, Ambrosino N. Early physiotherapy in the respiratory intensive care unit. Respir Med. 2005;99:1096–104.
29. Pelosi P, Tubiolo D, Mascheroni D, et al. Effects of the prone position on respiratory mechanics and gas exchange during acute lung injury. Am J Respir Crit Care Med. 1998;157:387–93.
30. Johnson KL, Meyenburg T. Physiological rationale and current evidence for therapeutic positioning of critically ill patients. AACN Adv Crit Care. 2009;20:228–40.
31. Morris PE, Goad A, Thompson C, et al. Early intensive care unit mobility therapy in the treatment of acute respiratory failure. Crit Care Med. 2008;36:2238–43.
32. Jin Y, Di J, Wang X. Early rehabilitation nursing in ICU promotes rehabilitation of patients with respiratory failure treated with invasive mechanical ventilation. Am J Transl Res. 2021;13:5232–9.
33. Gentil P, de Lira CAB, Coswig V, et al. Practical recommendations relevant to the use of resistance training for COVID-19 survivors. Front Physiol. 2021;12:637590.
34. Yu P, Wei Q, He C. Early rehabilitation for critically ill patients with COVID-19: more benefits than risks. Am J Phys Med Rehabil. 2020;99:468–9.
35. Hashem MD, Parker AM, Needham DM. Early mobilization and rehabilitation of patients who are critically ill. Chest. 2016;150:722–31.
36. Hodgson CL, Tipping CJ. Physiotherapy management of intensive care unit-acquired weakness. J Physiother. 2017;63:4–10.
37. Nydahl P, Ruhl AP, Bartoszek G, et al. Early mobilization of mechanically ventilated patients: a 1-day point-prevalence study in Germany. Crit Care Med. 2014;42:1178–86.
38. Baddeley RA. Physiotherapy for enhanced recovery in thoracic surgery. J Thorac Dis. 2016;8(Suppl 1):S107–10.
39. dos Santos RS, Donadio MV, da Silva GV, Blattner CN, Melo DA, Nunes FB. Immediate effects of chest physiotherapy on hemodynamic, metabolic, and oxidative stress parameters in subjects with septic shock. Respir Care. 2014;59:1398–403.

Sepsis Performance Improvement Programs: From Evidence Toward Clinical Implementation

30

M. Schinkel, P. W. B. Nanayakkara, and W. J. Wiersinga

30.1 Introduction

Since its launch in the early 2000s, the international Surviving Sepsis Campaign (SSC) has provided guidelines for the management of sepsis, most recently updated in 2021 [1]. The SSC aims to provide a standard of care for sepsis while increasing awareness among healthcare professionals and the general public. The goal is to reduce morbidity and mortality from sepsis and septic shock worldwide [2].

To facilitate the clinical implementation of the guidelines, the SSC bundles their recommendations into small groups of care processes that physicians should perform within a specific timeframe and that provides them with a concrete plan of action [1, 2]. Despite efforts to facilitate the successful implementation of the guidelines, adherence has been suboptimal, particularly regarding the microbiological

M. Schinkel
Center for Experimental and Molecular Medicine, Amsterdam UMC, Location Academic Medical Center, University of Amsterdam, Amsterdam, The Netherlands

Section General Internal Medicine, Department of Internal Medicine, Amsterdam Public Health Research Institute, Amsterdam UMC, Location VU University Medical Center, Amsterdam, The Netherlands

P. W. B. Nanayakkara
Section General Internal Medicine, Department of Internal Medicine, Amsterdam Public Health Research Institute, Amsterdam UMC, Location VU University Medical Center, Amsterdam, The Netherlands

W. J. Wiersinga (✉)
Center for Experimental and Molecular Medicine, Amsterdam UMC, Location Academic Medical Center, University of Amsterdam, Amsterdam, The Netherlands

Department of Medicine, Division of Infectious Diseases, Amsterdam UMC, Location Academic Medical Center, University of Amsterdam, Amsterdam, The Netherlands
e-mail: w.j.wiersinga@amsterdamumc.nl

J.-L. Vincent (ed.), *Annual Update in Intensive Care and Emergency Medicine 2022*, Annual Update in Intensive Care and Emergency Medicine,
https://doi.org/10.1007/978-3-030-93433-0_30

work-up and administration of appropriate antibiotics [3]. Non-compliance to the SSC guidelines seems most prominent among emergency medicine and internal medicine physicians [4].

In response to the low adoption rates of (SSC) sepsis guidelines, individual hospitals and organizations have introduced sepsis performance improvement programs. Usually, dedicated physicians or research teams lead these initiatives and use screening tools, process changes in sepsis care pathways, and sepsis educational programs to optimize adherence to the standard of care [5]. The latest update of the SSC guidelines recommends that all hospitals and health systems have sepsis performance improvement programs [1].

In this chapter, we discuss the literature on the use and benefits of sepsis performance improvement programs to improve protocol adherence and provide practical insights for the clinical implementation of such programs in your hospital.

30.2 Do 'One-Size-Fits-All' Care Bundles Improve Sepsis Outcomes?

Sepsis performance improvement programs aim to improve adherence to a guideline or protocol for sepsis care, and they are almost exclusively studied in the context of the SSC care bundles [5]. When one aims to improve compliance rates to any guideline, one should first be convinced that this is a goal worth pursuing. In the case of the SSC guidelines, this debate has been ongoing for many years, and this paragraph presents only a brief overview of this reflective and meaningful discussion [6, 7].

Expert panelists on sepsis have created the SSC bundles, spearheaded by the Society of Critical Care Medicine (SCCM) and European Society of Intensive Care Medicine (ESICM), and endorsed by numerous medical societies [1, 6]. However, the evidence base for these bundles and the timeframes in which they should be performed have been a matter of debate [7–9]. One prominent example concerns adherence to early goal-directed therapy (EDGT), an early form of bundled care that was associated with significantly lower in-hospital mortality rates (30.5% vs. 46.5% in the usual care group) in a randomized study of 263 patients with sepsis or septic shock presenting to the emergency department of a tertiary hospital in the United States [10]. However, these results were not replicated in subsequent large randomized trials and meta-analyses [11–13]. Furthermore, the value of individual bundle items, such as the 30 ml/kg fluid bolus and administration of antibiotics within 1 h to all patients, has been heavily debated because of conflicting results regarding the benefits [7, 14–16]. Moreover, fear exists that pressure to perform bundle items within a specific timeframe may promote harmful diagnostic tests and treatments, as was the case with the 2002 quality measure for the management of community-acquired pneumonia by the Centers for Medicare & Medicaid Services, which was later removed [9, 17].

Despite the limited evidence base that underlies some of the recommendations in the SSC bundles, the overall consensus, underscored by the endorsements from 35 international medical societies, seems to be that most of the care processes in the bundles will positively contribute to the management of the majority of sepsis patients [6]. Numerous observational studies have shown associations between improved bundle compliance and a reduction in mortality. An extensive 7.5-year study in 280 hospitals across Europe, South America, and the United States showed that overall mortality was significantly lower in high-compliance hospitals (29.0%) compared with low-compliance hospitals (38.6%) [18]. This study included 29,470 patients with sepsis or septic shock from emergency departments, regular wards, and intensive care units (ICUs) between January 1st 2005 and June 30th 2021. Notably, compliance was defined as high when sites completed the resuscitation bundle within 6 h for as few as 15% of their patients, suggesting that complete bundle adherence is only practical in a small subset of patients [18]. A similar project in Portugal studied the effects of adherence to the 6-hour bundle in 897 patients with community-acquired sepsis in 17 ICUs [19]. Among those 897 patients, the core bundle was only completed within 6 h in 12% of the patients. The highest compliance was seen for the administration of vasopressors (78%) and the collection of cultures before antibiotic treatment (77%). In comparison, the lowest adherence was seen for blood culture collection in general (48%) and administration of antibiotics (52%) [19]. Compliance with the complete bundle was associated with decreased 28-day mortality, with an adjusted odds ratio (OR) of 0.44 (95% confidence interval [CI] 0.24–0.80) in sepsis and 0.49 (95% CI 0.25–0.95) in septic shock. Other studies have found similar mortality benefits associated with improved SSC bundle adherence [20–22].

30.3 Sepsis Improvement Programs: What Is the Evidence?

Adherence to the SSC guidelines in hospitals and healthcare systems that have adopted them is still suboptimal [3, 5]. For example, a nationwide study in Finland showed complete guideline adherence in only 6 out of 92 ICU patients during the four-month study period, similar to rates found in other studies [5, 23]. Sepsis performance improvement programs may help improve compliance, and a 2015 systematic review and meta-analysis by Damiani and colleagues tried to quantify this effect [5]. The reviewers identified 50 observational studies with highly diverse improvement programs and study designs. Despite this heterogeneity, the meta-analysis showed that sepsis performance improvement programs were consistently associated with increased compliance with 6-hour (OR 4.12, 95% CI 2.95–5.76) and 24-hour (OR 2.57, 95%-CI 1.74–3.77) bundles and with reduced mortality (OR 0.66, 95%-CI 0.61–0.72). The mortality estimates are hard to interpret in this meta-analysis since they include in-hospital mortality as well as short- and long-term mortality.

Among the 50 studies included in the systematic review of Damiani et al., combinations of interventions using screening tools, process changes, and educational programs were independently associated with increased bundle compliance and reduced mortality [5]. It thus appears that having a sepsis performance improvement program in itself is more important than the specific content of the program. However, the best results were observed in programs with various simultaneous interventions for performance improvement and in hospitals where the initial compliance was lowest [5]. The following sections will discuss the most-studied interventions (implementation of sepsis screening tools, process changes in sepsis care pathways, and educational programs) and their effects in further detail.

30.3.1 Sepsis Screening Tools

A primary focus of many performance improvement programs is using screening tools to identify sepsis early. Correct treatment can be initiated earlier if sepsis is recognized sooner, which is expected to improve patient outcomes [2]. Three randomized controlled trials (RCTs) have studied whether the use of screening tools can improve patient outcomes in sepsis [24–26]. Downing et al. used an electronic health record (EHR) alert to detect sepsis early in medical and surgical wards, based on modified sepsis criteria including laboratory results and vital signs [24]. However, the alert did not result in improved performance measures or patient outcomes. Hooper and colleagues studied the effects of pager alerts whenever a patient in the medical ICU satisfied a modified version of the systemic inflammatory response syndrome (SIRS) criteria [25]. Again, the alerts did not result in any improved performance measures or decreased mortality rates. Only Shimabukuro and colleagues were able to show improvements in patient outcomes using automatically generated alerts in the EHR with their machine learning-based sepsis screening tool [26]. Among 142 patients in the US-based medical-surgical ICUs, the hospital length-of-stay (-2.30 days), ICU length-of-stay (-2.09 days), and in-hospital mortality (-12.3%, absolute) were all significantly lower in the intervention group that used the automated sepsis screening tool [26]. One explanation for why this study was able to find beneficial effects is that it was the only one of the three to combine the alert with a mandatory and immediate evaluation of the patient to specifically address the potential diagnosis of sepsis, which can be regarded as an additional process change.

A problem in sepsis screening is that there is a plethora of different risk scores and screening tools which are currently used, such as the SIRS criteria, Modified Early Warning Score (MEWS), National Early Warning Score (NEWS), and quick Sequential Organ Failure Score (qSOFA). The accuracy of these risk scores is highly variable in the emergency department, regular wards, and the ICU [27]. Several extensive studies and reviews have evaluated which screening tool is most effective for suspected infection or sepsis [27–31]. The NEWS and MEWS consistently show a balance between sensitivity and specificity, both usually ranging between 0.40 and 0.80 [27, 29]. SIRS is more sensitive than specific, and qSOFA more specific than sensitive. None of these instruments seems superior to the others in identifying sepsis across studies [27–31]. The SSC guideline consequently does not recommend using a particular tool [1]. Physicians should be aware of the benefits and limitations of the tools they use, and choices should be based on local preferences. The only exception is the use of qSOFA, which the guideline recommends against as a screening tool [1]. Although the qSOFA is highly specific, the poor sensitivity makes it unsuitable for screening purposes.

A limitation to all currently used tools is that they are susceptible to false positives because of the relatively low prevalence of sepsis, particularly in the general emergency department and ward populations [30]. Advanced computational approaches such as machine learning could provide a solution for this and may eventually replace the current, less complex risk scores. A systematic review and meta-analysis evaluating seven studies showed that machine learning algorithms outperform MEWS, SIRS, and qSOFA for sepsis prediction [32]. Additionally, monitoring through EHR systems with continuous data streams can detect sepsis even earlier than static risk scores. Van Wyk et al. showed this when their algorithm predicted sepsis onset in 377 ICU patients in the USA on average 205 min earlier than SIRS criteria would have [33]. However, many challenges still need to be overcome before safely introducing machine learning tools for sepsis into everyday clinical practice [34]. Some of these challenges were recently illustrated by the external validation of the Epic Sepsis Model, the machine learning-based screening tool for sepsis provided by the EHR vendor, Epic (Verona, WI, USA) [35]. This algorithm is widely adopted for sepsis screening, particularly in the USA. In a population of 2552 sepsis patients among 38,455 hospitalizations, the Epic Sepsis Model reached an area under the curve (AUC) of only 0.63 for sepsis recognition in an external validation [35]. Physicians using this tool evaluated an average of 109 patients based on sepsis screening alerts to detect only one case earlier than they would have without, putting a disproportionate burden on the healthcare system.

30.3.2 Process Changes in Sepsis Care Pathways

Several studies have examined the effect of sepsis performance improvement programs using process changes to improve adherence to the SSC care bundles. After identifying a patient who may have sepsis, the diagnostic work-up and treatments should be promptly initiated. The most critical process change in sepsis care pathways studied in this regard is the implementation of sepsis (response) teams. Instead of putting the responsibility to act on a sepsis screening alert on one consulting physician, who may already care for multiple patients, dedicated teams are created to respond to sepsis alerts collectively. A pre-post study by Viale et al. in Italian emergency departments showed that implementing a dedicated sepsis response team was associated with increased bundle adherence from 4.6% to 32%, improved appropriateness of the initial antibiotic therapy from 30% to 79%, and a hazard ratio of 0.64 (95% CI 0.43–0.94) for 14-day all-cause mortality [3]. In another study from Italy, these results were replicated in a multidisciplinary ICU [36]. In this setting, implementing a dedicated sepsis team was reported to be associated with a significant decrease in in-hospital mortality from 68% to 23%. Furthermore, the use of the dedicated sepsis team was significantly associated with decreased mortality in univariate logistic analysis (OR 0.28, 95% CI 0.10–0.79) [36]. However, the results of these studies should be interpreted cautiously, given their observational design and potential for confounding by indication.

Process changes other than implementing a dedicated sepsis team may also contribute to better bundle adherence when they improve the efficiency of the care workflow. Examples that have been extensively studied are printed or easily accessible protocols, standardized EHR order sets, daily auditing with weekly feedback, and nurse-driven sepsis protocols [5]. Nurse-driven sepsis protocols are a practical approach that acknowledges the essential role of nurses in the sepsis care pathways [37]. Their role is not formally described in the SSC guidelines, but they are often the first to triage patients and respond to their deteriorating condition. As an example, a Dutch study by Tromp et al. showed that a nurse-driven sepsis care bundle increased compliance with the complete bundle from 3.5% to 12.4% and the mean number of performed bundle elements within the appropriate timeframe from 3.0 to 4.2 [37]. Completion of four of the six individual bundle items, such as the measurement of serum lactate (23% to 80%) and the start of antibiotics within 3 h (38% to 56%), increased significantly. No significant changes in the in-hospital mortality rates or hospital length of stay were observed [37].

30.3.3 Sepsis Educational Programs

Arguably, increased sepsis awareness is one of the primary reasons for better patient outcomes through SSC care bundle use. Therefore, education is an essential aspect of sepsis performance improvement programs, as it helps raise awareness among healthcare professionals. The 2015 systematic review about sepsis performance improvement programs by Damiani et al. included 17 studies in which only educational programs were used [5]. These included educational materials, lectures, bedside teaching, and simulation training, among others. Many of these education-only programs showed significantly increased bundle adherence and decreased mortality rates. An early observational cohort study in the USA by Nguyen et al. studied the effects of a comprehensive sepsis education program in a small cohort of 96 patients with sepsis in their ICU [38]. A mortality rate of 45% was observed when the compliance with SSC care bundles was high, but was 73% when SSC guidelines were largely disregarded ($p = 0.006$). Another example of the effects of educational programs is the more extensive study by van Zanten and colleagues, which also reduced the limitations of the observational approach by using control groups and propensity score matching [22]. Implementation of educational programs in 52 participating hospitals was associated with an absolute increase of 23.6% in SSC bundle adherence and an absolute decrease in mortality rates of 5.8% in 8031 ICU patients with sepsis during the study period. No such associations were found in 8387 ICU patients in 30 non-participating hospitals over the same period.

30.4 The Road Ahead

The discussion about the precise value of the SSC care bundles and the care processes within them will inevitably continue [6, 7]. Standardized expert care recommendations are indispensable for a syndrome with a mortality rate as high as it is in sepsis. However, such recommendations are often challenging to develop given the heterogeneity of sepsis and the weak and often contradicting evidence for its different treatment modalities [1, 13, 39]. Still, bundle adherence has consistently been associated with improved patient outcomes. An unanswered question is whether improved patient outcomes are caused by the items in the care bundles, by increased awareness irrespective of bundle adherence, or whether they are just artifacts of confounding by indication. Well-controlled trials could potentially find a definitive answer to this question, further determining what matters most while implementing sepsis performance improvement programs. Such a trial will, however, be hard to carry out and needs sophisticated methodological design.

Sepsis improvement programs are associated with improved protocol compliance and can be helpful to improve protocol adherence when a hospital or healthcare system implements either the SSC sepsis guidelines or their version of a protocol for sepsis detection and treatment. Therefore, these programs should be used in any hospital with low adherence rates to local protocols. The program should ideally consist of various simultaneous interventions to promote bundle compliance optimally [5]. Those interventions can be sepsis screening tools, process changes in sepsis care pathways, and sepsis educational programs. However, the goal should never be to mandate 100% guideline adherence but to leave room to deviate from standardized protocols when appropriate.

In our university medical center, we initiated a sepsis performance improvement program in 2021. As an illustration, we provide the details about this program, including early lessons learned from the implementation process in Box 30.1. The flowchart for our sepsis response team set-up is visually presented in Fig. 30.1. A major takeaway is that the engagement of only a few clinical leaders per department seems insufficient in an emergency department's dynamic and continuous environment. Furthermore, the involvement of patient representatives is important when initiating a sepsis performance improvement program, as the values and perspectives of the main stakeholder should not be overlooked. In high-pressure situations, such as acute care for patients with suspected sepsis in the emergency department, treatment of the patient's physical state is prioritized over the mental state. However, systematically addressing important questions the patient may have could alleviate much of the mental stress they will likely experience. In Box 30.2, we summarize important questions to address from the viewpoint of a sepsis survivor who has been involved with our sepsis performance improvement program.

Box 30.1 An example from the emergency department: creating a sepsis performance improvement program in a large university medical center. The different phases of implementing a sepsis performance improvement program in the Amsterdam University Medical Center

Pre-implementation phase:

- Retrospective and prospective evaluation of the current situation to identify opportunities for improvement. We noted:
  - Sequential ED consultations by various specialists, which delayed appropriate care.
  - Non-urgent triage codes in (elderly) patients with suspected sepsis.
- Involvement of patient representatives.

Interventions:

- Screening tool selected: MEWS (already in use and thus easy to incorporate).
- Process changes: Initiation of a sepsis response team, standardized notes and EHR order sets, daily audit and weekly feedback.
- Education: Launch of a dedicated website, pocket cards, talks at morning hand-over.

Lessons learned so far:

- Early challenges include behavior change and trust among all stakeholders that the new workflow will be efficient and may improve outcomes.
- The engagement of only a few clinical leaders per department seems insufficient for successful implementation, especially in the dynamic environment of an ED.

ED emergency department, *ICU* intensive care unit, *MEWS* Modified Early Warning Score, *EHR* electronic health record

Box 30.2. Essential aspects of emergency department sepsis care from the patient's point of view. A summary of aspects to address during the evaluation of and conversation with a patient who may have sepsis

- Acknowledge the signs that a patient is worried and take them seriously
- Communicate about the word "sepsis" and what it means
- Communicate the urgency that the potential sepsis is recognized
- Inform the patient about the use of a sepsis team or sepsis protocol
- Inform the patient about the plan of action, including possible tests, treatments, and other decisions to be made over the following hours
- Inform the patient about the effects/symptoms that can be expected from the treatment or progression of the syndrome

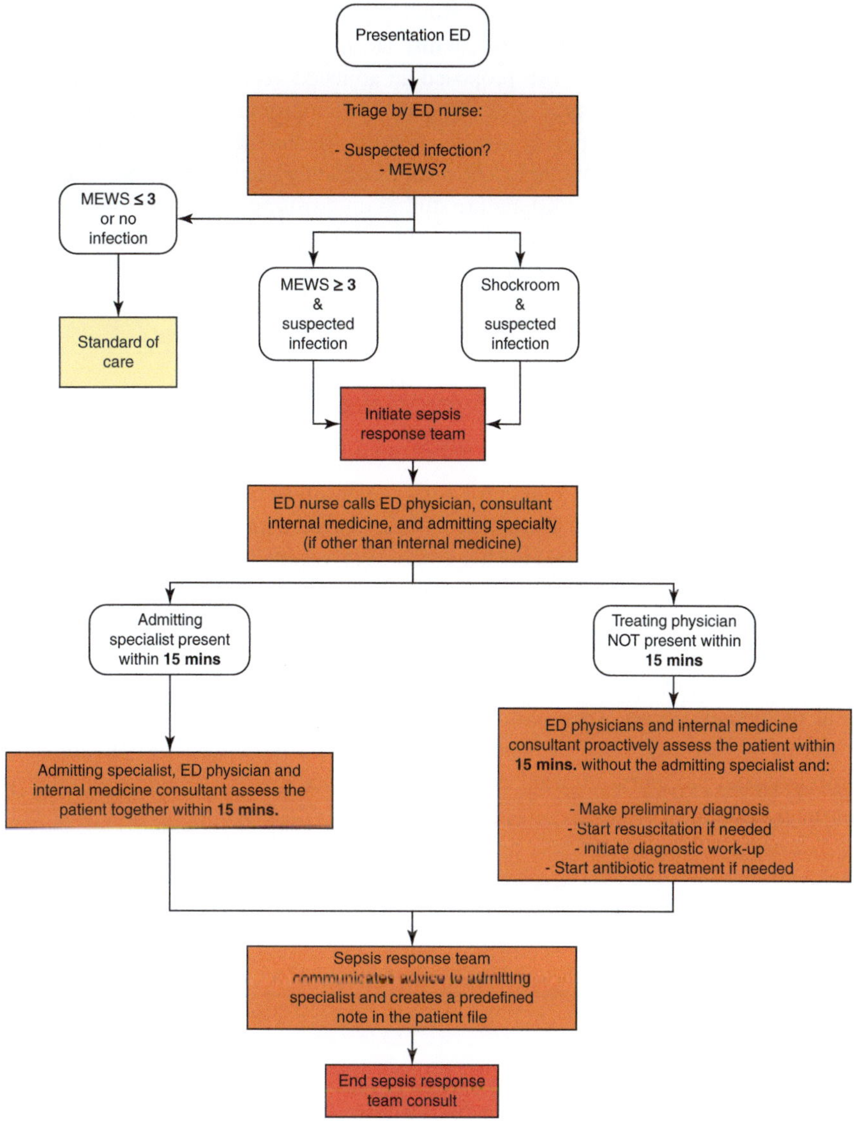

Fig. 30.1 Flowchart of sepsis response team involvement in a large teaching university medical center. A practical example from Amsterdam University Medical Center including all aspects from early detection to the diagnostic work-up and treatment decisions. *ED* emergency department, *MEWS* Modified Early Warning Score

Finally, most studies investigating the benefits of bundled care and sepsis performance improvement programs used mortality reduction as an endpoint [5]. Already in 2005, an International Sepsis Forum (ISF) colloquium provided a broad set of outcome measures that sepsis studies can use beyond survival as the only and ultimate goal of sepsis care [40]. Nevertheless, the literature is still dominated by the pursuit of short-term survival benefits. During the coronavirus disease 2019 (COVID-19) pandemic, the ISF proposed an adjusted version of the original outcome set, which was adopted globally [40, 41]. Improving outcome parameters such as resource use, duration of invasive treatments, and the development of organ dysfunction that requires higher levels of care, suddenly became extremely valuable in a resource-scarce setting [42]. Future studies on sepsis performance improvement programs and sepsis care bundles should similarly expand the core set of outcome measures to capture these additional benefits. In the era of shared decision-making and patient-centered care, we should acknowledge that there is more to life than death [43].

30.5 Conclusion

Sepsis performance improvement programs can optimize compliance to sepsis care protocols, which have been associated with improved patient outcomes in various studies. These programs should ideally combine screening tools, process changes in sepsis care pathways, and educational programs to create awareness about sepsis care. The consequent gains through swift and adequate recognition of sepsis can be used to diagnose and treat patients accurately and timely according to (SSC) care protocols and deliberately think about when it is necessary to deviate from the general recommendations. Trust and behavior change are essential aspects of implementing sepsis care bundles. These aspects can be reinforced by performance improvement programs but need time. Engaging a large group of multidisciplinary clinical leaders for sepsis improvement programs seems essential for their success.

Acknowledgments This work is supported by an innovation grant from the Amsterdam UMC. We would also like to thank Idelette Nutma, patient representative and sepsis survivor, for contributing to this work.

References

1. Evans L, Rhodes A, Alhazzani W, et al. Surviving sepsis campaign: international guidelines for management of sepsis and septic shock 2021. Intensive Care Med. 2021;47:1181–247.
2. Dellinger RP. The future of sepsis performance improvement. Crit Care Med. 2015;43:1787–9.
3. Viale P, Tedeschi S, Scudeller L, et al. Infectious diseases team for the early management of severe sepsis and septic shock in the emergency department. Clin Infect Dis. 2017;65:1253–9.
4. Djurkovic S, Baracaldo JC, Guerra JA, Sartorius J, Haupt MT. A survey of clinicians addressing the approach to the management of severe sepsis and septic shock in the United States. J Crit Care. 2010;25:658.e1–6.
5. Damiani E, Donati A, Serafini G, et al. Effect of performance improvement programs on compliance with sepsis bundles and mortality: a systematic review and meta-analysis of observational studies. PLoS One. 2015;10:e0125827.
6. Levy MM, Rhodes A, Evans LE, et al. COUNTERPOINT: should the surviving sepsis campaign guidelines be retired? No. Chest. 2019;155:14–7.

7. Marik PE, Farkas JD, Spiegel R, et al. POINT: should the surviving sepsis campaign guidelines be retired? Yes. Chest. 2019;155:12–4.
8. Gilbert DN, Kalil AC, Klompas M, Masur H, Winslow DL. IDSA position statement: why IDSA did not endorse the surviving sepsis campaign guidelines. Clin Infect Dis. 2017;45:486.
9. Spiegel R, Farkas JD, Rola P, Kenny JE, Olusanya S, Marik PE, Weingart SD. The 2018 surviving sepsis Campaign's treatment bundle: when guidelines outpace the evidence supporting their use. Ann Emerg Med. 2019;73:356–8.
10. Rivers E, Nguyen B, Havstad S, et al. Early goal-directed therapy in the treatment of severe sepsis and septic shock. N Engl J Med. 2001;345:1368–77.
11. The ProCESS Investigators. A randomized trial of protocol-based care for early septic shock. N Engl J Med. 2014;370:1683–93.
12. The ARISE Investigators and the ANZICS Clinical Trials Group. Goal-directed resuscitation for patients with early septic shock. N Engl J Med. 2014;371:1496–506.
13. Angus DC, Barnato AE, Bell D, et al. A systematic review and meta-analysis of early goal-directed therapy for septic shock: the ARISE, ProCESS and ProMISe Investigators. Intensive Care Med. 2015;41:1549–60.
14. Alam N, Oskam E, Stassen PM, et al. Prehospital antibiotics in the ambulance for sepsis: a multicentre, open label, randomised trial. Lancet Respir Med. 2018;6:40–50.
15. Andrews B, Semler MW, Muchemwa L, et al. Effect of an early resuscitation protocol on in-hospital mortality among adults with sepsis and hypotension: a randomized clinical trial. JAMA. 2017;318:1233–40.
16. Rothrock SG, Cassidy DD, Barneck M, et al. Outcome of immediate versus early antibiotics in severe sepsis and septic shock: a systematic review and meta-analysis. Ann Emerg Med. 2020;76:427–41.
17. Schinkel M, Nannan Panday RS, Wiersinga WJ, Nanayakkara PWB. Timeliness of antibiotics for patients with sepsis and septic shock. J Thorac Dis. 2020;12(Suppl 1):S66–71.
18. Levy MM, Rhodes A, Phillips GS, et al. Surviving sepsis campaign: association between performance metrics and outcomes in a 7.5-year study. Crit Care Med. 2015;43:3–12.
19. Cardoso T, Carneiro AH, Ribeiro O, Teixeira-Pinto A, Costa-Pereira A. Reducing mortality in severe sepsis with the implementation of a core 6-hour bundle: results from the Portuguese community-acquired sepsis study (SACiUCI study). Crit Care. 2010;14:R8.
20. Miller RR, Dong L, Nelson NC, et al. Multicenter implementation of a severe sepsis and septic shock treatment bundle. Am J Respir Crit Care Med. 2013;188:77–82.
21. Castellanos-Ortega Á, Suberviola B, García-Astudillo LA, Holanda MS, Ortiz F, Llorca J, Delgado-Rodríguez M. Impact of the surviving sepsis campaign protocols on hospital length of stay and mortality in septic shock patients: results of a three-year follow-up quasi-experimental study. Crit Care Med. 2010;38:1036–43.
22. Van Zanten ARH, Brinkman S, Arbous MS, Abu-Hanna A, Levy MM, De Keizer NF. Guideline bundles adherence and mortality in severe sepsis and septic shock. Crit Care Med. 2014;42:1890–8.
23. Varpula M, Karlsson S, Parviainen I, Ruokonen E, Pettilä V. Community-acquired septic shock: early management and outcome in a nationwide study in Finland. Acta Anaesthesiol Scand. 2007;51:1320–6.
24. Downing NL, Rolnick J, Poole SF, Hall E, Wessels AJ, Heidenreich P, Shieh L. Electronic health record-based clinical decision support alert for severe sepsis: a randomised evaluation. BMJ Qual Saf. 2019;28:762–8.
25. Hooper MH, Weavind L, Wheeler AP, et al. Randomized trial of automated, electronic monitoring to facilitate early detection of sepsis in the intensive care unit. Crit Care Med. 2012;40:2096–101.
26. Shimabukuro DW, Barton CW, Feldman MD, Mataraso SJ, Das R. Effect of a machine learning-based severe sepsis prediction algorithm on patient survival and hospital length of stay: a randomised clinical trial. BMJ Open Respir Res. 2017;4:e000234.

27. Nannan Panday RS, Minderhoud TC, Alam N, Nanayakkara PWB. Prognostic value of early warning scores in the emergency department (ED) and acute medical unit (AMU): a narrative review. Eur J Intern Med. 2017;45:20–31.
28. Liu VX, Lu Y, Carey KA, et al. Comparison of early warning scoring systems for hospitalized patients with and without infection at risk for in-hospital mortality and transfer to the intensive care unit. JAMA Netw Open. 2020;3:e205191.
29. Goulden R, Hoyle MC, Monis J, et al. QSOFA, SIRS and NEWS for predicting inhospital mortality and ICU admission in emergency admissions treated as sepsis. Emerg Med J. 2018;35:345–9.
30. Yu SC, Shivakumar N, Betthauser K, et al. Comparison of early warning scores for sepsis early identification and prediction in the general ward setting. JAMIA Open. 2021;4:1–6.
31. Usman OA, Usman AA, Ward MA. Comparison of SIRS, qSOFA, and NEWS for the early identification of sepsis in the emergency department. Am J Emerg Med. 2019;37:1490–7.
32. Islam MM, Nasrin T, Walther BA, Wu CC, Yang HC, Li YC. Prediction of sepsis patients using machine learning approach: a meta-analysis. Comput Methods Prog Biomed. 2019;170:1–9.
33. Van Wyk F, Khojandi A, Kamaleswaran R. Improving prediction performance using hierarchical analysis of real-time data: a sepsis case study. IEEE J Biomed Heal Informatics. 2019;23:978–86.
34. Schinkel M, Paranjape K, Panday RSN, Skyttberg N, Nanayakkara PWB. Clinical applications of artificial intelligence in sepsis: a narrative review. Comput Biol Med. 2019;115:103488.
35. Wong A, Otles E, Donnelly JP, et al. External validation of a widely implemented proprietary sepsis prediction model in hospitalized patients. JAMA Intern Med. 2021;181:1065–70.
36. Girardis M, Rinaldi L, Donno L, Marietta M, Codeluppi M, Marchegiano P. Venturelli C (2009) effects on management and outcome of severe sepsis and septic shock patients admitted to the intensive care unit after implementation of a sepsis program: a pilot study. Crit Care. 2009;135:1–8.
37. Tromp M, Hulscher M, Bleeker-Rovers CP, et al. The role of nurses in the recognition and treatment of patients with sepsis in the emergency department: a prospective before-and-after intervention study. Int J Nurs Stud. 2010;47:1464–73.
38. Nguyen HM, Schiavoni A, Scott KD, Tanios MA. Implementation of sepsis management guideline in a community-based teaching hospital – can education be potentially beneficial for septic patients? Int J Clin Pract. 2012;66:705–10.
39. Singer M, Deutschman CS, Seymour CW, et al. The third international consensus definitions for sepsis and septic shock (Sepsis-3). JAMA. 2016;315:801.
40. Marshall JG, Vincent JL, Guyatt G, et al. Outcome measures for clinical research in sepsis: a report of the 2nd Cambridge colloquium of the international sepsis forum. Crit Care Med. 2005;33:1708–16.
41. Marshall JC, Murthy S, Diaz J, et al. A minimal common outcome measure set for COVID-19 clinical research. Lancet Infect Dis. 2020;20:e192–7.
42. Schinkel M, Virk HS, Nanayakkara PWB, van der Poll T, Wiersinga WJ. What sepsis researchers can learn from COVID-19. Am J Respir Crit Care Med. 2021;203:125–7.
43. Hartzband P, Groopman J. There is more to life than death. N Engl J Med. 2012;367:987–9.

Index

A
Acid-base balance, 183
Acute brain injury, 302, 317
Acute circulatory failure, 174
Acute coronary syndrome, 278
Acute kidney injury (AKI), 203, 213, 223, 237, 325
Acute respiratory distress syndrome (ARDS), 13, 53, 75, 101, 116, 130, 161, 173
Advanced life support, 273
Aerobic glycolysis, 71
Aerosol, 81
Albumin, 16, 224
Alzheimer's disease, 291
Anakinra, 33
Anesthesia, 334
Angiotensin II, 264
Angiotensin converting enzyme (ACE) inhibitors, 102, 224
Angiotensin receptor blockers, 224
Antibiotic resistance, 25, 374
Anticoagulation, 88, 213
Antimicrobial stewardship, 370
Arterial compliance, 252
Artificial intelligence (AI), 353, 369
Atrial natriuretic peptide, 229

B
Bicarbonate, 187
Biomarkers, 30, 230, 265, 285, 373
Blood pressure, 260
Bundles, 397

C
Calcium, 186
Capillary leakage, 176
Carbon monoxide, 9
Cardiac arrest, 266, 273, 285, 323, 355
Cardiac rehabilitation, 388
Cardiac surgery, 224, 334
Cardiopulmonary bypass, 226
Caspase-1, 20
Cellular metabolism, 3
Chloride, 188
Closing pressure, 56
Coagulopathy, 175
Cognitive impairment, 309
Continuous renal replacement therapy (CRRT), 203, 213
Contrast-enhanced ultrasound, 237
Coronary angiography, 278–280
Coronavirus disease 2019 (COVID-19), 13, 29, 39, 81, 101, 173, 345, 394
Cuff leak test, 138

D
Damage associated molecular patterns (DAMPs), 5, 14, 32, 131, 302
D-dimer, 102
Deep learning, 358
Defibrillation, 275
Delirium, 140, 334
Dengue hemorrhagic fever, 24
Density spectral array, 338
Dexmedetomidine, 227
Diaphragm function, 129
Diaphragm-protective ventilation, 133
Diastolic arterial pressure, 252
Diastolic shock index, 252

J.-L. Vincent (ed.), *Annual Update in Intensive Care and Emergency Medicine 2022*, Annual Update in Intensive Care and Emergency Medicine,
https://doi.org/10.1007/978-3-030-93433-0

Disseminated intravascular coagulation (DIC), 14
Doxycycline, 20
Dysbiosis, 322
Dysphagia, 139

E
Echocardiography, 61, 166, 175, 250
Edema, 151
Electroencephalogram (EEG), 285
Electroencephalography, 334
Electrolytes, 183
End-expiratory occlusion test (EEOT), 168, 178, 252
Endotracheal tube (ETT), 137
Enteral nutrition, 311
Epinephrine, 276
Erythropoietin, 71, 225
Extracorporeal cardiopulmonary resuscitation, 277
Extracorporeal membrane oxygenation (ECMO), 39
Extravascular lung water (EVLW), 178
Extubation, 144

F
Fatty acid metabolism, 4
Fecal microbiota transplantation, 312
Federated learning, 362
Filter life, 213
Fission, 6
Flow-controlled ventilation, 117
Fluid administration, 151
Fluid balance, 152
Fluid overload, 151
Fluid responsiveness, 156, 162, 176, 252
Fluid resuscitation, 151
Forecasting, 370
Fusion, 6

G
Glial fibrillary acidic protein, 293
Glycolysis, 4
Granulocyte monocyte colony stimulating factor (GM-CSF), 87
Great Oxidation Event, 68
Gut-associated lymphoid tissue, 310

H
Hemoadsorption, 40
Hemodynamic monitoring, 250
Hemodynamic resuscitation, 64
Hemorrhagic stroke, 308
Heparin, 88, 214
Heterogeneity, 357
Heterotopic ossification, 393
Homocysteine, 307
Hydroxychloroquine, 83
Hypercalcemia, 187
Hyperchloremia, 188
Hyperkalemia, 186
Hypermagnesemia, 186
Hypernatremia, 185
Hyperphosphatemia, 187
Hypoalbuminemia, 224
Hypocalcemia, 187, 207
Hypochloremia, 188
Hypokalemia, 185
Hypomagnesemia, 186
Hyponatremia, 185
Hypoperfusion, 249
Hypophosphatemia, 187
Hypotension, 249, 259
Hypothalamic–pituitary–adrenal axis, 304
Hypovolemia, 174
Hypoxemia, 130, 176
Hypoxia, 72
Hypoxic brain injury, 287, 294
Hypoxic pulmonary vasoconstriction (HPV), 104, 176

I
ICU-acquired weakness, 140
Immune homeostasis, 13
Immunomodulation, 82
Immunoparalysis, 3
Immunosuppression, 14
Infection, 378
Inflammasomes, 18, 31, 304
Inflammation, 72
Inflammatory response, 40
Influenza, 21
Interferon, 5, 90
Interleukin (IL)-1β, 5
Interleukin (IL)-18, 5
Intra-aortic balloon pump, 227
Intracerebral hemorrhage, 308
Intraosseous, 277
Ischemic preconditioning, 227
Ischemic stroke, 308
Itaconate, 6
Ivermectin, 87

L
Lactate, 69, 253, 263
Laryngotracheal stenosis, 141
Larynx, 137
Leukodepletion, 226
Levosimendan, 321, 326
Lung edema, 176
Lung-protective ventilation, 133

M
Machine learning, 354, 369, 401
Magnesium, 186
Mechanical ventilation, 113, 131, 138, 152, 163, 228
Metabolic acidosis, 188
Metabolic alkalosis, 188
Metformin, 9
Microbial dysbiosis, 301
Microbiome, 301, 322
Microbiota, 301
Microbubbles, 238
Microcirculation, 237
Microthrombi, 175
Minimally invasive extracorporeal circulation, 226
Mitochondria, 3, 70
Mitochondrial DNA, 4
Mitochondrial function, 22
Mitochondrial transplantation, 8
Mitogen-activated protein kinase pathways, 23
Mitophagy, 4, 6
Monitoring, 353
Motor-sensory potentials, 334
Mottling score, 253
Mucokinetics, 91
Multiple organ dysfunction, 317

N
N-acetylcysteine, 225
Near-infrared spectroscopy (NIRS), 334
Nebulized therapy, 82
Nephrocalcinosis, 187
Neurofilaments, 290
Neurogenic stunned myocardium, 320
Neuromonitoring, 333
Neuron-specific enolase, 286
Neuroprognostication, 280
Nitric oxide (NO), 9, 209
NLRP3 inflammasome, 5, 19, 32, 309
Norepinephrine, 259, 264
Nosocomial pneumonia, 138
Nowcasting, 371
Nuclear factor-kappa B (NF-κB), 14, 22
Nutrition, 311

O
Operating room (OR), 168, 334
Optic nerve sheath diameter, 334
Organ cross-talk, 317
Organ injury, 17
Osmolality, 183
Outcome measures, 406
Oxidative phosphorylation, 4
Oxyhemoglobin dissociation curve, 69

P
Parenteral nutrition, 311
Passive leg raising (PLR), 161, 178
Pathogen-associated molecular patterns (PAMPs), 14, 40, 302
Patient self-inflicted lung injury (P-SILI), 129
Pattern recognition receptors (PRRs), 5, 14
Pendelluft, 134
Percutaneous coronary intervention, 278
Performance improvement programs, 400
Perfusion pressures, 260
Pharmacokinetics (PK), 83
Pharmacometrics, 374
Phenotypes, 250, 356
Phosphate, 187
Physiotherapists, 385
Pneumonia, 18, 81
Pneumoperitoneum, 169
Potassium, 185, 207
Precision medicine, 25
Pressure sores, 392
Probiotics, 312
Prognostication, 280
Prone position, 168, 178
Pulmonary arterial compliance, 58
Pulmonary artery catheter, 64, 179
Pulmonary blood flow, 53
Pulmonary edema, 154
Pulmonary hypertension, 60
Pulmonary shunt, 176
Pulmonary vascular permeability index (PVPI), 178
Pulmonary vascular resistance, 54
Pulmonary vasodilators, 92
Pulse oximetry, 68

Pulse pressure variation (PPV), 161, 177, 252
Pupillometry, 334

Q
Quality assessment, 364
Quality of life, 274

R
Reactive oxygen species, 4
Recruitment maneuvers, 116
Regional citrate, 214
Regional wall motion abnormalities (RWMAs), 208
Rehabilitation, 385
Reinforcement learning, 357, 360
Remdesivir, 86
Renal replacement therapies (RRT), 203, 213
Renin, 266
Renin-angiotensin system, 261
Respiratory failure, 29
Resuscitation, 262
Risk scores, 400

S
S100 calcium-binding protein B, 290
Sedation, 345
Seizures, 345
Sepsis, 13, 237, 259, 369, 397
Sepsis response team, 401
Septic shock, 174, 249, 262
Severe acute respiratory syndrome coronavirus-2 (SARS-CoV-2), 53, 81, 102, 173
Shock, 173, 238, 259
Short-chain fatty acids, 312
Sodium, 206
Sodium bicarbonate, 225
Soluble urokinase plasminogen activator receptor (suPAR), 32
Somatosensory evoked potentials, 334
Spinal cord injury, 310, 390
Spontaneous breathing, 132, 163
Spontaneous breathing trial (SBT), 152
Standardization, 361
Statins, 224
Status epilepticus, 345
Steroids, 90, 224
Strain, 114, 132
Stress, 114, 131
Stress-induced cardiomyopathy, 320
Stroke, 389
Stroke volume, 252
Stroke volume variation (SVV), 161
Subarachnoid hemorrhage (SAH), 309
Subphenotypes, 25
Succinate, 6
Surfactant, 92–93
Surviving Sepsis Campaign, 173, 262, 397
Syndrome of inappropriate antidiuretic hormone secretion (SIADH), 185

T
Takotsubo cardiomyopathy, 320
Tau protein, 293
Temperature management, 280
Tetracyclines, 13
Tidal volume, 114
Tidal volume challenge, 162, 177
Tissue plasminogen activator (tPA), 89
Transcranial Doppler, 334
Transfusion, 228
Transpulmonary pressure gradient, 51, 53
Transpulmonary thermodilution, 178
Traumatic brain injury, 306, 326
Trimethylamine-N-oxide, 305

U
Ubiquitin C-terminal hydrolase L1 (UCH-L1), 292
Ultrafiltration, 204

V
Vasodilatory shock, 259
Vasopressin, 262, 265, 276
Vasopressors, 260
Ventilation/perfusion (V/Q) mismatch, 175
Ventilator-induced diaphragm dysfunction (VIDD), 133
Ventilator-induced lung injury (VILI), 21, 114, 129
Vibrating mesh nebulizer, 83
Vocal folds, 138

W
Weakly supervised classification, 362
Weaning, 152

MIX
Papier aus verantwortungsvollen Quellen
Paper from responsible sources
FSC® C105338

If you have any concerns about our products,
you can contact us on
ProductSafety@springernature.com

In case Publisher is established outside the EU,
the EU authorized representative is:
Springer Nature Customer Service Center GmbH
Europaplatz 3, 69115 Heidelberg, Germany

Printed by Libri Plureos GmbH
in Hamburg, Germany